SHOULDER INJURIES IN SPORT

EVALUATION, TREATMENT, AND REHABILITATION

Jerome Vincent Ciullo, MD
Medical Director, Sports Medicine Center of Metro Detroit
Troy, Michigan

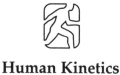

Human Kinetics

Library of Congress Cataloging-in-Publication Data

Ciullo, Jerome V.
  Shoulder injuries in sport : evaluation, treatment, and
rehabilitation / Jerome Vincent Ciullo.
      p.   cm.
  Includes bibliographical references and index.
  ISBN 0-87322-651-8
  1. Shoulder--Wounds and injuries. 2. Sports injuries. I. Title.
RD557.5.C58   1996
617.5'72044--dc20   95-41120
                                                    CIP

ISBN: 0-87322-651-8

Figures 12.1, 12.2, 12.8, 12.9, 12.10, 12.11, 12.12, and 12.13 were adapted from "Swimmer's Shoulder" by J.V. Ciullo, 1986, *Clinics in Sports Medicine*, **5**(1), 125-126. Copyright 1986 by W.B. Saunders Co. Adapted by permission.

Acquisitions Editor: Richard Washburn; **Developmental Editors:** Nanette Smith, Mary Fowler; **Assistant Editors:** Henry Woolsey, Lynn M. Hooper; **Editorial Assistants:** Coree Schutter, Jennifer Hemphill; **Copyeditor:** Karen Bojda; **Proofreader:** Pamela Johnson; **Indexer:** Theresa Schaefer; **Typesetter and Layout Artist:** Sandra Meier; **Text Designer:** Robert Reuther; **Art and Photo Coordinator:** Denise Lowry; **Photo Editor:** Boyd LaFoon; **Cover Designer:** Jack Davis; **Photographer (interior):** Jerome V. Ciullo, MD; **Illustrator:** William Loechell; **Printer:** Edwards Brothers

Printed in the United States of America   10 9 8 7 6 5 4 3 2

Human Kinetics
Web site: www.humankinetics.com

United States: Human Kinetics, P.O. Box 5076, Champaign, IL 61825-5076
1-800-747-4457
e-mail: humank@hkusa.com

Canada: Human Kinetics, 475 Devonshire Road, Unit 100, Windsor, ON N8Y 2L5
1-800-465-7301 (in Canada only)
e-mail: humank@hkcanada.com

Europe: Human Kinetics, P.O. Box IW14, Leeds LS16 6TR, United Kingdom
+44 (0)113-278 1708
e-mail: humank@hkeurope.com

Australia: Human Kinetics, 57A Price Avenue, Lower Mitcham, South Australia 5062
(08) 82771555
e-mail: liahka@senet.com.au

New Zealand: Human Kinetics, P.O. Box 105-231, Auckland Central
09-309-1890
e-mail: humank@hknewz.com

To my wife, Susan, my partner and my best friend, who keeps me organized and whose love and encouragement along with that of my children, Jeremy, Courtney, and Zachary, have allowed me to complete this book. Yes, the library is finally picked up, and we have more time to spend together as a family.

Contents

Preface

The shoulder is a unique joint that sacrifices stability to gain motion for athletic performance; its function is to allow positioning of the hand through space. Shoulder function is of prime importance to most sport activity. Balancing, stability, and motion leave the shoulder vulnerable to injury, particularly with the repetitive trauma and high demands of sport activity. Repetition in training and competition may produce pure injury patterns that are easier to understand in relation to specific aspects of sport. With identification comes the understanding needed to treat injury, which carries over from the athletic arena to the industrial or household setting.

The importance of assessing and treating sports injuries has led to a number of books geared toward specific audiences such as orthopedic surgeons, primary care physicians, athletic trainers, or physical therapists. Treatment of the injured athlete's shoulder, however, is not a mutually exclusive concern. The orthopedist, family practitioner, generalist, physiatrist, or specialty physician assumes the role of team physician, working with physical therapists, athletic trainers, and medical consultants in treating the injured athlete's shoulder. There is presently no book that adequately addresses the needs of all these team members in order to provide a common frame of reference and to provide better treatment for shoulder injuries. This book is intended to fill that gap.

The aim of the following sections of the book is to give a common framework, yet the importance of each section may vary according to the area of expertise of the reader. Details of the surgical approach are provided for the orthopedic surgeon to demonstrate means that have been found effective in dealing with the shoulder. Although the specifics of surgery may not be as important to the athletic trainer or physical therapist, the extent of what can be done has relevance to the aggressiveness and timing of the rehabilitative effort. Likewise, exercises and methods of rehabilitation available to the athlete may vary in usefulness depending on the surgeon's or treatment physician's methods of management. A goal of this book is to open the channels of communication between the different members of the sports medicine team.

In the first part of the book relevant anatomy and kinesiology of the shoulder are highlighted.

ix

Structural analysis is presented in an effort to highlight what is normal, how injuries occur, and how injuries are to be dealt with. The importance of obtaining a proper medical history and of identifying injury type is outlined. The principle of *triad degeneration* is emphasized to demonstrate the interrelationship of neuromuscular integration, stability, and arthrosis. Clinical assessment is next dealt with to present a common method of assessment and clinical testing that may enhance communication between different disciplines.

Analytic tools of X-ray, enhanced radiographic studies, and alternative diagnostic tools are presented in an effort to better understand injury patterns as well as to identify the severity of injury, indicating the magnitude of intervention. Arthroscopy is described as a diagnostic tool and as a method of surgical intervention for the shoulder.

Part II discusses specific injury patterns. The most common injuries—sprains and strains—have chapters of their own and are dealt with in some detail due to their frequence in sports injuries. Less common shoulder problems are cited because they seriously impede ultimate shoulder function in athletics. Inflammation and fibrosis about the shoulder and neurovascular injuries are subdivided to help identify specific injury patterns that may seriously hamper the shoulder's athletic function. Assessment and treatment of fractures and arthritis about the shoulder that have developed from shoulder athletic trauma in injury are further emphasized.

In Part III specific principles of shoulder rehabilitation are dealt with. Specific shoulder exercises are presented, and modalities of treatment are advocated in relation to the level of athletic tissue trauma. Finally, returning the athlete with an injured shoulder to sporting activity is discussed in relation to the treating specialist, the athlete's coach, and the injured athlete himself or herself. Additional reading and references are cited.

In reading this book, the therapist, trainer, and physician become more aware of what is available to them, through their association in the common effort of treating the injured athlete's shoulder appropriately. This book does not focus on the bench research that is becoming more and more prevalent in the technical journals. Instead, it emphasizes methods of analysis and treatment that have been found clinically useful in treating the injured athlete's shoulder. Teamwork and common understanding of the team physician, specialist, athletic trainer, and therapist will lead to better prevention, treatment, and recovery from athletic shoulder injury.

Acknowledgments

Thanks to Ernest A. Codman, who wrote a book about the shoulder in 1934 that continues to educate and inspire many physicians and surgeons who came after him. He proved himself wrong when he said, "most medical books are scarcely more enduring than shooting stars, in fact many are obsolete by the time they are published."

Thanks to Carter R. Rowe, who personified professional ethics and taught the fine points of shoulder examination and technical aspects of surgery. He said, "close the fascia, preserve the anatomy . . . as courtesy to the next fellow."

To Bertram Zarins, who taught me the importance of dedication and organization: "If a fellow physician writes a letter and asks a question, it is your obligation to reply; teaching each other is our professional obligation."

To Douglas W. Jackson, who was the living example of the Greek *Whole Man* concept, demonstrating that you can be a successful physician and surgeon; find time for research, athletics, and even seeking little critters on the bottom of Mezcal, while making sure that the family comes first; and

still remain the perfect educator. He taught, "work hard and teach freely; repetition, repetition, repetition—reputation."

To Joseph L. Posch, who repaired my hand, taught me, and helped to start me in practice; whose compassion for his patients and dedication to his family and to his profession remain an inspiration for all of his students. "People are like jelly donuts; a bad one was never made."

To Edwin Guise, my residency director, who taught me the importance of listening to the patient. "The patient will always tell you what is wrong," he said. "You have to listen and tie in the clinical finding to come up with the proper diagnosis and means of treatment."

And to my parents: my mother for her gentle prodding toward the medical profession; and to my dad, a carpenter, who taught me more about the use of orthopedic equipment in his shop than I learned during my residency. He taught his apprentices: "If the only tool you have is a hammer, then everything looks like a nail." This philosophy holds true in comparison of open versus arthroscopic surgery!

To the individuals who taught me and reinforced the concept of team effort, who remain as role models, and have proven the concept that "you are only as good as the people you surround yourself with":

Athletic Trainers: Rose Snyder (Center for Athletic Medicine/Henry Ford Hospital), Kent Falb (Detroit Lions), Jim Pengali (Boston Bruins), Tom Healion (New England Patriots), Kevin Downey (Michigan Panthers), Jennifer Stone (1983 US Olympic Swim Trials), Jeff Rokop (Sports Medicine Center of Metro Detroit), Bob Ogar (Cranbrook Schools), Emanuel "Manny" Murua (Detroit Wheels Soccer), Bill Murray (Detroit Vipers Hockey), and especially Robert "Doc" White (Wayne State University), and Mike Abdenour (Detroit Pistons).

Physical Therapists: Brad Wilson (Center for Athletic Medicine Henry Ford Hospital/Sports Medicine Center Harper Hospital), Bill Dwight (Harper Hospital Sports Medicine Center/Dwight Orthopaedics), Debbie Nadel (Sports Medicine Center of Metro Detroit), Ron Brickey (Rehabilitation Specialist Top of Troy), and Arnie Kander (Strength and Conditioning Coach Detroit Pistons).

Coaches: David Ferris (Wayne State University Football), Mark Zalin (Cranbrook Schools Athletic director/Head Coach), Jim Stanley (Michigan Panthers), and Doug Collins (Detroit Pistons).

Team Physicians: Ed Guise (Detroit Lions), Doug Jackson (Long Beach State), Bert Zarins (New England Patriots/Boston Bruins), and especially Ben Paolucci (Detroit Pistons—25 years!).

Consultants: David Lustig (Neurology), Ed Burke and Richard Singer (Hand Surgeons), Alexander Iwanow (Physiatry), Ron Little (Orthopaedics), Alvin Crawford (Pediatric Orthopaedics), Miguel Schmitz (Orthopaedics), Walter Kubinski (Team Dentist Detroit Vipers).

Support Staff: Kevin Kacer (Equipment Manager Detroit Pistons), Rich Matthews (Equipment Manager Detroit Vipers), Bill Nyeholt (Equipment Manager Detroit Pistons), John Wirth (Exercise Physiologist Wayne State University), Greg Stevens (Exercise Physiologist Center for Athletic Medicine), Albert King (Bio-Engineer Wayne State University), David Viano (Bio-Engineer General Motors).

Team Management: Al Taubman (Owner Michigan Panthers), William Davidson (Owner Detroit Pistons/Vipers), Tom Wilson (President Detroit Pistons/Vipers), Nancy Bontumasi (Executive Assistant Detroit Pistons/Vipers), Billy McKinney (VP Detroit Pistons), Rick Sund (VP Detroit Pistons), Matt Dobek (Public Relations Detroit Pistons).

And to the athletes who have proven the concepts presented in this book.

And finally, thanks to Julie Lukasik for her typing (and retyping) of this manuscript, and William Loechell for the precise medical illustration of this book.

God bless all of you. This book would never have been completed without your influence or what you have shared. I can only pray that the concepts presented here, like the ideas published by Codman, will help to stimulate interest, understanding, and better management of shoulder pathology in the future.

Part I

*Analyzing and Diagnosing
Shoulder Injuries*

The shoulder is the most complex joint in the body. Athletic performance is predicated on neuromuscular integration, muscular strength, and structural integrity. Analysis of injury is the first step in treatment, and proper treatment leads to the ultimate potential return of function. In chapter 1 shoulder anatomy is highlighted. One must understand what is normal before trying to assess the abnormal. Chapter 2 deals with medical history and identification of injury type. The concept of *triad degeneration* is emphasized. Specific clinical examination techniques are presented in chapter 3. Analytic diagnostic tools are presented in chapter 4. Finally, in chapter 5, the role of arthroscopy in diagnostic assessment of the shoulder and in surgical intervention is presented.

1

Introduction to Shoulder Anatomy

By understanding what is normal, the clinician can better define injuries of the shoulder. Knowledge of what may be considered optimal performance due to neuromuscular integration can help define variances seen in injury or that may lead to injury. Understanding the shoulder's anatomy will help the clinician both to understand the parameters of injuries and to communicate the extent of injury to colleagues on the sports medicine team. This should lead to earlier identification of injury patterns, earlier treatment, and earlier return to sport.

Theory and Phylogeny

The shoulder is unique among joints in sacrificing stability to provide mobility. As humans have assumed an upright stance, the upper extremity has become free to position the hand through space for foraging or industrial activity as well as for propelling objects for offensive or defensive maneuvers. This has led to military activity and its corollary, sport activity—the "civilized" method of showing physical superiority.

Codman (1934) has stated that the shoulder was not designed for overhead function. Nevertheless, evolutionary changes, in conjunction with an upright stance, have freed the upper extremities for overhead use. There have been radical phylogenetic changes as the *fore* limb evolved into the *upper* limb (Figure 1.1).

Four-legged animals utilize the crossed-extensor reflex or cross-pattern gait in order to ambulate (Figure 1.2, a and b). The humeral head is positioned directly under the scapuloglenoid socket. The internal and external scapular muscles have equivalent bulk, and the joint works primarily as a hinge in ambulation. As prehension and a biped gait codevelop, the glenoid socket is no longer found to cover the humeral head well. The acromion enlarges both to cover the humeral head and

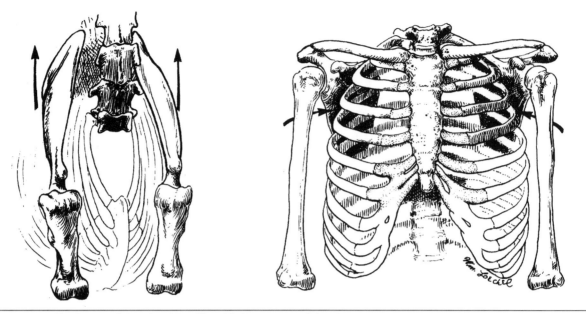

Figure 1.1 Evolution of the shoulder. The AP dimension of the thorax narrows as the scapula rotates back. The *forelimb* becomes the *upper limb*; thus the glenohumeral joint changes from a hinged joint to one allowing circumduction.

to provide a mechanical advantage of leverage. There is a concurrent shift in muscle structure to contain the shoulder in the socket and to maintain the humeral head's instant center of rotation, preparing it for overhead activity. Gravity no longer assists an overlying glenoid socket to contain the humeral head, and again, the acromion enlarges in conjunction with the sliding mechanism under the coracoacromial arch to serve the same purpose—containment. As the anterior-posterior (AP) diameter of the chest narrows in the upright stance, the scapula rotates from being directly at the side to being around toward the back, so that the humeral socket is now angled 45°, increasing functional ability of the upper extremity and essentially allowing developmental change from a hinged joint to a universal joint.

Bones, Joints, Capsules, Ligaments, and Extensions

To position the hand through space in sport activity, the muscles act primarily on the three bones of the shoulder complex: clavicle, scapula, and humerus. These three bones are interconnected through a series of joint ligaments, capsules, and intra-articular extensions that allow mobility yet provide significant stability to this linkage and leverage system. Two sliding mechanisms are also

involved—the *scapulothoracic*, providing substantial mobility, and the subacromial and infraclavicular *supraspinatus outlet*, which contains the shoulder and helps maintain the normal axis of rotation while providing a mechanical advantage in elevation (Figure 1.3). The scapulothoracic mechanism is usually most active in the lower and upper thirds of abduction, as well as retraction, protraction, and outward rotation of the lateral scapula. The supraspinatus outlet sliding mechanism is normally used in the midthird of lateral abduction, in forward flexion, and midway in functional abduction. If there is something wrong with one of these mechanisms, the other commonly will be overused to compensate.

Sternoclavicular Joint

Skeletal attachment of the upper extremity to the axial skeleton is provided through the sternoclavicular joint. The convex proximal clavicle attaches to a very shallow sternomanubrial fossa, and stability is provided almost entirely by ligamentous structures. There is a complete intra-articular disk that separates the joint into two compartments. This disk is anchored by the manubrial ligament superiorly and directly to the first rib below. The joint is encapsulated by the anterior and posterior sternoclavicular ligaments, and the clavicle is further anchored to the first rib by inferior, anterior, and posterior costoclavicular ligaments (Figure 1.4). The intra-articular free disk arrangement of

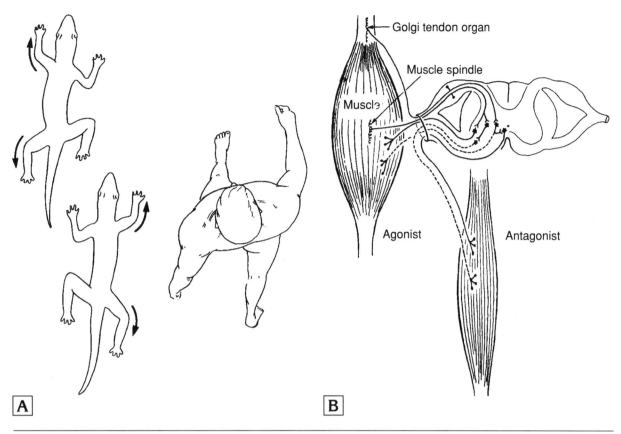

Figure 1.2

[A] Crossed-extensor reflex. Reciprocal innervation is important in locomotion as well as athletic performance. Neuromuscular integration of concentric and eccentric contracture is the basis of athletic performance.

[B] Neuromuscular integration. With contraction the muscle spindle is activated and, through central integration, leads to balancing muscular co-contraction eccentrically or inhibition of the antagonist. This integration is the basis of proprioceptive neuromuscular facilitation (PNF), kinetic chain, and (along with the viscoelastic component) plyometric exercises in rehabilitation.

From "Track and Field" by J.V. Ciullo and D.W. Jackson. In *Sports Injuries: Mechanisms, Prevention and Treatment* (p. 216, 217) by R.C. Schneider, J.C. Kennedy, and M.L. Plant (Eds.), Baltimore: Williams and Wilkins. Copyright 1985 by Williams and Wilkins. Reprinted by permission.

this joint allows 30° of elevation, 30° of anterior-posterior flexion, and approximately 45° of rotation along the functional axis, the range in which the shoulder is usually engaged, in line with the scapula. Although the sternocleidomastoid is found in the front of this joint and the sternohyoid and sternothyroid muscles behind, these are a thin barrier to the posterior structures of the subclavian and jugular veins, innominate artery, and trachea. In radiographic analysis of athletic trauma to this area, it is important to remember that the proximal clavicular apophysis does not fuse in many cases until the age of 25.

Clavicle

The clavicle itself is a relatively flat S-shaped bone proximally convex anteriorly and distally concave anteriorly. It works as a lever to provide stability to the upper extremity through the insertion of the subclavius muscle inferiorly, the trapezius muscle distally and superoposteriorly, the posterior origin of the sternocleidomastoid and sternohyoid medially, the pectoralis major origin medially, and the deltoid origin inferoanteriorly in the distal third. Medially and posteriorly the subclavian vein and artery, as well as the brachial plexus, lie in close proximity. The coracoclavicular ligaments further stabilize the distal clavicle to allow the bone to function as a mechanical strut (Figure 1.5).

Acromioclavicular Joint

The clavicle attaches to the scapula through the acromioclavicular (A/C) joint. This joint generally has an open-front V-shaped configuration, the closest contact being directly posterior, often seen on axillary film. A horseshoe-shaped disk with a very thin veil between the two ends or thicker anterior cartilage normally fits in this V-shaped joint.

Anterior and posterior stability clinically appears to be controlled at the joint by anterior and posterior capsular ligaments (Figure 1.4). Superior and inferior stability is controlled primarily through the conoid and trapezoid coracoclavicular ligaments. The V-shaped configuration of the joint

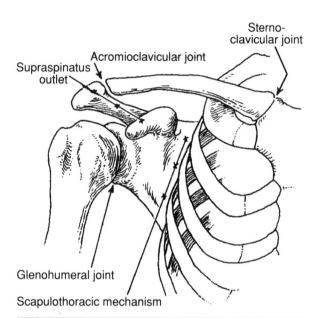

Figure 1.3 The shoulder's joint and sliding mechanisms.

allows anterior compression through the disk or cartilage as the arm is elevated and horizontally flexed (the plane perpendicular to the body at shoulder level from medial to lateral). This allows smoother scapulothoracic rotation on the ribs where scapulothoracic slide is the greatest in the initial 20° to 40° of elevation. If the anterior capsular ligament is injured, the clavicle may sag back with no apparent change on routine X-rays. If the anterior and posterior capsular ligaments are slightly injured, the clavicle may sag back on axillary X-ray with no apparent change on routine AP X-ray. With both the anterior and posterior ligaments transected, distraction may be seen so that this joint may look wider than the opposite side. If the conoid and trapezoid ligaments are transected, then superior and inferior relationships change so that there is a step-off deformity at this joint. Rotation is also integral to this joint and allows for scapular protraction and retraction, and assists in activity such as reaching behind the back.

There is no real physis at the end of the clavicle; length is due to progressive enchondral ossification at the articular cartilage end. It appears clinically that the articular cartilage at the end of the clavicle or even the intra-articular disk in the joint, when present, undergoes a process of enchondral ossification with overuse and injury, which may increase stability but decrease function.

Scapulothoracic Motion Plane

The scapula is a relatively thin sheet of bone that functions primarily to stabilize the shoulder

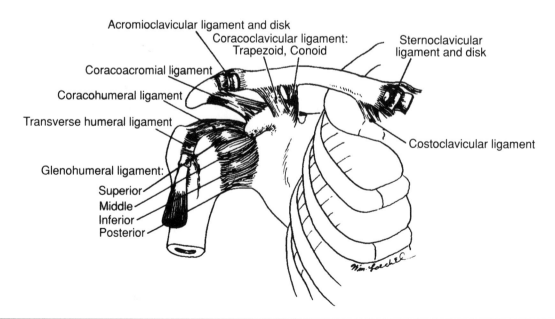

Figure 1.4 The shoulder's capsular and ligamentous anatomy.

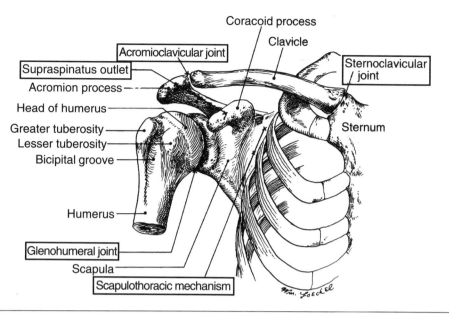

Figure 1.5 The shoulder's bony anatomy.

through muscular and ligamentous attachments. Tissue planes under the scapula normally allow this bone to ride smoothly on the rib cage when the other joints and musculotendinous relationships remain intact. This sliding mechanism usually allows for one third of normal elevation of the arm, primarily in the upper and lower ranges.

Scapular Glenoid Socket

The glenoid is an extension of the scapula and provides an articular socket for the humerus. Again, in an upright stance the humeral head is not well covered by the glenoid, and stability must be obtained by other means, including the glenoid labrum, a superior suspensory mechanism, a hydraulic fit, the corkscrew configuration of the joint capsule, an intact muscular system that balances and contains the joint, the shape of the acromion, and the superior curve of the glenoid socket. Stretching, thinning, or tearing tissue involved (capsule, tendon, labrum, or articular cartilage) can unbalance the shoulder and accelerate degenerative arthritis.

The glenoid socket appears kidney-bean shaped. The smaller superior aspect is curved upward approximately 5° to provide a keel or superior buttress-type mechanism to help contain the shoulder. It has a common growth center with the coracoid, being a later evolutionary addition. Saha (1983) has pointed out that there are three anterior-to-posterior configurations of the glenoid socket: type A, the humeral surface with a radius of curvature smaller than that of the glenoid, leading to a circular glenoid contact area; type B, in which the humeral and glenoid surfaces have similar curvatures and larger surface area contact; and type C, in which the humeral head has a radius of curvature larger than the glenoid, with contact surface limited to the periphery. Saha further stated that the concave glenoid surface is approximately one-quarter the size of the convex humeral head. However, the glenoid labrum varies in appearance and configuration, being extremely large in some individuals and almost nonexistent in others. When the glenoid labrum and the glenoid articular surface are measured together, it appears that at least 75% of the humeral head articular cartilage is covered in the normal state regardless of the anatomic variance; that is, when the glenoid articular surface is small, the labrum is correspondingly larger. Congenital variance from such patterns may lead to instability.

Glenohumeral Joint

Approximately two thirds of the motion in elevation is accomplished at the glenohumeral articulation. The articular cartilage is normally smoother than glass. It has no blood supply and is essentially maintained through a sponge-like mechanism. When pressure is put on it, it eliminates its waste products, and when pressure is taken off, joint fluid and associated nutritional factors are absorbed (Kennedy, 1979). Overall, this may produce negative pressure or a vacuum phenomenon to keep the shoulder in its socket. With an intact labrum and proper muscle balance, the joint fluid provides a hydraulic fit that assists in holding the joint together. A small recess in the anterior capsule or opening of the subscapular bursa above the leading edge of the subscapularis muscle can hold extra joint fluid to help regulate this hydraulic mechanism. A tear in the joint capsule or the rotator cuff can eliminate negative pressure, especially when coupled with axillary nerve injury and associated dysfunction of the deltoid muscle, as in a stretch or a contusion to the axillary nerve. This can allow inferior sag or *pseudosubluxation* of the humeral head, which is a common posttraumatic finding (Figure 1.6).

The glenohumeral capsule has approximately three anterior thickenings and one less-substantial posterior thickening that work as structural bands to stabilize the joint. Originating from the soft tissue at the base of the coracoid and attaching to the labrum at the superoanterior aspect of the glenoid, the superior glenohumeral ligament, when intact, helps prevent inferior subluxation of the shoulder and superior toggle that contributes to wear into the rotator cuff. When functioning properly, this ligament, along with the posterior joint capsule,

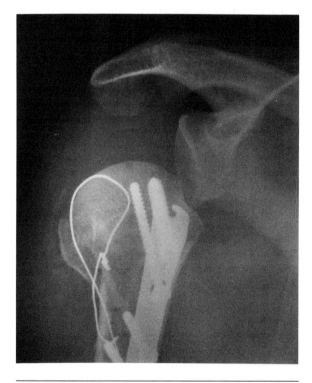

Figure 1.6 Pseudosubluxation of the humeral head. A 4-week-old, 3-part fracture in a 34-year-old jogger underwent osteoclasis and open reduction internal fixation. Postoperatively, after traction to the axillary nerve and exposure through the rotator cuff breaking the hydrostatic seal, pseudosubluxation developed but completely resolved within 3 weeks.

helps provide stability against anterior and particularly posterior subluxation. The middle glenohumeral ligament is quite variable, ranging from a broad expanse connecting the superior to inferior capsule, to a thin band or to nonexistence. When present, it functions to limit external rotation in lower range abduction. The inferior glenohumeral ligament is even more restrictive of motion, preventing displacement as the shoulder swings out of joint around an axis provided by the superior glenohumeral ligament and long biceps tendon. A posterior band can extend from the inferior portion of the inferior capsular ligament. It is thin and quite variable.

Humeral Head Stabilizers

The humeral head is also held in the socket by the short rotators, primarily the infraspinatus and teres minor posteriorly and the two muscles with separate innervations that make the subscapularis anteriorly (Figure 1.7). These muscles work in concert to help hold the humeral head down so that the supraspinatus and deltoid can work as a force couple in elevation (Lucas, 1973). This muscular humeral head depression cannot be overemphasized. Without such balance, up-riding of the humeral head sandwiches the cuff between the humerus and acromion, causing muscular erosion and increased capsular sprain. As the supraspinatus thins and the infraspinatus and subscapularis upper fibers weaken, their function as humeral head depressors may be neutralized or reversed. This causes further friction against the undersurface of the acromioclavicular (A/C) joint and progressive hypertrophy to distribute force through a larger surface; the spurring further erodes into the cuff, and the cycle worsens. Factors that help prevent superior migration of the humeral head are the shape of the acromion, the coracoacromial ligament, the biceps tendon, the thickness of the supraspinatus, the web of ligaments originating from the coracoid process, and isometric tensioning of the muscle surrounding the joint.

Coracoid Anchoring Mechanism

Structures about the coracoid process are a key factor in glenohumeral stability. A web of tissue at the superior aspect of the joint provides a *pivot point* for proprioception and stabilized rotation while the inferior capsule maintains stability in abduction external rotation.

In one of ten individuals the pectoralis minor exists as a slip of tissue over, or has a digastric muscle belly extending from, the coracoid process

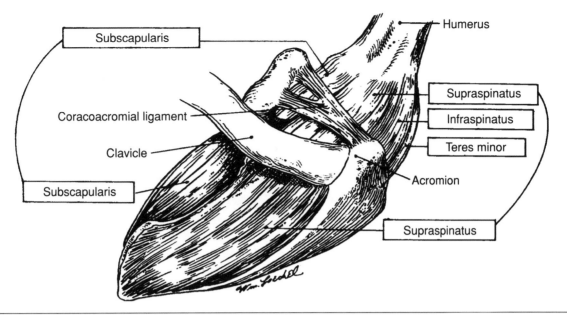

Figure 1.7 The rotator cuff.

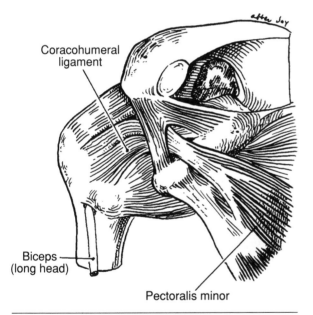

Figure 1.8 An anomalous slip of the pectoralis minor over the coracoid merging with the coracohumeral ligament is occasionally seen. This gives evidence of the evolutionary nature of the shoulder's suspensory system; the slip eventually developed into a separate coracohumeral ligament.

(Figure 1.8). The distal slip exists as the coracohumeral ligament, which anchors on both sides of the biceps tendon but primarily to the greater tuberosity in most individuals; this also explains the inverted Y shape of the coracoacromial ligament, which accommodates passage of a not uncommon slip of tendon over the coracoid. The

coracohumeral ligament extra-articularly and the coracoglenoid and superoglenohumeral ligaments intra-articularly stabilize the superior biceps and labrum and provide an anchoring point for stability (Figure 1.9).

When this superior suspension system is intact, an undamaged inferior glenohumeral ligament works as a tether by allowing corkscrew tightening of the capsule in abduction and external rotation. When this suspension mechanism is not intact, the shoulder is not contained properly. It wobbles, leading to increased stretching of the superior components, laxity of inferior components, abrasion of the rotator cuff against the undersurface of the acromion, transmission of force through the acromion into the A/C joint, and progressive attritional changes within all these structures.

Subacromial Sliding Mechanism

Tissue moving within the subacromial space, or supraspinatus outlet, must be considered another sliding mechanism for shoulder motion. There is a small bursal sac under the acromion (Figure 1.10). Because the shoulder was not designed primarily for overhead use, the bursal cross-striations wear out early or coalesce following hemorrhage, causing bands that snap in circumferential motion. Peripheral thickening of the remaining bursa can also cause a snapping phenomenon as well as increased friction affecting scapulohumeral rhythm in elevation. As the residual wall of the subacromial bursa

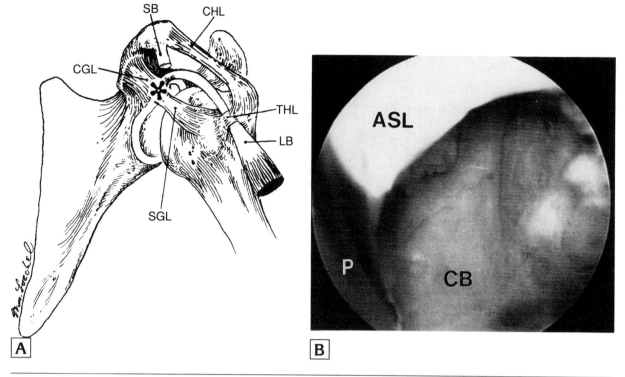

Figure 1.9

[A] Superior suspensory system. The coracoglenoid ligamentous tissue (CGL), superior glenohumeral ligament (SGL), long biceps tendon (LB), pivot point (*), coracohumeral ligament (CHL), transverse humeral ligament (THL), and short biceps tendon (SB) are shown.

[B] Detachment of tissue at the anterior-superior quadrant hampers the proprioceptive function of this tissue and destabilizes the pivot point. Displacing detached anterior superior labrum (ASL) with a probe (P) exposes the coracoid base (CB) demonstrating detachment of coracoglenoid soft tissue.

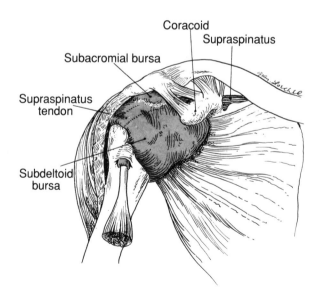

Figure 1.10 Subacromial and subdeltoid bursal anatomy. Starting as one structure, the subacromial area clears out, leaving a thickened rim separating the subdeltoid area and possibly binding the motion plane.

thickens, it may tether the rotator cuff to the acromial edge, particularly posteriorly, and limit motion. This will wall off the subdeltoid area, making it a separate space. Progressive wear of the muscle tissue will allow superior migration of the humerus and accelerate degenerative change.

If there is instability of the glenohumeral articulation, the body's attempt to maintain the humeral head in the socket may increase acromial periosteal thickness due to stress and traction at the anterior lip of the acromion, thus dampening or decreasing abnormal anteroposterior motion. Traction at the deltoid origin may also enlarge this spur. This, however, leaves a spur that will *impinge* against the supraspinatus insertion at the greater tuberosity and may lead eventually to a full-thickness rotator cuff tear or attritional changes in the muscle leading to focal necrosis, calcific tendinitis, or reactive adhesions.

Humeral Shaft

The humerus itself not only provides one of the articular surfaces of the glenohumeral joint, but also allows an area of attachment for many muscles that work in shoulder motion. Seen arthroscopically, just outside the humeral intra-articular metaphyseal area, there is a ring for bony attachment of ligaments and muscles. The humeral head is found to be retroverted about 30°, and this primarily allows the arm to be elevated away from the body in a direct line with the scapular body, much as it did in earlier evolutionary stages when the scapula was directly at the side.

The long head of the biceps tendon passes between the two tuberosities through the supraspinatus muscle and is anchored in place by the coracohumeral ligament, coalescing to become a transverse humeral ligament over the biceps tendon. This allows the biceps, in conjunction with the coracohumeral superior glenohumeral ligament suspensory system, to provide an anchoring mechanism to help retain the humeral head in the socket; generated static tension leads to a resultant force toward the center of the joint. The lesser tuberosity is the insertion point of the upper and lower subscapularis tendons, which work together with the infraspinatus and teres minor muscles inserting into the greater tuberosity to help hold the shoulder down.

The coracobrachialis initiates from the coracoid process, inserting on the medial aspect of the humerus midlength; the deltoid initiates at the outer aspect of the scapular spine, acromion, and clavicle insert on the lateral midpoint of the humerus. Both these muscles aid in elevation, assisting in scapulohumeral rhythm. The pectoralis major inserts laterally to the intertubercular sulcus, whereas the latissimus dorsi and teres major insert medially; they work together to provide extrinsic stabilization of the shoulder.

Musculotendinous Anatomy

Less than 25 sets of muscles are commonly given credit for moving the shoulder linkage mechanism. This is not at all accurate, because almost every muscle in the body contributes to holding the humeral head over the glenoid socket (Figure 1.11, a and b). This is accomplished through leaning and tilting, use of the crossed-extensor reflex system, bending the spine, and propping the shoulder to essentially balance the humeral head over the glenoid socket. All of the body's muscles are involved in use of the shoulder. For example, it is not uncommon that a pitcher or thrower develops shoulder pain following a knee or lower extremity injury. The amplification of force in the upper extremity accomplished by motion in the lower extremity can be jeopardized by lower extremity injury. This may demand more force to be generated in the upper extremity leading to ultimate system breakdown in the shoulder.

The individual involved in karate soon learns that delivering a punch is most effective by concentrating on pulling back the opposite hand and twisting the pelvis as the contralateral knee is locked forward and the punch delivered. The energy amplification system mandates an effective linkage system throughout the body for athletic performance. Nevertheless, certain muscles can be isolated that move the shoulder and allow the hand to be positioned through space. These muscles work as stabilizers, spacers, prime movers, and assistant movers.

Muscles about the shoulders work as passive restraints or spacers to position the humeral head at its instant center, allowing other muscles to be placed at their optimal length for shoulder movement. Length tension curves follow the anatomical patterns presented in a healthy state and help produce a joint reaction force to stabilize the shoulder and provide the correct center of rotation for functional mobility.

The prime movers of the glenohumeral joint consist of the short rotator cuff muscles and the external cap muscle of the deltoid. We will explore how these muscles and others about the shoulder work together in force-couple arrangements to stabilize the shoulder and to allow a strong elevation of the humeral head against the glenoid socket. Body tilt and tightening of many muscles throughout the body help assist in normal shoulder action and energy amplification in throwing and other sport activity.

Supraspinatus

The *supraspinatus* originates in the scapular supraspinatus fossa and inserts at the top of the humeral greater tuberosity. Its function is to elevate the humerus, and it is innervated by the suprascapular nerve, which is of C5-6 origin.

Infraspinatus

The *infraspinatus* originates in the scapular infraspinatus fossa and inserts below the supraspinatus on the greater tuberosity. Rather than elevating the humeral head, it actually depresses and holds it in place as a passive stabilizer to posterior subluxation while providing 60% of the external rotation force of this joint. It is also innervated by a branch of the suprascapular nerve.

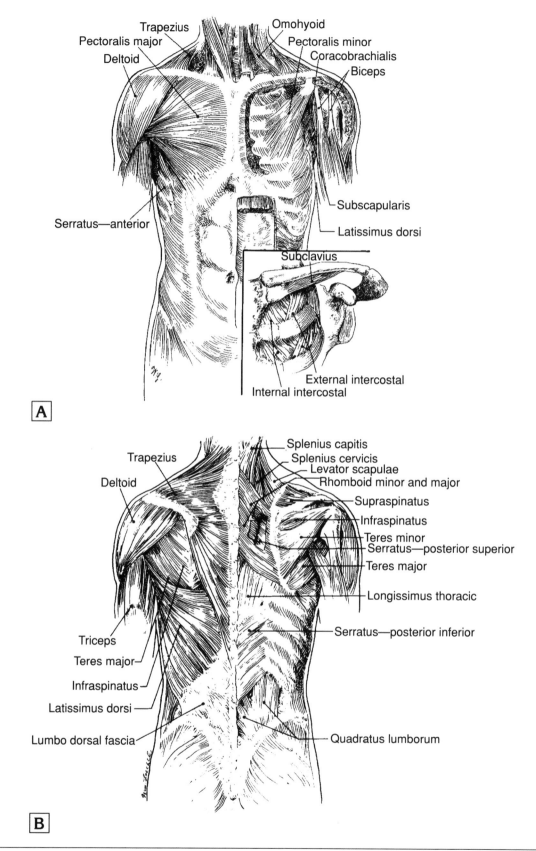

Figure 1.11

[A] The shoulder's ventral muscular anatomy.

[B] The shoulder's dorsal muscular anatomy.

Teres Minor

The *teres minor* originates in the midlateral scapula, inferiorly and laterally to the infraspinatus, and provides approximately 40% of external rotation strength at this joint by its insertion into the greater tuberosity under the infraspinatus. It is innervated through the posterior branch of the axillary nerve, of C5-6 origin.

Deltoid

The *deltoid* muscle works in conjunction with the rotator cuff in force-couple arrangement and aids in elevation of the arm above 90° through its insertion on the deltoid tubercle of the lateral humerus. The deltoid originates in its anterior head along the lateral third of the clavicle, in its medial head along the acromion, and in its posterior head along the posterior scapular spine. Its innervation is the axillary nerve of C5-6 origin. Along with the supraspinatus, the middle head helps in elevation of the humerus at all times. The middle and anterior heads work together to elevate the arm in the scapular plane, that is, in a direct line with the scapula.

Trapezius

The *trapezius* itself originates from the occiput, ligamentum nuchae, and the spinous processes of vertebrae C7 through T12. The muscle inserts in the distal one third of the upper clavicle, the lower scapular spine and scapula, as well as the lower base of the scapula. This muscle is important in scapular rotation and retraction, with upper fibers pulling on the lateral scapular angle for elevation. The trapezius and periscapular muscles assist in elevating the shoulder. Trapezial innervation is through accessory cranial nerve 11 and C1 through C4.

Rhomboid Minor and Major

The *rhomboid minor* originates from the ligamentum nuchae and vertebrae C7 and T1, and inserts on the posterior portion of the superomedial angle of the scapula. The *rhomboid major* originates at T2 through T5 and inserts into the entire posteromedial edge of the scapula below its spine. The rhomboids together retract and elevate the scapula. They are innervated by the dorsal scapular nerve, primarily C5.

Levator Scapulae

The *levator scapulae* originates in the transverse processes and posterior tubercles of vertebrae C1 through C4 to insert on the superior angle of the scapula. It acts to elevate the superior angle and works closely with the serratus anterior to produce upward rotation. It is innervated by part of the dorsal scapular nerve C4 and deep branches of C3 and C4.

Serratus Anterior

The *serratus anterior* has three sections originating from the anterolateral ribs. The first section from ribs 1 and 2 progresses to the superior angle of the scapula. The second section, originating from ribs 2 through 4, inserts on the anteromedial border of the scapula. The third section, originating from ribs 2 through 9, inserts on the inferior angle of the scapula. The primary function of the serratus anterior is to hold the scapula down during upward rotation, that is, to prevent scapular winging. This muscle is innervated by the long thoracic nerve, C5, C6, and C7, and, because of its angulated course across the second rib, is prone to injury from compression in this area or depression of the shoulder.

Pectoralis Minor

The *pectoralis minor* originates from the second through fifth ribs on the anterior chest wall and primarily inserts on the medial coracoid. In 2% of cases it exists as a digastric muscle, one on each side of the coracoid, and 8% of the cases have anomalous slips over the top of the humerus through the interval in the inverted Y shape of the coracoacromial ligament. This seems to be an evolutionary carry-over, because in birds and other small animals, the pectoralis minor is the sixth muscle of the rotator cuff, the subscapularis being counted as two.

The vestigial remnant of this muscle is in fact the coracohumeral ligament, but other slips exist as the coracoclavicular ligament, coracoglenoid ligament, and coracoscapular ligaments. These ligaments are evolutionary changes that provide a pivot point at the superior aspect of the glenoid and, along with the sliding mechanism of the biceps, stabilize the glenohumeral joint in the upright position. Through its attachment to the coracoid the pectoralis minor further functions to depress the scapulae when it is upwardly rotated or to center the scapulae as the lateral angle is depressed. It depresses the scapulae with upward motion and is an important part of the superior suspensory system. It is innervated by the medial pectoral nerve, C8, T1.

Subclavius

The *subclavius* originates from the first rib and inserts on the inferior medial third of the clavicle. It crosses the sternoclavicular joint and stabilizes this joint in overhead activity such as military press and narrow-grip incline bench pressing. It is supplied neurologically by the nerve to the subclavius, C3 through C8, primarily C5.

Teres Major

The *teres major* originates on the posterior surface of the scapula at the inferior aspect of the lateral border. It has a common tendinous insertion with the latissimus dorsi at the medial edge of the bicipital groove, which is a landmark in continuity with the lesser tuberosity. In the common insertion there is a spiral turn of 180°, such that the posterior latissimus dorsi twists to insert anteriorly to the teres major. The teres major adducts, extends, and internally rotates the arm against resistance. It is innervated by the lower subscapular nerve, C5 and C6.

Pectoralis Major

The *pectoralis major* originates from the medial half of the clavicle and inserts into the lateral edge of the bicipital groove in its upper portion. The middle portion originates from the sternomanubrium and the upper two thirds of the sternal body on ribs 2 through 4 to insert behind the clavicular portion in the lateral bicipital groove. The pectoralis major originates inferiorly from the lower distal sternal body, ribs 5 and 6, and the external obliquus fascia. These fibers also insert along the lateral edge of the bicipital groove but rotate 180° so that they insert superiorly on the common insertion. This is a balancing muscle, with the clavicular portion participating in forward flexion together with the deltoid, while the lower portion works directly against this in forward flexion. Segments work together to depress the lateral angle of the scapula and for adduction across the glenohumeral joint, whereas the clavicular section is most active in horizontal abduction across the front of the body. The upper sternal portion is innervated by the medial pectoral nerve, C7-8 and T1, and the clavicular portion is innervated by the lateral pectoral nerve, C5 through C7.

Latissimus Dorsi

The *latissimus dorsi* originates from the inferior angle of the scapula, the lower four ribs, the dorsal spines T7 through L5, the sacrum, and the iliac crest. It inserts into the medial edge and floor of the bicipital groove. It is innervated by the thoracodorsal nerve, C6 and C7, and functions to cause inward rotation and adduction of the humerus and to assist in inferior pull of the scapula.

Coracobrachialis

The *coracobrachialis* originates from the coracoid process in common with the short head of the biceps as the conjoined tendon to insert on the anteromedial midhumerus. It assists in adduction and flexion of the glenohumeral articulation and is innervated by a branch of the musculocutaneous nerve lateral cord, C5 and C6.

Biceps Brachii

The *biceps brachii* has two heads. The long head originates from the superoposterior glenoid labrum and acts as a stabilizer and humeral head depressor, part of the pivot point or superior suspensory mechanism around which the humeral head spins. The short head originates from the coracoid tip in common with the coracobrachialis in the lateral aspect of the conjoined tendon. The short head contains the subscapularis and yields further stability. There is not much tendon excursion near the shoulder, because the main function is to provide guided stability. Excursion is primarily at the elbow, where the distal tendon laterally inserts on the posterior radial tuberosity, and the medial insertion is through the lacertus fibrosus and into the muscle fascia of the volar forearm. The biceps stabilizes the glenohumeral joint while providing flexion and supination at the elbow. It is innervated by C5 and C6 components of the musculocutaneous nerve.

Triceps

The *triceps* has a long head that is extra-articular and reinforces the inferior capsule of the glenohumeral joint. Like the biceps, the major excursion is in extension at the elbow, and it is innervated by the C6 through C8 fibers of the radial nerve.

Motion Analysis

Every athletic endeavor is different; there are different rules, motions, and stresses with every sport. Even within each sport, positional variation can significantly change stress as in pitching, catching, midfield, outfield, and batting activities in baseball. Any injury can occur in any sport, but certain patterns become sport specific. As a team physician it is important to learn as much as you can about the biomechanics of the sport with which you are dealing to anticipate common injuries while observing the game or in postgame ER or office management, and to allow you to work with the coach and trainers in injury prevention.

Basic Throw

Overhead activity in many sporting events has three common elements: cocking, acceleration, and follow-through. How propulsion of an object is accomplished, however, is markedly different from sport to sport. The overhead throw in baseball is decidedly different from the underhand softball pitch, which in fact more resembles bowling, curling, or horseshoe pitching. Even throwing a javelin directly overhand varies significantly from fastball pitching because the arm is locked out in a certain position of rotation for a longer period of time and because lower-extremity energy amplification is done through running rather than a whipping rotation of the contralateral leg in a relatively stationary position. The golf swing and track and field hammer throw events, although appearing similar in many ways, lead to significantly different stresses on the shoulder due to the weight involved and the differences in impact versus release of the object projected. Tennis and racquetball vary considerably in horizontal flexion-to-extension activity versus vertical elevation and depression motions. Swimming, like gymnastics and handball, causes considerably more weight bearing on the

shoulder and leads to different repetitive forces and therefore different injury patterns.

Throwing is a complex energy amplification system in which 50% of the power of the throw is generated from the back musculature, and the throw itself is accomplished by combined motion of the trunk segments, scapulothoracic joint, and glenohumeral joint. Imbalance and faulty technique can easily lead to breakdown of structures about the shoulder.

The activity of throwing a ball is divided into three phases: *cocking* (80%), *acceleration* (2%), and *follow-through* (18%). Each phase can be subdivided for better analysis.

Cocking. The cocking phase is subdivided into three activities (Pappas, Zawacki, & Sullivan, 1985): wind-up, early cocking, and late cocking (Figure 1.12). While the capsule is being preloaded in abduction and external rotation to store energy, the contralateral leg is whipped in front of the body as an essential component of the linkage system to provide energy amplification through the cross-extensor reflex. Through the linkage system, the trunk rotates from the hips upward in order to position the shoulder. With the shoulder capsule preloaded in abduction and external rotation, the subscapularis anteriorly and the infraspinatus posteriorly must balance the humeral head in the socket while the supraspinatus/deltoid force couple elevates the arm and depresses the humeral head. There is no forward motion of the arm in this phase, which merely positions the shoulder for delivery.

Acceleration. Acceleration is provided by release of energy stored in the viscoelastic component of the shoulder capsule when the infraspinatus, teres minor, and supraspinatus muscles

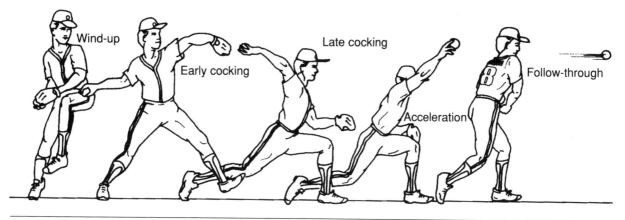

Figure 1.12 Motion analysis: pitching.

Adapted from "Biomechanics of Baseball Pitching: A Preliminary Report" by A.M. Pappas, R.M. Zawacki, and T.J. Sullivan, 1985, *American Journal of Sports Medicine*, **13**, pp. 216-222, and "The Shoulder in Sports" by F.W. Jobe, J.E. Tibone, C.M. Jobe, and R.S. Kvitne, in *The Shoulder* (pp. 962, 982) by C.A. Rockwood and F.A. Matsen, 1990, Philadelphia: W.B. Saunders.

relax. The shoulder is quickly derotated as ball release occurs (between 40° to 60° of external rotation), the elbow flexes and then quickly extends, the wrist starts an extension and moves to neutral, and the forearm pronates just before ball release.

Follow-Through. As the acceleration stage ends, the subscapularis and pectoralis major are already firing to produce the internal rotation force necessary to decelerate the arm, initiating the follow-through phase, which continues until the throwing motion ends. Initially, the posterior shoulder and periscapular musculature fire in conjunction with a force couple of the biceps tendon. Continuing internal rotation and horizontal flexion put stress across the A/C joint, while muscles about the shoulder are all active to hold the shoulder in the

socket, thus preventing stretch of the infero-anterior joint capsule. The body continues to rotate in order to catch up with the arm.

Swim Stroke

In swimming there are two main phases, which Richardson, Jobe, and Collins (1980) have subdivided into three substages each for purposes of stroke analysis of freestyle, butterfly, and back-stroke (Figure 1.13). Separate subphases have been set up for breaststroke. Overhead pull-through is initiated with the hand entry phase when the humerus is externally rotated and abducted to 180° while the biceps is firing to flex the elbow. The subscapularis begins to fire as the upper limb makes contact with the water surface. Body roll,

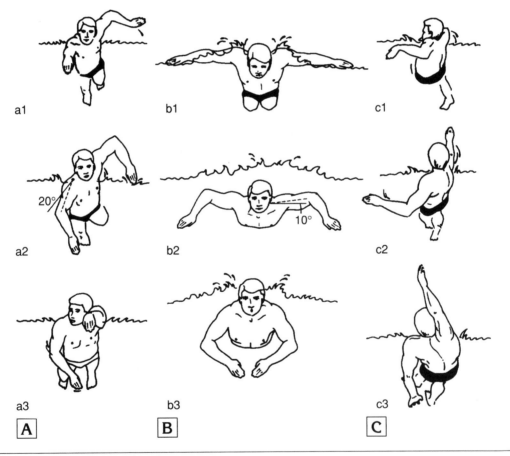

Figure 1.13 Motion analysis: swimming.

   [A] Freestyle. Right arm: (1) hand entry, (2) mid-pull-through, (3) end of pull-through; left arm: (1) elbow lift, (2) midrecovery, (3) hand entry.

   [B] Butterfly. (1) midrecovery, (2) mid-pull-through, (3) end of pull-through.

   [C] Backstroke. Right arm: (1) hand lift, (2) midrecovery, (3) hand entry; left arm: (1) hand entry, (2) mid-pull-through, (3) end of pull-through.

Adapted from "The Shoulder in Competitive Swimming" by A.B. Richardson, F.W. Jobe, and H.R. Collins, 1980, *American Journal of Sports Medicine*, **8**, pp. 159-163.

which begins here, is an important factor in energy amplification and prevention of stress on the shoulder. During mid-pull-through phase with the arm at 90° of abduction and changing from external to internal rotation, the latissimus dorsi is firing at its peak, when body roll is at maximum. Latissimus and subscapularis contraction continue through the pull-through phase until the arm is in a fully abducted and internally rotated position, as the body regains horizontal positioning. The clavicular head of the pectoralis major is also active during this motion. At this point the middle deltoid increases activity through the entire recovery phase when the arm is abducted over the head (Nuber, Jobe, Perry, Moynes, & Antonelli, 1986). Initiating the recovery phase with elbow lift, the supraspinatus and infraspinatus as well as serratus anterior muscles activate and remain active until the reinitiation of the pull-through phase. The hand and shoulder lead the elbow to diminish the occurrence of impingement of the supraspinatus. However, in fatigue when the elbow starts leading the hand, impingement of the supraspinatus increases; it also increases on the breathing side when body roll continues and increased abduction must compensate (Ciullo & Stevens, 1989). Breathing from one side alone can unbalance the energy amplification system and lead to stress on the shoulder, commonly resulting in impingement.

Golf Swing

Golf is not a power sport but one of form and technique. The golf swing is nonphysiologic, and overusing the shoulder for energy amplification developed through trunk rotation easily leads to shoulder injury. The swing can be analyzed in three stages: *take-away, impact,* and *follow-through* (Figure 1.14). The shoulder in this sport works basically as a stabilizer. It is the linkage mechanism and cross-extensor reflex that primarily allow rotation of the shoulders, chest, hips, and lower extremities during the take-away, which consists of the setup until the top of the backswing. In this stage back, wrist, elbow, and neck tendinitis are common, but shoulder strain is not unless a preexisting impingement exists.

In the impact phase the swing is initiated, with the subscapularis, pectoralis major, and latissimus dorsi activated into the acceleration phase. At impact significant compression occurs into the wrist, and valgus impact into the medial aspect of the back leg. Compression injuries often involve these structures, and injury, including carpal fractures and carpal tunnel syndrome, is not uncommon. The ball is hit while the body is pivoting, and the spine initially rotates rather than the shoulders (McCarroll, 1985).

The follow-through is accompanied by a weight shift to the nondominant side. Even if follow-through is done properly, overuse leads to pain at the lower back and hip area. Bending the elbows too much, poor weight shift, or poor stance can lead to increased stress on the shoulders and therefore increased risk of injury.

Variance in Style

Even within a single sport, the style of performance may lead to significantly different injuries. In throwing a javelin, an athlete utilizes full acceleration and a sudden stop to generate a significant force for throwing. A crossover step is used, with

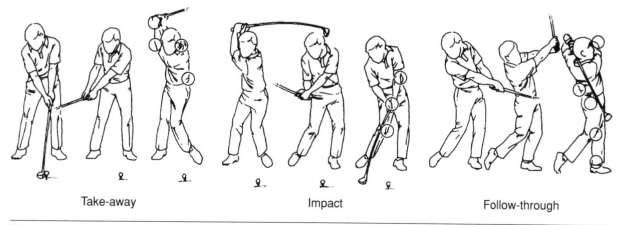

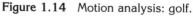

Take-away   Impact   Follow-through

Figure 1.14 Motion analysis: golf.

Adapted from ''Golf'' by J.R. McCarroll. In *Sports Injuries: Mechanism, Prevention and Treatment* (pp. 290-294) by R.C. Schneider, J.C. Kennedy, and M.R. Plant (Eds.), 1985, Baltimore: Williams and Wilkins.

the body in front of the javelin to maximize forward momentum, and the shoulders are kept in line with the direction of the throw. The body rotates, and the javelin is brought close to the ear, through the center of gravity where the elbow leads the hand in the throw. The javelin is then whipped forward.

In the Finnish javelin-throwing style the cross step is low, and the throw at the frontal stance position is generated through the abdominal muscles (Figure 1.15a). Energy amplification is maximized by using a rapid series of crossover steps to achieve acceleration in the approach to the throwing position. The javelin is thrown over the shoulder using rotation to whip the javelin forward; a side-arm throw generating more supraspinatus and teres minor shoulder force

can lead to strain of these muscles and must be avoided.

Americans, accustomed to throwing a baseball from center field, have developed a less smooth and more hopping motion in throwing the javelin (Figure 1.15b). The crossover technique is not as smooth, and the shoulders are kept in line with the throw, which hurls the javelin directly over the shoulder from an abducted, externally rotated position forward, emphasizing pure muscle force in the overhand throw and utilizing stored energy in the joint capsule. This style is less energy efficient than the former and leads to increased supraspinatus strain and capsular sprain injuries.

In either style the deltoid fibers fire first, followed by supraspinatus, infraspinatus, teres minor, and finally subscapularis activity. The

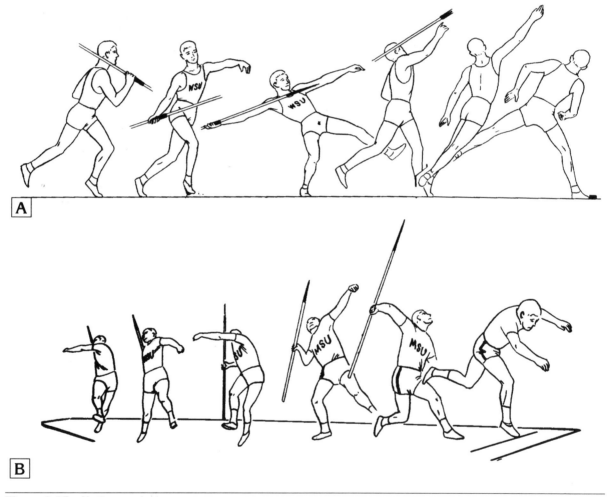

Figure 1.15 Motion analysis.

[A] Finnish-style javelin approach.

[B] American-style javelin approach.

From "Track and Field" by J.V. Ciullo and D.W. Jackson. In *Sports Injuries: Mechanisms, Prevention and Treatment* (p. 245) by R.C., Schneider, J.C. Kennedy, and M.L. Plant (Eds.), 1985, Baltimore: Williams and Wilkins. Copyright 1985 by Williams and Wilkins. Reprinted by permission.

throw must be made through the center of gravity as the weight shifts forward, otherwise imbalance occurs and injury is common. Muscle balance must be achieved; imbalance leads to injury, specifically glenoid labrum tear, often around the superior labrum. Warm-up is necessary to help prevent back and triceps muscle injury due to uncoupling energy amplification and muscular coordination necessary in the throw. In the javelin throw, inefficient warm-up means less flexibility, which can lead most commonly to shoulder impingement or occasionally to elbow sprain injury.

Summary

The shoulder is an important joint for sport participation and activities of daily living. To determine normal function versus dysfunction or injury,

underlying anatomy must be understood. Structural interrelationships and neuromuscular balance must be understood for both analysis and reassessment during rehabilitation. Methods of injury prevention such as stretching and strengthening may become evident during examination of imbalances related to the diseased state. The medical team managing the athlete's shoulder must understand the anatomy and demands of the sport to best serve the athlete's needs.

There are significant differences in shoulder utilization in various sports. The forces and resultant injury sustained during an overhead throw in baseball are not the same as those sustained in a sidearm pitch, an overhead football pass, an underhand softball pitch, a lateral rugby throw, a punch in boxing, or a forearm block in karate. Effective sport activity depends on the proper balance of strength and flexibility (Figure 1.16). For athletes who are in different sports, in different events, or

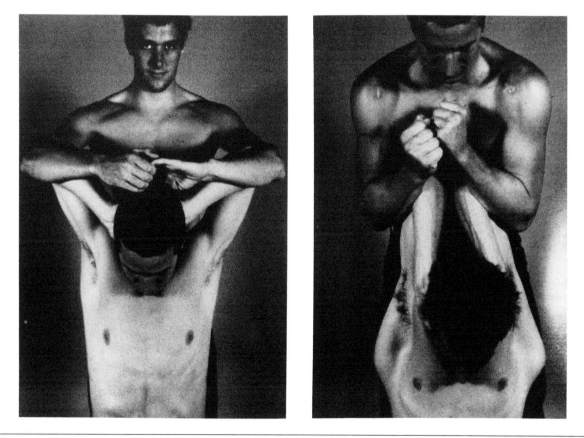

Figure 1.16 Optimal flexibility varies considerably. These two teammates underwent similar training programs through high school and college. Variance of flexibility may lead to variance of technique, selection, or profiling of sport. The athlete being stretched in the first picture was a national champion in the freestyle stroke; the athlete being stretched in the second picture, a national champion in the butterfly stroke. Performance is the product of flexibility, strength, and neuromuscular integration.

even within the same sport, individual variance may lead to different styles of achieving maximal performance. Motion analysis is important in identifying improper technique. Warm-up, stretch, and strengthening are used in conjunction with proper form to prevent injury. These same factors are important to analyze to help prevent reinjury when recovered athletes return to sport activity.

2

Stating the Problem

In diagnosis of a shoulder injury, the patient always tells the examiner what is wrong. It is important to avoid preconceived notions, otherwise the proper diagnosis may be missed. The history, physical examination, X-rays, and correlative studies must be balanced together in order to come up with a working diagnosis. With a diagnosis in hand, the proper therapeutic measures can be initiated. At the same time, the cause of the problem must be sought, because the healed patient should not be sent back to the same injury-producing environment, ill prepared due to improper biomechanics or fatigue, so that he or she will be destined to return to the clinic with the same or a related injury.

The fact that the patient may be suffering from shoulder pain secondary to another cause must not be forgotten. Preexisting goiter or diabetes may have a significant effect on inflammatory states or adhesive capsulitis, thus clinical response may be much slower. Steroid usage in arthritis, asthma, and inflammatory connective tissue states may not only hamper healing but may also interefere with normal preoperative and postoperative case management.

In this chapter we will consider the factors and questions relevant in obtaining a medical history. The concept of referred pain is covered, because many clinical entities will present with symptoms common to those found in shoulder pathology and must be differentiated. How to classify injury is then covered, because this helps communicate injury patterns and rehabilitative needs to colleagues. Last, the concept of triad degeneration is presented to emphasize the interrelated nature of injury. Early diagnosis, intervention, and even prevention become the goals of treating the athlete's shoulder.

Medical History

Overall, the patient's own history is the most important factor in differential diagnosis. It helps to establish whether the pain is coming from the shoulder itself or is referred in nature. It is important to determine whether the instability of the shoulder occurs only with trauma or is something that the patient can easily reproduce with or without pain.

The patient's chief complaint, age, and dominant handedness are of importance. These give a baseline for the rest of the examination. For example, the dominant arm in throwing activity usually has 15° more external rotation and an internal rotation of two less vertebrae behind the back when compared to the nondominant arm; such motion variance would be considered normal. Age and activity level may have a lot to do with the patient's expectations. One must try to determine exactly what those expectations are. They will vary from demands on the shoulder related to recreational activity, fitness activity, or, in the master athlete, even competitive activity. What the patient expects from treatment is also important.

Activity Level

Whether the patient presents with an occupational injury that interferes with recreational sports or a sport injury that interferes with the patient's performance at work must be established up front. The physician must understand whether occupational or sport activity is the situation that must be analyzed and corrected. Also, whether litigation is involved is important. There is nothing more disturbing than going through the work-up and having the case canceled the day before surgery because it is "in dispute."

Whether the athlete is involved in more than one sport is important, as is the sport the athlete considers his or her primary sport. Frequently activities in one sport lead to selective hypertrophy or relative atrophy of muscles, stretching of tissue, and so on, which can lead to fatigue or mechanical imbalance in another sport. It is important to know what the athlete is capable and not capable of doing. Past history must be elicited, such as general medical health, medications, psychological history, family history, previous orthopedic assessment and tests, as well as surgery. For example, a history of previous neck surgery may help determine that the shoulder problem may be referred pain from the preexisting neck problem and may lead to a different line of diagnostic testing and treatment.

Preexisting Injury

Preexisting orthopedic problems may disclose whether the patient has excessive ligamentous laxity or an underlying congenital handicap. Whether the patient considers the problem an acute or a chronic complaint makes a significant difference.

An acute injury can often be managed by nonsteroidal anti-inflammatory medication, a short period of rest, or initial selective exercises. One would not wish to rush prematurely into expensive diagnostic tests that may be made unnecessary over a few days' or weeks' time due to the body's ability to heal. However, if this is a chronic problem, then diagnostic testing may be immediately necessary. One should inquire about what tests have been done so that they are not repeated. If previous surgery has been done, obtaining surgical dictations is important, because there is often considerable difference between what the patient believes was done and what has actually been done. Obviously, the patient's statement that he or she had been treated "successfully" in the past and that this is a "new injury" cannot be medically substantiated without the aid of previous medical reports.

Listening to the Athlete

The physician who considers him- or herself a "sports medicine expert" may easily jump to the conclusion that the patient must have a certain sort of injury because of participation in a certain sport, for example, a high school swimmer with an impingement problem of the shoulder. Don't fall into that trap. Let the patient speak and take the time to listen. He or she will say something that will tie into the clinical examination and that will identify the problem, teach the examiner something about the shoulder, and help the subsequent assessment of future patients. Then it becomes the examiner's responsibility to communicate learned information to colleagues so that the field of sports medicine is enhanced and more athletes and patients will benefit.

One must inquire about the characteristics of the pain. Is it night pain that is made worse by lying on the joint, which would implicate an A/C joint problem, or is it night pain made worse by not lying on it, allowing distraction and escape of joint fluid and implicating a rotator cuff problem? Is it pain made worse with activity (implicating a tendinitis), pain associated with turning one's head to the opposite direction (implicating an underlying neck problem or brachial plexopathy), or pain associated with certain positions, such as abducted external rotation, which might implicate capsular laxity? Is it pain following activity (stage 1 tendinitis; Blazina, Kerlan, Jobe, Carter, & Carlson, 1973), during activity (stage 2 tendinitis), or interfering with performance (stage 3 tendinitis)? Is it pain with horizontal flexion activity, such as tennis, not found in overhand pitching or overhead basketball activity, which might implicate an A/C joint problem? The "burning pain" of calcific tendinitis or cervical nerve radiculopathy is quite a bit different than the "dull toothache" type of pain experienced with partial- or full-thickness rotator cuff tearing.

Is a shoulder pain developed well out of proportion to the initiating insult? For example, suppose a recreational runner's husband lost his job the same day that her running partner moved to another state and she bumped her shoulder into a clothing rack at the local department store; since then she has had swelling in the arm with temperature change, significant atrophy, osteopenia from disuse, and constant pain. This is not a candidate for surgical intervention alone. A diagnosis of reflex sympathetic dystrophy is suggested, and psychological intervention is a necessary initial part of management.

What does the patient perceive the problem to be? If the patient tells the examiner that it feels as if the shoulder has moved out of joint, he or she may have an instability problem. Remember, the patient is right; the days when an X-ray was necessary to document that the shoulder was out of place before treating it for instability are no more. Listening carefully to what the patient perceives as the mechanism of injury is important. Tying this to the clinical examination can direct the physician to the proper tests needed for documentation and diagnosis. If the patient has a difficult time explaining the problem, it is often quite interesting to ask the spouse (if any), who may be able to explain the loss of certain motions and activities. The patient must also be questioned about changes in appearance and function.

Inability to reach overhead frequently means a rotator cuff problem has occurred. Inability to reach behind the back, however, may implicate an A/C joint problem, or *posterior capsulitis*—adhesions between the rotator cuff and deltoid muscle or progressive thickening of the residual subacromial bursal wall, which limits supraspinatus slide under the acromion. The patient commonly attributes the problem to some initial injury when pain developed in the shoulder, and then a few days or weeks later, "something gave in the shoulder and there has been an inability to lift since." In this situation, the rotator cuff tear may have been initiated with the first trauma, the remaining fibers allowing continued function over the next few weeks; the tear may subsequently propagate with activities as trivial as tossing a baseball or as significant as being involved in a

motor vehicle accident. Whether this secondary event was the "cause" or "aggravation" may have legal implications not immediately obvious at the time of the initial clinical presentation. Accurate documentation is mandatory.

History of recent illness or trauma is important in the differentiation of viral plexitis from a traumatic nerve root avulsion. Implications, expected outcome, and work-up are significantly different; the history is the key.

Referred Pain

The examiner must always be aware of *referred pain patterns*; structural problems in one part of the body can lead to symptoms in another part of the body, and effective treatment must be for the primary problem rather than the secondary pain (Figure 2.1). Pain is often referred to the superomedial angle of the scapula from upper cervical nerve root problems. Nerve irritation from the lower cervical spine is referred to the inferior border of the scapula. Irritation of the diaphragm from a hiatal hernia or fluid collection at the base of the lung can be referred through the phrenic nerve to the superomedial angle of the scapula, the trapezius muscle, and the midclavicular area. Heart disease may cause pain radiating down the left shoulder to the ulnar aspect of the upper arm, but don't be fooled. Although the descending and transverse aortic arch, if diseased, will have pain radiating to the left shoulder, the ascending arch can have pain radiating to the right shoulder. Intrascapular pain is common with poor posture; however, it is also a source of referred pain from pancreatic and gastric problems. Pain can be referred generally to the periscapular area of either shoulder with hepatic disease, subphrenic abscess, ruptured abdominal viscus, ulcer, gallbladder disease, and even pulmonary infarction.

If the pain pattern is somewhat atypical in an older patient with a long history of smoking, with or without Horner's syndrome, make sure that you get a chest X-ray to rule out an apical or pancoast tumor, in which shoulder pain may be the only presenting symptom.

When the complaint of pain is well out of proportion to clinical findings, don't be afraid to enlist the help of a pain clinic. This may help the patient deal with anxiety, eliminate the need for multiple expensive diagnostic tests, and at least suggest whether or not a prolonged period of physical therapy or possible surgical intervention would have

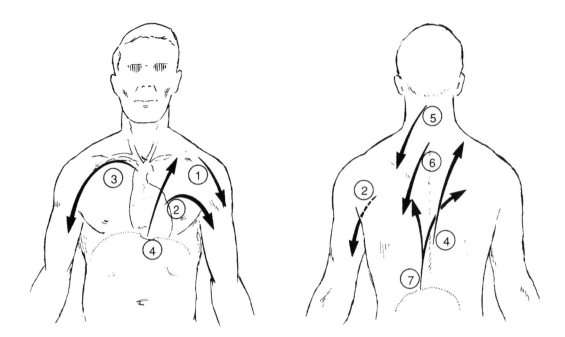

Figure 2.1 Referred pain patterns. (1) A/C, glenohumeral, or cuff disease to root of deltoid; (2) cardiac down left arm; (3) ascending aortic arch down right arm; (4) peridiaphragmatic visceral to midclavicle, midtrapezoid, or superior midscapula; (5) upper cervical to upper medial scapula; (6) lower cervical to lower midscapula; (7) visceral to periscapular area.

any chance of success. Always remember that the patient may be plagued with more than one problem, and due to the body's linkage system, each must be dealt with in order to achieve an effective cure.

Injury Type

Most athletic shoulder injuries are due to soft tissue injury. They most often may not be documented by routine shoulder X-ray and, in the early phase, most likely will respond to anti-inflammatory medication, stretching, and exercise progressing toward the return to sport activity.

Sprain

A *sprain* is an injury to the tissue immediately surrounding a joint that helps to stabilize that joint (Figure 2.2). This tissue includes the capsule, ligaments, and, in the case of the shoulder, the labrum. In this regard, a *separation* or disruption of the acromioclavicular joint is a sprain injury to the acromioclavicular capsule or surrounding ligaments, just as stretching of the capsule of the glenohumeral joint yields laxity leading to *subluxation* (partial displacement of the humeral head from the glenoid socket) or *dislocation* (total disruption of the humeral head from the glenoid socket).

Strain

A shoulder *strain* consists of an injury to the musculotendinous unit, whether this is a hole in the rotator cuff tendon itself or separation of the musculotendinous portion of the biceps. This type of injury can occur any place along the musculotendinous unit, including a bony avulsion of the origin, intratendinous separation, musculotendinous disruption, or intramuscular tear. Just as in a sprain, it can occur from repetitive overuse or from a single traumatic event overriding the viscoelastic component of energy absorption and leading to a tissue tear.

Arthritis

Arthritis is another component of injury. Normally, the joint surface is covered with articular cartilage that is smoother than glass. It has no innate blood supply, and nourishment is achieved as if the tissue were a sponge. Pressure on the cartilage releases waste products, and removal of pressure allows absorption of joint fluid, which contains nutritive substances (Kennedy, 1979). If for any reason the cycle of use is interfered with, the cartilage will soften (chondromalacia or grade 1 arthritis), will blister and break (grade 2 arthritis), will fissure down to bone and thin somewhat (grade 3 arthritis), or will be lost, exposing bare bone (grade

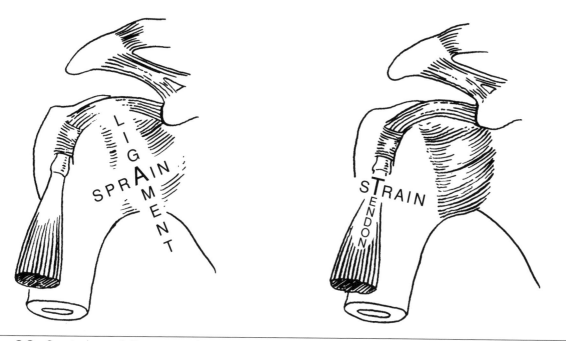

Figure 2.2 Sprain (capsuloligamentous) versus strain (musculotendinous) injury.

4 arthritis). Trauma can accelerate this process or shred tissue, as can an underlying metabolic state such as diabetes, gout, chondrocalcinosis, or immobilization. When cartilage flakes off, it stimulates the synovial joint lining, which may hypertrophy and cause a pannus of tissue to grow across the articular cartilage, causing increased pain, which limits motion and interferes with cartilage nutrition. This can also occur with certain disease states such as rheumatoid arthritis, pigmented villonodular synovitis, and infection. All of these speed up the cycle and accelerate arthritis. Putting too much stress on the shoulder, as may occur in handball, gymnastics, and carrying weights while jogging, can wear out articular cartilage as well. The best defense against progressive arthritis change is, first, maintenance of motion so that the entire articular surface can maintain nutrition and, second, preservation of strength so that muscles may work as shock absorbers to diminish stress on the joint surface.

Fractures

Fractures are broken bones either from a stress situation with minor breakdown, which may not show up on initial X-ray, or from major displacement, which should show up on X-ray. Improper healing leads to abnormal wear patterns and abnormal stresses, progressively breaking down the linkage system of the shoulder.

Triad Degeneration

In the shoulder more than in any other joint, the principle of triad degeneration becomes most important (Figure 2.3). Three factors of *joint stability and mobility*, *muscular balance* (integration and strength), and *joint surface articular integrity* must be well balanced in order to prevent injury or to compensate for injury. If these are not balanced, then a degenerative cycle involving joint laxity, muscular imbalance, and articular wear develops and becomes progressively more difficult to manage. Degeneration of one factor leads to progressive breakdown of the others.

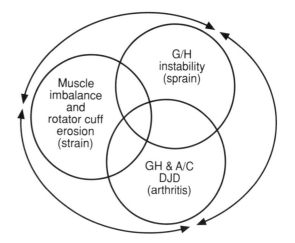

Figure 2.3 Disease triad: cyclic relationship of instability, strain/imbalance, and arthritis.

If the joint capsule has been stretched, then the extrinsic muscles about the shoulder must be relied upon to balance the shoulder to prevent progressive wear and tear. As a protective mechanism, posture may change, and certain muscles may be overused while others are underutilized, leading to dysfunction, impingement, periscapular muscle spasm, and neck pain. Without a strong subscapularis anteriorly to contain the shoulder, repetitive dislocation or subluxation episodes could occur, leading to further stretching of the joint capsule, further immobilization of the joint due to apprehension and lack of humeral head depression, loss of normal cartilage nutrition, and progressive arthritis. Inflammation combined with inactivity leads to fibrosis. Decreased humeral depression linked with postural change leads to impingement, traumatic wear, and inflammation of the supraspinatus.

With significant trauma in an initial dislocation, a notch may occur in the back of the humeral head (Hill-Sachs lesion) or to the inferoanterior rim of the glenoid (Bankart lesion), which will be discussed in chapter 6. Small fragments of torn labrum or loose bodies formed at the time of fracture can progressively erode against the joint surface, leading to early arthritis, which paradoxically may temporarily yield some stability to the joint by providing a friction fit rather than a hydraulic fit. Degeneration progresses nevertheless.

If a pitcher has stronger internal rotators than external rotators, it may be that the humeral head is not well contained in the socket at the end of the throw, and capsular tissue will stretch in the posterior aspect of the joint in follow-through. The fact that the weak posterior musculature does not keep the humeral head depressed may mean that the humeral head rides a little higher, eroding into the supraspinatus tendon. In this case the humeral head will ride progressively higher, eventually wearing into the biceps and through the rotator cuff, leading to a cuff tear, as well as to the associated arthritis within the joint due to joint incongruity and a clinical condition of end-stage impingement that is difficult to manage. Pressure against the biceps may cause it to develop partial detachment of its superior labral base, interfering significantly with the normal force-couples and normal motion patterns. The key to prevent progressive degeneration is correct early management or prevention.

Summary

The patient will always tell the examiner what is wrong, so it is important to listen carefully. The clinician must understand classification of injury patterns for documentation and for appropriate referral for further work-up or rehabilitation. The extent of the injury may increase with repetitive athletic trauma or overuse, but early identification may limit the extent of injury. Instability may lead to impingement, and vice versa. Both these problems could lead to arthritis, which in itself may limit mobility, lead to further muscle weakness, and accelerate breakdown, decreasing the speed of recovery and impairing postinjury performance. Although common terms become the springboard for communication in the rehabilitative effort, common clinical examination techniques, the subject of the next chapter, also aid in communication.

3

Clinical Examination Techniques

After obtaining a history, physical examination is the next step in assessment of the injured athlete's shoulder. Visual assessment may identify changes in motion patterns that have developed to prevent irritation of injured tissue. Tissue injury causes painful inflammation. Palpation and tests designed to stress specific anatomic sites can help identify the injured tissue. Even the occurrence of pain within the range of motion can help determine injured structures.

The patient may state that it hurts to place the shoulder in a certain range. Subjective findings such as this can be elicited either actively by having the athlete move his or her own shoulder or passively when the examiner moves the shoulder. Nevertheless, when pain occurs in certain ranges of motion, clinically correlating with stress of specific anatomic structures, such findings are considered objective medically.

One must identify the problem before seeking relevant therapeutic measures. This chapter presents a logical and orderly method of observation and objective and subjective clinical testing to help identify the structural problems of the injured athlete's shoulder.

Inspection

Watching the patient dress or undress may yield important clinical information; however, this practice makes most patients uncomfortable and should be avoided. Nevertheless, the shoulder cannot be examined without being uncovered. Rather than paper or expensive cloth gowns, sleeveless T-shirts are recommended because they don't come open like hospital gowns, so the patient is less self-conscious about traveling through the clinic for X-ray or therapy if necessary. A patient can be instructed to come to the clinic dressed in a sleeveless T-shirt, which would avoid the expense of providing the examining attire.

There are many ways to examine the shoulder. The examiner must find a method that is logical, that he or she is comfortable with, and that will be adhered to so that relevant information is not left out. The examiner first observes the patient from the front, looking for asymmetry from side to side that might be either posttraumatic or congenital. Asymmetry may mean previous fracture, muscle atrophy, or abnormal bony prominences from malunion, nonunion, or arthritis. Have the patient attempt range of motion bilaterally, that is, both arms at the same time, in an effort to see what is normal or difficult for him or her, to assess smoothness of scapulohumeral motion, and to see when pain is initiated *prior* to palpation, which could bring on pain and considerably minimize active motion. It is important to keep in mind which shoulder is affected in order to ascertain whether similar findings are present in the opposite side or whether restricted motion is normal compared to the opposite nonpainful shoulder.

Evaluate the patient while he or she is sitting. Look for scars from previous surgery, depigmentation, or subcutaneous atrophy, which might be associated with previous cortisone injection, and look at how the patient positions his or her arm. Poor posture may allow forward rolling of the scapula and put considerable stress on the trapezius and periscapular muscles, leading to pain at the superomedial scapular angle or spasm of the levator scapulae muscle. The way the patient holds his or her arm toward the body may correlate with the acuteness of the trauma, posture problems, or possible coexistent swelling of that extremity, including the fingers. Swelling or mottling of the skin might implicate disuse or a reflex sympathetic dystrophy. Deltoid atrophy may correlate with axillary nerve injury. Combined or isolated supraspinatus or infraspinatus atrophy may correlate with suprascapular nerve compression. Ecchymosis may be associated with avulsion trauma, such as in a pectoralis major rupture.

Recording Clinical Findings

Because of the universal positioning ability of the shoulder, measurement standards have varied considerably in various textbooks in the past. Strict forward flexion and strict abduction have been measured, but these are not the most normal or significant motions of the shoulder. In fact, *functional abduction* is both the most common and a more significant motion to measure. An office

examination must be thorough and systematic, producing information in a manner that can be communicated to other medical professionals through the written record. Conforming to recent standards set by the Society of American Shoulder and Elbow Surgeons (see the form on pp. 39 and 40) will facilitate the communication of data.

Recording Range of Motion

After inspection, the range of motion is determined by asking the patient to "follow the leader." The examiner makes a certain motion and asks the patient to do the same on his or her own. Next the examiner passively moves the neck and upper extremities and notes the differences between active and passive motion. Scapular rotation is done in conjunction with examination of the neck, spine, and ribs. Symptoms of cervical radiculopathy could overlap with shoulder symptoms. Neck examination must be part of the shoulder exam. Flexion, extension, and rotation of the neck are recorded (Figure 3.1).

Scapulothoracic function is assessed by elevation and depression of the shoulder (or shoulder shrug), protraction/flexion, and retraction/extension (Figure 3.2). Motions that are perhaps more functional than strict abduction or forward flexion include *scapular elevation*, or shrugging one's shoulders; *scapular rotation*, used in reaching on a horizontal plane across the midline in front of the body; *scapular protraction*, rolling the scapula forward while reaching behind one's back; and *scapular retraction*, needed to reach behind one's head. Rotation of the clavicle at the acromioclavicular (A/C) joint also allows the clavicle to act as a lever as elevation continues. Nevertheless, scapular motion and rotation through the A/C joint are hard to measure or establish in physical examination, even though these components are essential to normal function. Loss of normal sliding of the supraspinatus within its outlet due to a rough surface; thickened bursa; subdeltoid adhesions; or protrusion of bone from the A/C joint, clavicle, or acromion will lead to overuse of this scapulothoracic sliding mechanism.

Arthritis at the A/C joint will diminish normal motion through this joint—that is, horizontal flexion, hyperabduction, and reverse extension (Figure 3.3)—and will also lead to overuse of the scapulothoracic mechanism. Soft tissue interposition into the glenohumeral joint—such as a superior labral anterior-to-posterior (SLAP) lesion,

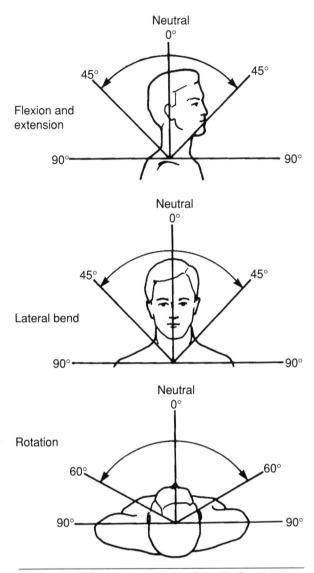

Figure 3.1 The clinical range of cervical motion.

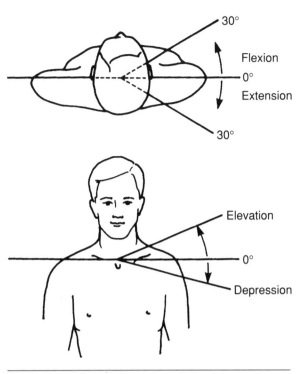

Figure 3.2 The clinical range of shoulder girdle motion.

Bankart lesion, or loose body—or postural changes and muscle imbalance all lead to decreased use of the central aspect of the shoulder (i.e., the A/C joint, glenohumeral joint, and supraspinatus sliding mechanism) and an overuse leading to pain at the two ends, less commonly at the sternoclavicular joint and more commonly at the scapulothoracic mechanism.

Scapulothoracic overuse of the upper trapezial and levator scapulae muscles leads to pain at the superomedial angle of the scapula, spasm of the levator scapulae muscle, tenderness of the rhomboids, and neck pain with atypical migraine headaches due to overuse of the muscles attaching behind the ear. Scapular rotation is markedly affected by posture and protraction of the scapula; scapular rotation leading to a forward slump of the shoulder

must be noted. Lateral rotation of the scapula should be recorded at the inferior tip if markedly different from the unaffected shoulder (Figure 3.4).

The patient is asked to attempt functional abduction, that is, bilateral, palm-down elevation in line with the scapula as far as possible even with pain. Forward flexion is next attempted, palm down, palm up, then both again; any difference is noted. Strict abduction is then attempted while the examiner looks for a painful arc (Kessel & Watson, 1973). Even with a frozen shoulder, 40° of abduction is usually possible due to scapulothoracic motion, often that associated with a shoulder shrug. If there is pain between 80° and 120° during palm-down elevation that is gone during palm-up elevation, then rotation cuff tendinitis exists.

Above 120° and below 80°, A/C joint leverage is most effective in positioning the upper extremity and hand in space, and there is more room in the supraspinatus outlet as the cuff drops away from the elevated scapula. In the midrange, 80° to 120°, the supraspinatus slides under the confines of the coracoacromial ligament, A/C joint, distal clavicle, and acromion. If the patient cannot lift the shoulder in this midrange but can lift the opposite side, there is very possibly a full-thickness rotator cuff tear or adhesions between the deltoid and rotator cuff freezing the motion plane, as will be discussed in

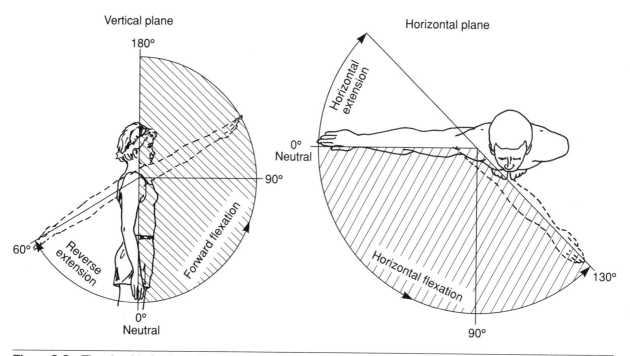

Figure 3.3 The shoulder's clinical range of flexion/extension.

chapter 8. Abduction pain above 120° palm up or palm down implicates the A/C joint as a problem.

More pain in midrange abduction palm up than palm down clinically correlates with early adhesive capsulitis, bursal adhesions caught in the supraspinatus fossa behind the scapular spine or between the deltoid and rotator cuff, synovitis in the posterior recess of the shoulder, or glenohumeral joint capsular laxity coexisting with rotator cuff tendinitis. The primary entity to be treated should be the subluxation so that joint instability will be minimized and secondary tendinitis eliminated. A subluxation-reduction test, described subsequently, is useful to delineate this.

Horizontal flexion causes pain behind the scapular spine with adhesive capsulitis and at the A/C joint with A/C joint arthritis. Pain that is found in midrange palm-down abduction but eliminated palm-up is due to a swollen or bruised supraspinatus, which is moved out of the way in palm-up abduction (Figure 3.5). The patient attempts to externally rotate his or her arm at the side to see if there is a difference between the affected and unaffected shoulders in active and passive motion (Figure 3.6).

Next, move behind the patient and look for dimpling around the shoulder that correlates with subluxation or previous cortisone injection. Muscle wasting of the infraspinatus may be clinically evident. Internal rotation is best assessed from this

position by asking the patient to reach behind his or her back along the spine to see how high he or she can reach (Figure 3.6). Check the affected side against the unaffected side; although it is useful to estimate that one side can reach to T5 and the other side to T10, a clinically reproducible method of recording is more useful. This is easily assessed by palpating the number of spaces between the spinous processes directly posterior; this information is easy to record in your office notes. A 10-vertebrae difference on one assessment but only 5 on a subsequent exam may indicate that adhesive capsulitis is resolving and motion is improving. Subscapularis function, the ability to lift the hand off the back, can be assessed at this time.

Move the arm through a passive range of motion when the active range is judged incomplete to find if loss of motion is due to stiffness or pain inhibition. Passive mobility should be tested in functional elevation, forward flexion, or abduction if any of these were restricted actively or seemed to be limited due to significant pain. The difference between active and passive motion should be recorded.

Objective Clinical Tests

Placing the arm in certain positions will stress different areas of the shoulder. The patient may complain of pain associated with certain positions. Because some may argue that the athlete may have

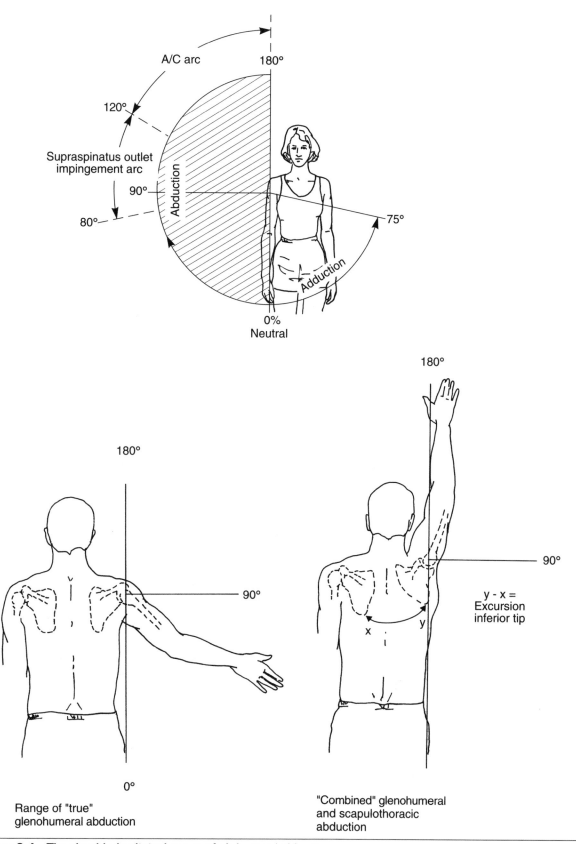

Figure 3.4 The shoulder's clinical range of abduction/adduction.

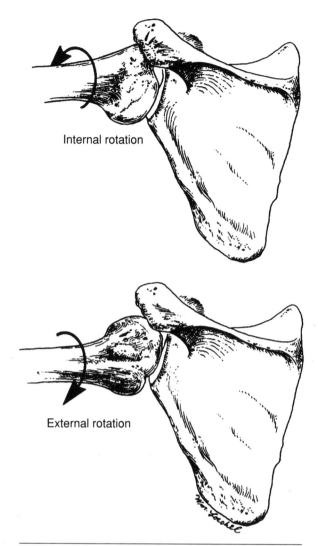

Internal rotation

External rotation

Figure 3.5 Impingement of the greater tuberosity. The rotator cuff's insertion is trapped in true impingement against the acromion in midrange abduction but is cleared with external rotation (palm-up abduction).

learned to complain when the shoulder is stressed in certain ways for secondary gain, such as avoiding an athletic event or strenuous practice, consistent findings on various tests will help affirm diagnosis and take the findings out of the subjective realm.

Initial Laxity Testing

While behind the patient, the examiner can easily assess the external rotation at 90° of one side versus the other. The examiner tests each shoulder independently by placing the palm of his or her hand in the back of the glenohumeral joint and assessing limits of external rotation. Going beyond neutral yields significant information. The patient may not

allow this, or may wince when this motion occurs, which are positive *apprehension signs* showing that the joint capsule is loose (Rowe & Zarins, 1981). A positive result may indicate that the humeral head is sliding out anteriorly and particularly inferiorly, causing abrasion of the rotator cuff against the acromion, compressing the ulnar nerve and causing numbness in the two ulnar digits, or just causing apprehension because the patient does not want the humeral head to pop out of the socket. Two other factors may also become apparent by doing this maneuver. You may feel the shoulder slide forward or find grinding as the apprehension test is done, which may or may not be associated with apprehension. This indicates some soft tissue wear—such as Bankart lesion or capsular avulsion at the inferoanterior rim of the glenoid—or that the humeral head is merely sliding out of the socket. From this abducted, externally rotated position, the arm can be moved into internal rotation, and feeling a click usually correlates with soft tissue interposition due to a labral tear in the superoanterior quadrant (Figure 3.7). This is similar to a McMurray maneuver in the knee.

Acromioclavicular Versus Impingement Pain

Move back in front of the patient, and palpate the A/C joint to find whether it is tender and whether pain is made worse with forced horizontal flexion and forced hyperabduction, which implicates A/C joint arthritis. Moving the distal clavicle anteriorly and posteriorly with the fingertips may elicit pain with acromioclavicular joint sprain. Palpate over the coracoid tip and the coracoacromial ligament, and then do an impingement test at 90° of forward flexion and internal rotation to see whether the pain in this area is worsened (Hawkins & Kennedy, 1980), a positive sign that the rotator cuff is injured (Figure 3.8).

SLAP Lesion Test

From a 90° forward-flexed position, adduct the arm an additional 30° in the horizontal plane and internally rotate (Figure 3.9). If the patient complains of pain radiating down the biceps tendon area, even from the back of the joint, be highly suspicious that the superior labrum is detached or is loose in association with superior capsular laxity and is being caught in the joint with this maneuver (Ciullo, 1989a; Figure 3.10, a and b). This has been described in the past as a test for posterior subluxation, and in fact this position can produce posterior

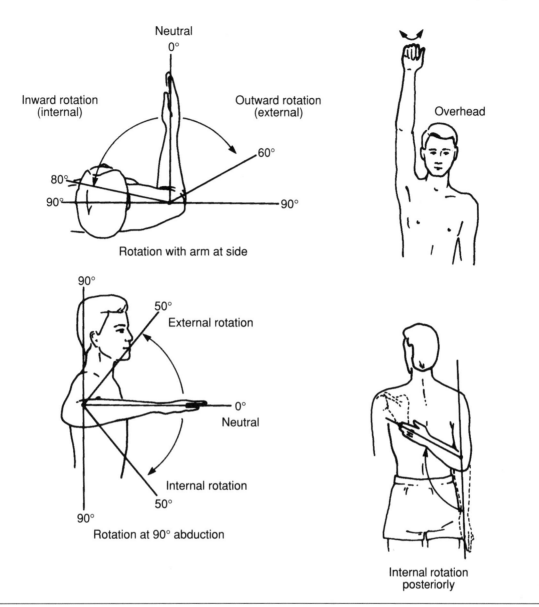

Figure 3.6 The shoulder's clinical range of rotation.

subluxation either actively or passively, but this posterior subluxation is not often symptomatic. Structures at the top of the joint (important posterior stabilizers) are either loose or worn, or the superior labrum and biceps complex are loose and interposed in the joint with or without a pathognomonic click with this maneuver.

Strength Testing

With the patient's arm down at the side and the elbow bent at 90°, the examiner places one hand on the patient's elbow, holding it in, and the other on the patient's wrist, and tests external rotation strength against resistance of the infraspinatus, teres minor, and posterior deltoid musculature.

The patient then places the bent elbow behind the back and brings the hand away from the body to test for isolated subscapularis function. A more isolated infraspinatus test is to bring the arm at the side to 30° of abduction and to test externally rotated abduction against resistance. Bringing the bent elbow behind the back with the arm still at the side tests for more isolated posterior deltoid strength. Bringing the arms up to 45° of abduction against resistance can test for middle deltoid strength. The arms are then brought into the position of functional abduction (Figure 3.11), thumbs down toward the ground, to test for supraspinatus strength (Jobe & Jobe, 1983). Bringing the arms in forward elevation about 90° against resistance checks for anterior deltoid strength. Resistance of

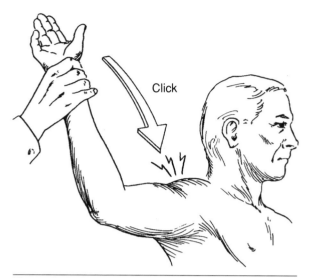

Figure 3.7 Functional subluxation *click test.*

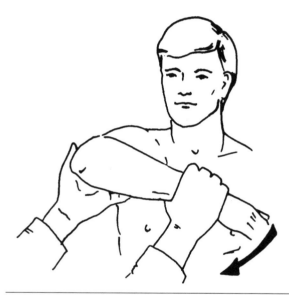

Figure 3.8 Hawkins's *impingement test* for rotator cuff tendinitis.

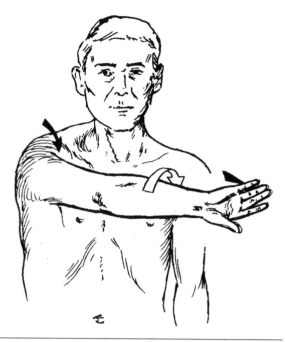

Figure 3.9 *SLAP lesion test* indicating injury to the superior suspensory system.

extension and flexion at the elbow tests for triceps and biceps function, respectively. Shoulder shrug against resistance tests for trapezial strength, for levator scapulae strength, and somewhat for rhomboid major and minor strength. Strength deficits should be noted in the office records, graded from 0 to 5, or from paralysis to normal function, respectively (Table 3.1).

Additional Laxity Tests

With the arm directly at the side, hold the elbow and pull down on the arm, comparing the affected arm to the unaffected arm (Warren, 1983). If the shoulder can be pulled out of joint, with a sulcus demonstrated under the acromion, you are dealing with an extremely loose joint, most likely a multi-directional instability (Figure 3.12). The fact that such findings may occur bilaterally in an athlete, even on an asymptomatic side, means that there is merely inherent laxity or progressive stress that has led to symmetrical laxity. This is not uncommon in sports such as swimming. The fact is, however, that once pain is associated with such laxity, the laxity is no longer considered physiologic and must be treated.

In another laxity test, the examiner stands behind the patient and asks the patient to pull the shoulder blades back to test rhomboid major and minor function. The examiner places his or her hand on the scapula and then twists the 90°-abducted arm into external rotation, the standard *apprehension test* (Figure 3.13a). Still holding the clavicle and scapular spine in one hand, the examiner's other hand surrounds the humeral head (Figure 3.13b). This is often difficult in an obese patient; however, the examiner will develop a clinical feel for how far he or she is able to move the shoulder out of the socket (Hawkins & Boker, 1990). More than 50% is abnormal in any direction. Next, the patient rests a straight-armed elbow on the examiner's shoulder so that the examiner can use both hands to push down on his 90°-abducted shoulder (Figure 3.13c), first directly inferiorly, then anteriorly, and then posteriorly for complete assessment of instability (Hawkins & Boker, 1990).

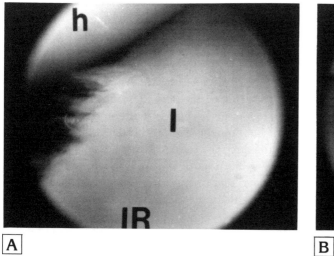

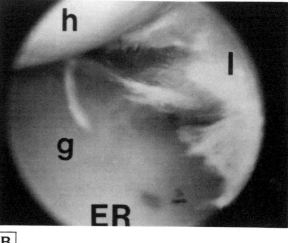

Figure 3.10 Detached superior labrum.

[A] Catching in the joint with horizontal flexion and internal rotation.

[B] Released in external rotation (h = humerus, g = glenoid, l = labrum, IR = internal rotation, ER = external rotation).

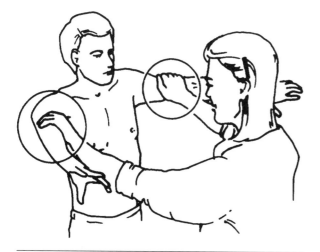

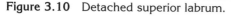

Figure 3.11 Jobe's *supraspinatus test* for rotator cuff tendinitis.

The patient then lies down supine on the examining table. The examiner sits down, preferably on a rolling stool, grasping the clavicle and scapular spine in one hand with the thumb and the fingers, respectively. With the opposite hand's thumb anteriorly and fingers posteriorly in the axilla, the examiner attempts to translate the humeral head anteriorly to posteriorly or circumferentially with the arm at 30°, 60°, and 90° of abduction in neutral and in 40° and 80° of external rotation. Remember, up to 50% translation in the glenohumeral joint can be considered normal; however, because of the corkscrew-type capsular fiber orientation, it should tighten toward external rotation so that

Table 3.1 Neuromuscular Functional Strength Assessment

Grade	Definition
0 ("Zero")	No palpable voluntary muscle contraction
1 ("Trace")	Slight voluntary muscle contraction but no active joint motion
2 ("Poor")	Functional voluntary range of motion with gravity eliminated (e.g., supine forward flexion)
3 ("Fair")	Functional range of motion against gravity, but unable to resist examiner
4 ("Good")	Functional range of motion against gravity, able to resist examiner, but can be overcome
5 ("Normal")	Functional range of motion against gravity, full resistance against examiner

Note. Assumes no structural blockage, such as arthritic or fracture deformity, soft tissue or loose body interposition, arthrofibrosis, or adhesive capsulitis.

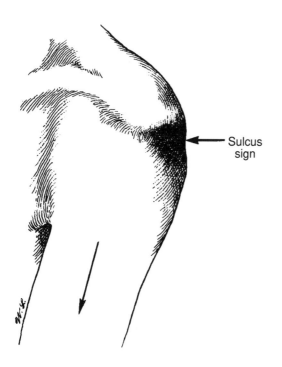

Figure 3.12 Warren's *sulcus sign.*

initial anterior laxity will be resolved in external rotation. If laxity persists or is increased in external rotation, then this is the best test for capsular stretching inferoanteriorly and for release of the suspensory structures superiorly. A large dimple in the front of the shoulder superiorly caused by testing at 80° abduction with neutral or full external rotation shows that there has been disruption of the superior suspensory mechanism, which increases both the likelihood of a poor response to physical therapy and the need of surgical correction, particularly if grinding is associated.

With the patient supine, trapping the scapula on the examining table and keeping the arm at 90° of abduction, the examiner can perform an apprehension test. With shoulder laxity, the patient may demonstrate extreme apprehension. The examiner can reduce a subluxated shoulder by placing his or her palm on the top of the shoulder and pushing it back into the socket, a procedure that I have used clinically since 1983 and have called a *containment maneuver* (Figure 3.14). When pain is relieved in external rotation and abduction while the hand is

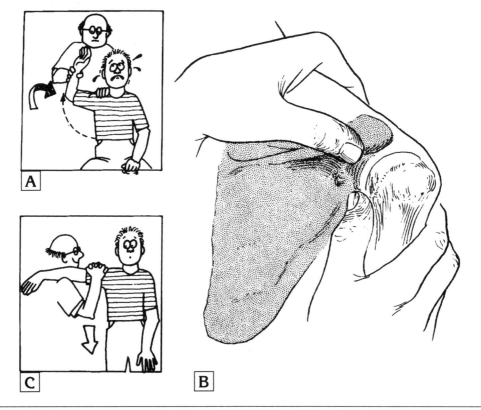

Figure 3.13 Glenohumeral clinical laxity tests.

[A] Rowe's *apprehension test.*

[B] Hawkins's *load and shift test.*

[C] Feagin's *downward traction apprehension test.*

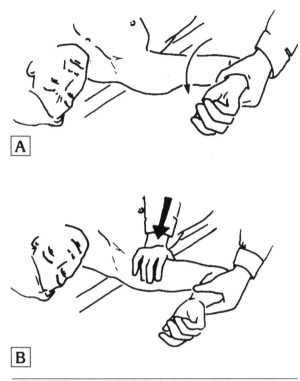

Figure 3.14 *Containment maneuver.*

[A] Apprehension with abduction in external rotation.

[B] Pain is minimized with anterior pressure or "containment" of the humeral head, but returns when the examiner's hand is released.

on the front of the shoulder and is again reproduced when the hand is removed, the impingement findings are most likely secondary to the looseness of the joint, and instability rather than tendinitis is the primary concern to be treated conservatively or surgically.

Tests for Scapular Winging

With the palms flat and fingertips toward each other, the patient is asked to push his or her weight off from the wall, a wall push-up. Scapular winging, when the medial edge of the scapula rotates outward, usually designates neurologic injury, leading to decreased function of the serratus anterior or trapezial fibers, but can also be associated with structural problems of the central shoulder—supraspinatus sliding mechanism, glenohumeral joint, or A/C joint dysfunction. When the central portion of the shoulder is not working properly, overuse of the scapulothoracic mechanism to provide motion through protraction can mimic serratus palsy, leading to a condition called *pseudowinging*. This may clinically indicate the need for an EMG to aid in differential diagnosis.

Thoracic Outlet Testing

Thoracic outlet syndrome must also be ruled out because symptoms about the shoulder often overlap those of instability. Scar tissue or stretch about the shoulder capsule often leads to neurovascular symptoms radiating down the arm, particularly while reaching overhead. If there is a complaint of radiating pain down the arm, if the pulse decreases in abducted external rotation (a *Wright maneuver* in the upper range and an *Adson maneuver* in the lower range) and if there is also a complaint of fatigue while opening and closing the hand overhead (a *Roos maneuver*), then thoracic outlet syndrome or compression of the neurovascular structures as they leave the thoracic cage must be suspected and treated accordingly (Figure 3.15). This is particularly true when there is no clinical laxity to anterior, posterior, or inferior manual translational testing. With signs of instability, however, particularly when combined with clinical signs of rotator cuff tendinitis and posterior tenderness at the superomedial angle associated with scapulothoracic overuse, treatment of the underlying subluxation through postural retraining, muscle balancing, and even surgery may completely eliminate the secondary scapulothoracic symptoms, which may be due to postural change associated with the generalized shoulder dysfunction.

Provocative Steroid Injection Testing

Many orthopedists will add select injections to the clinical examination to help define the role of the A/C joint or tendinitis in the subacromial area as part of the pathologic pattern. This is a shotgun approach and adds little to what can be found clinically without such injections.

The routine use of steroids to decrease painful conditions about the shoulder should be avoided. Steroid injection may in fact decrease inflammation due to tendinitis, arthritis, synovitis, or injury. Inflammation, however, is part of the healing response, and by decreasing inflammation, although pain may be relieved, the healing response is diminished as well.

Kennedy and Willis (1976) have shown that steroid injection unravels the collagen in capsular and ligamentous substance, leaving that tissue weak for 4 to 6 weeks following such injection. The pain may be diminished, but steroid injection also decreases its protective function, and the tissue may in fact be more prone to injury. One or two selective extra-articular injections may be useful and perhaps not cause too much damage, but the athlete

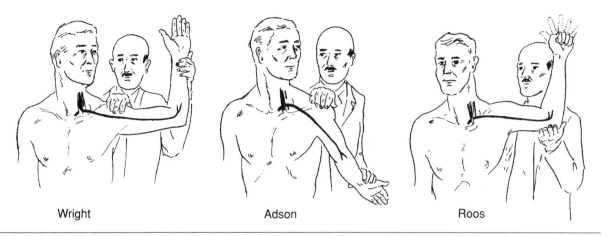

| Wright | Adson | Roos |

Figure 3.15 Clinical tests in assessment of thoracic outlet syndrome.

must be warned of potential complications and is actually more injury prone for the next 4 to 6 weeks. Repetitive cortisone injections should be condemned. Not only is pain diminished, so is the healing response, leaving the athlete at risk of future injury.

clinical process of inspection, palpation, and subjective and objective analysis, the athlete's shoulder pathology can be more clearly identified. With identification, specific treatment options become apparent.

Summary

In order to treat a problem correctly, the actual problem must be identified. Using a systematic

Form 3.1
Society of American Shoulder and Elbow Surgeons
Basic Shoulder Evaluation Form

Name _____ Shoulder R/L _____

Date of examination _____

(Circle choice)

I. **Pain** (5 = none, 4 = slight, 3 = after unusual activity, 2 = moderate, 1 = marked, 0 = complete disability, and NA = not available) _____

II. **Motion**
    A. Patient sitting (enter motion or NA if not measured)
       1. Active total elevation of arm _____ degrees.
       2. Passive internal rotation.
          (Circle segment of posterior anatomy reached by thumb)
          (Enter NA if reach restricted by limited elbow flexion)

1 = Less than trochanter	8 = L2	15 = T7	(# of vertebrae
2 = Trochanter	9 = L1	16 = T6	less than opposite
3 = Gluteal	10 = T12	17 = T5	side = _____)*.
4 = Sacrum	11 = T11	18 = T4	*Dominant side is
5 = L5	12 = T10	19 = T3	usually 2
6 = L4	13 = T9	20 = T2	vertebrae less
7 = L3	14 = T8	21 = T1	

       3. Active external rotation with arm at side _____ degrees.
       4. Passive external rotation at 90 degrees abduction _____ degrees.
          (enter NA if cannot achieve 90 degrees of abduction)
    B. Patient supine
       1. Passive total elevation of arm _____ degrees.
       2. Passive external rotation with arm at side _____ degrees.

III. **Strength** (5 = normal, 4 = good, 3 = fair, 2 = poor, 1 = brace, 0 = paralysis, and NA = not available) (Enter numbers below)
     A. Anterior deltoid _____
     B. Middle deltoid _____
     C. External rotation _____
     D. Internal rotation _____

IV. **Stability** (5 = normal, 4 = apprehension, 3 = rare subluxation, 1 = recurrent dislocation, 0 = fixed dislocation, and NA = not available) (Enter numbers below)
     A. Anterior _____
     B. Posterior _____
     C. Interior _____

V. **Function** (4 = normal, 3 = mild compromise, 2 = difficulty, 1 = with aid, 0 = unable, and NA = not available) (Enter numbers below)
    A. Use back pocket (if male); fasten bra (if female) _____
    B. Perineal care _____

(continued)

Form 3.1 *(continued)*

   C. Wash opposite axilla _____

   D. Eat with utensil _____

   E. Comb hair _____

   F. Use hand with arm at shoulder level _____

   G. Carry 10 to 15 lb with arm at side _____

   H. Dress _____

   I. Sleep on affected side _____

   J. Pulling _____

   K. Use hand overhead _____

   L. Throwing _____

   M. Lifting _____

   N. Do usual work _____ (Specify type of work) _____

   O. Do usual sport _____ (Specify sport) _____

VI. **Patient Response**

   (Circle choice)

   (3 = much better, 2 = better, 1 = same, 0 = worse, and NA = not available/applicable)

Total elevation of the arm is measured by viewing the patient from the side and using a goniometer to determine the angle between the arm and the thorax.

4

Analytic Tools

Clinical examination helps to identify injured structures; however, examination is not always enough to indicate the extent of injury and the type of intervention necessary to allow the injured athlete's shoulder to regain maximal performance. Pain tolerance is one intervening factor. Many athletes underestimate their problems and may be considered to have a high pain tolerance. It would be a mistake to allow such an athlete to participate in an aggressive rehabilitation program that might in fact make the problem worse. At the opposite end of the spectrum, the individual with a low pain tolerance may be overemphasizing his or her injury from a clinical perspective, and objective testing might avoid unnecessary surgical intervention. The in-between patient is more common; that is, examination may be equivocal and diagnostic testing indicated.

In this regard, various analytic tools become important in assessment of the injured athlete's shoulder. These will help determine the extent of injury and indicate the type of intervention. Obviously, minor structural damage indicates more conservative management, such as flexibility and strengthening exercises, working with the trainer, or an organized physical therapy program. More complicated structural tissue damage may indicate the need for surgical intervention. Objective studies range from electrical measurement of neuromuscular function to radiographic assessment of bones and soft tissue. The purpose of this chapter is to introduce the tools that are best used to assess the injured athlete's shoulder and to compare their relevance.

Four-View X-Ray Series

A three-view anterior-posterior (AP) X-ray series of the shoulder in internal rotation, neutral, and external rotation is still routine throughout much of the United States. This is an archaic X-ray series, popularized in the 1930s for looking for calcific tendinitis, and is not adequate to properly assess the athlete's shoulder. As in any other joint, at least two views, at 90° to each other, are important for assessment. Four views are recommended to assess the athlete's shoulder.

AP Modified Grashey View

A modified Grashey true AP view is taken angled out 15° to 20° to compensate for retroversion of the glenohumeral joint as well as for the carrying angle of the scapula on the rib cage. This is routinely angled down 15° to look for an acromial spur at the inferoanterior edge of the acromion. The hand is placed behind the back in internal rotation to look for notching in the back of the posterolateral humeral head, a Hill-Sachs lesion that correlates with subluxation. Loose bodies, fragmentation of the inferoanterior edge of the glenoid, or calcification slightly medial to the inferoanterior rim of the glenoid due to capsular stripping and periosteal new bone formation is found in about 15% of subluxating shoulders with this view (Figure 4.1, a-d).

On the AP view, if there is less than 6 mm between the humeral head and the acromion, which is considered normal with the X-ray taken 30 in. from the patient, and therefore a break in Maloney's line at the inferior glenoid, then thinning of the rotator cuff or tearing may be suspected. It is interesting that in some patients the normal humeral acromial interval on the standard AP film (Figure 4.2a) can be altered merely by the patient's actively pushing him- or herself out of a chair, causing the humeral head to "buttonhole" through the defect (Figure 4.2b).

A/C Joint Zanca View

Next, an AP film angled upward 10° with 5 kV decreased penetration is taken to assess the normally posteriorly closed V shape of the A/C joint (Zanca, 1971; Figure 4.3, a-d).

Sclerosis on both sides of the joint, calcification of the disk, loose bodies in the joint, distal clavicular erosion, or complete loss of the joint is best assessed on this view, which is done in external rotation (Figure 4.4, a-d). This view helps identify calcium deposits in the supraspinatus, which are best defined with decreased roentgenographic penetration, unless the patient is obese, in which case normal penetration may be necessary. Trabecular mound atrophy and sclerosis of the outer cortical rim of the greater tuberosity, associated with impingement, may be seen here.

Posterior-Anterior Scapular Y View

The third view is a posterior-anterior (PA) scapular Y view angled down 15° to assess the relationship of the humeral head to the glenoid socket in dislocation and the shape of the acromion in impingement (Figure 4.5, a-d). This view can give considerable information about traction spur formation within the coracoacromial ligament or deltoid origin, calcific tendinitis, decreased space between the humeral head and the acromion, clavicular intrusion into the subacromial space, and calcific deposits. Unfortunately, postural change due to pain or habit may make this view difficult to reproduce.

Type I (flat), II (curved), and III (hooked) changes of the acromion on this view (Figure 4.6a) have been associated with rotator cuff pathology, with Type III having the highest correlation (Bigliani, Morrison, & April, 1986). By changing the caudal angle between 5° and 25°, a patient without an acromial hook can appear to change on the AP film from a Type I to a Type III, due to optical projection (Figure 4.6b).

Positional variance and posture may have a lot to do with the projection of a hook on this view, so one must interpret it carefully. Impingement can often be documented by contact of the acromion against the soft tissue shadow of the rotator cuff (Figure 4.7a); impingement can also be due to contact of the inferior clavicle (Figure 4.7b). Acromial typing is not necessarily a progressive nor a hereditary phenomenon, because such curves or hooks are rarely found before 16 years of age. In fact, these patterns may not even be stable, as Type II curves may progress toward Type I, or Type III toward Type II (Figure 4.7, c and d). Therefore, it is the amount of penetration into the supraspinatus outlet more than the type that becomes the determining factor in the development of impingement.

Modified Lawrence Axillary View

The fourth view is a modified Lawrence axillary view. The patient is placed in a supine position, and the shoulder is not propped. The arm is brought as far in abduction and external rotation as is comfortable to the patient. The X-ray cassette is then brought into the neck and elevated 30° off the point of the shoulder (Figure 4.8, a-d). The X-ray tube is placed next to the table, shooting perpendicular to the plate, parallel to the floor, and directly through the axilla.

Even in acute trauma when the shoulder is in a sling, merely placing a small foam wedge under the elbow to elevate it forward provides a position that gives considerable information about the relationship of the humeral head to the glenoid socket.

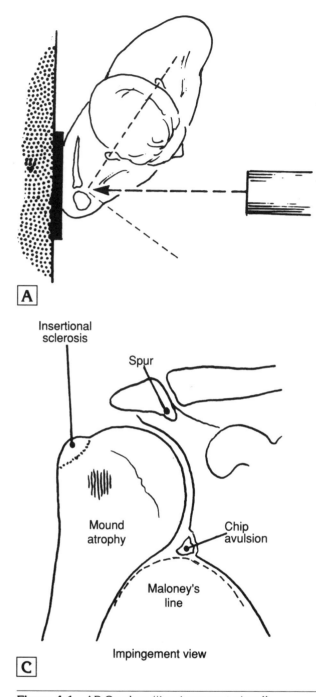

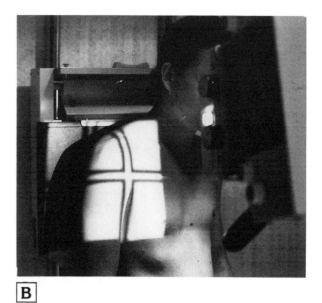

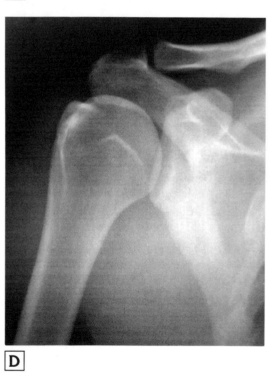

Figure 4.1 AP Grashey "impingement view."

   [A] Position drawing.

   [B] Clinical positioning.

   [C] X-ray drawing.

   [D] Clinical X-ray.

There is no reason why this *axillary trauma view* cannot be obtained in any emergency setting (Ciullo, Koniuch, & Teitge, 1982; Figure 4.9). Also, this supine axillary view is useful if the orthopedist wishes to do radiographic stress analysis of the shoulder for anterior and posterior subluxation (Ciullo, Koniuch, & Teitge, 1984; Figure 4.10). This view also is the best for defining nonunions, apophyseal lines, or physeal stress reactions within the acromion (Figure 4.11).

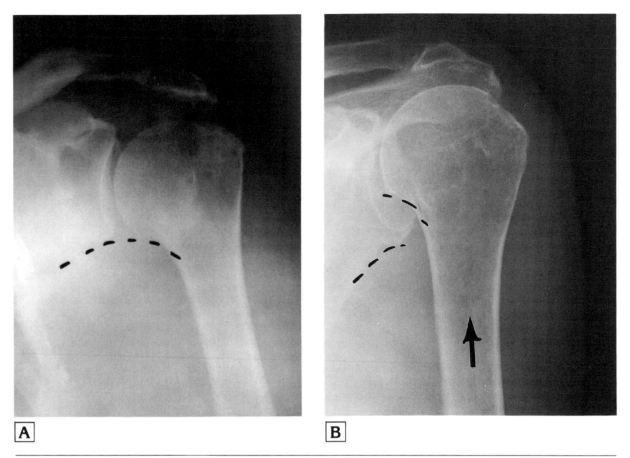

Figure 4.2 Maloney's line.

[A] Normal acromial humeral distance where inferior scapular neck and humeral neck make a round arch in a sitting, elderly tennis player.

[B] Arch is disrupted with superior migration of the humeral head when pushing up out of a chair as the humerus "buttonholes" through the rotator cuff rupture.

Computerized Tomography and Arthrography

Remember that most athletic injuries to the shoulder are soft tissue injuries and, at least acutely, will not show changes on standard X-rays. *Computerized tomography* (CT) traditionally has been used to assess bony changes. Fracture (Figure 4.12) and bony erosion (Figure 4.13) are not well established on routine X-rays but are better identified with CT technique. The standard *arthrogram* (Figure 4.14), obtained by injecting contrast material within the joint, has traditionally been used to assess the presence of a rotator cuff tear (Figure 4.15). By combining these two techniques, a computer-enhanced, low-radiation, multilayer study yields significant soft tissue information.

The CT-arthrogram is useful in assessing the rotator cuff but primarily assists in identification of capsular and labral pathology (Figure 4.16, a-e). If rotator cuff tearing and possible need for repair is the only concern in an older patient, then an arthrogram by itself may be 80% to 95% effective in affirming large tears. Superior migration of the humeral head, interposition of scar tissue, adhesive capsulitis, or upward deltoid pull on the humerus may seal the hole and yield false negative results. If there is a question of labral pathology, then a CT-arthrogram is the procedure of choice, but with a coexisting cuff tear dye may leak out, and detail of the labral tissue may be lost. A CT-arthrogram is usually done as a double-contrast test. Wear of the glenoid, fractures, and loose bodies are best assessed by the CT-arthrogram scan, which remains the "gold standard," giving more information than the MRI. Labral pathology, including tearing, detachment, and flattening, as well as bony pathology, capsular stripping or tearing, and capsular redundancy or inadequacy are assessed well with CT augmentation.

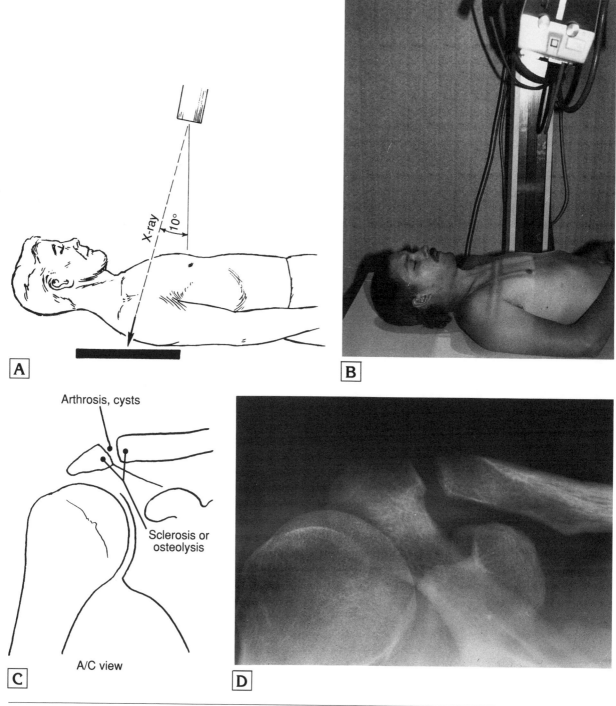

Figure 4.3 A/C joint Zanca view.

[A] Position drawing.

[B] Clinical positioning.

[C] X-ray drawing.

[D] Clinical X-ray.

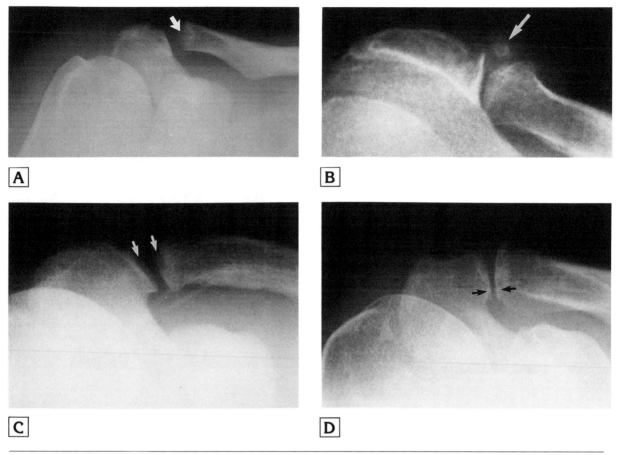

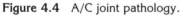

Figure 4.4 A/C joint pathology.

[A] Osteolysis.

[B] Loose body.

[C] Early arthritis with early enchondral ossification of articular cartilage.

[D] Late arthrosis.

Anterior displacement of the labrum is best assessed with the anterior structures relaxed in internal rotation and the elbow at the side (Figure 4.16a), whereas posterior detachment of the labrum is best assessed through posterior relaxation provided in external rotation (Figure 4.16c). The radiologist must be aware of this procedure because it will add another 5 min to a normally 25-min examination. A blush of dye within the labral substance cephalad to the coracoid is pathognomonic of a SLAP lesion (Figure 4.17, a and b). The joint is scanned by 3- to 4-mm slices, which are then computer enhanced to minimize the amount of radiation exposure to the patient.

Bone Scan

The *bone scan* may be used to define situations of increased synovitis, particularly posteriorly in the shoulder, as well as calcific tendinitis, which may not be demonstrated on routine shoulder X-ray, and arthritic changes in both the glenohumeral joint and the A/C joint (Figure 4.18, a and b).

Some clinicians will not operate on an A/C joint unless there are changes on the bone scan. However, inflammatory hot spots may only indicate early disease; burned-out arthritis or late arthrosis may no longer be hot. Changes tend to be bilaterally symmetrical and may not demonstrate significant variance; for this reason the bone scan is found to be relatively unimportant in the work-up of the shoulder. A triphase bone scan, however, is extremely important in attempting to diagnose reflex sympathetic dystrophy, with a blush on the early phase considered 99% diagnostic. Increased activity may be found without X-ray changes in early osteolysis. Increased activity with heterotopic bone after resection may indicate the need to postpone further debridement to avoid reaccumulation of bone.

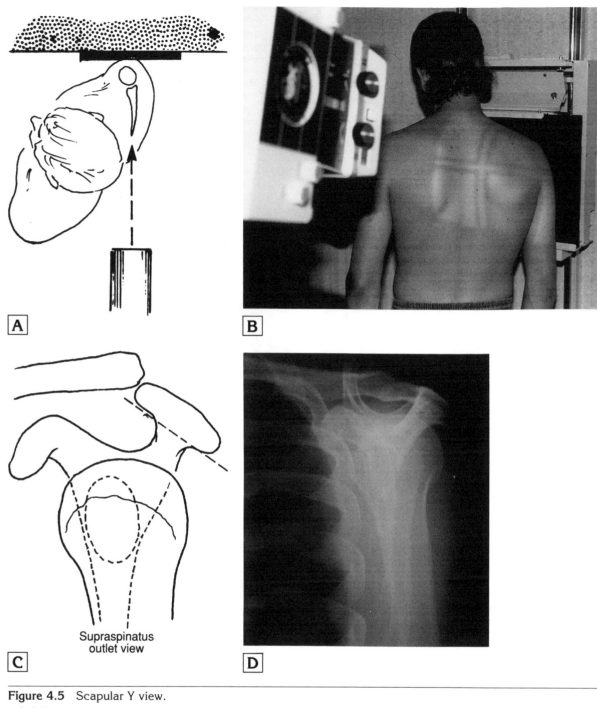

Figure 4.5 Scapular Y view.
  [A] Position drawing.
  [B] Clinical positioning.
  [C] X-ray drawing.
  [D] Clinical X-ray.

Ultrasound

Ultrasonography is a noninvasive technique that can give considerable information about the shoulder, specifically if a rotator cuff tear or wear is suspected (Figure 4.19). Occasionally, biceps tendon inflammation with subluxation can be found (Figure 4.20). However, a learning curve of at least 50 cases is necessary. The test is radiologist dependent

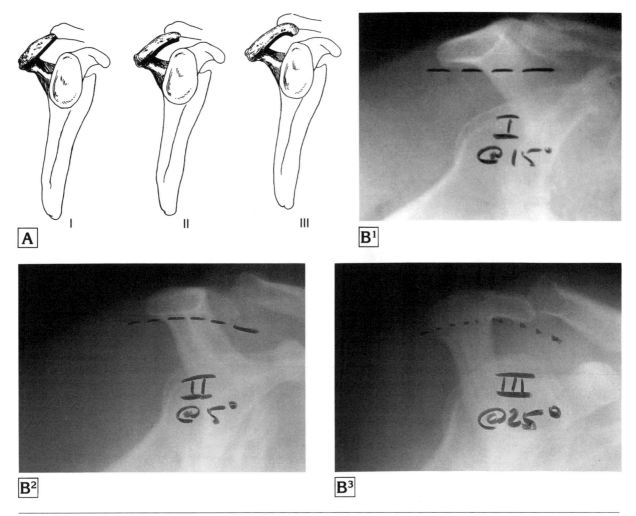

Figure 4.6 Acromial slope patterns.

  [A] Bigliani Types I-III.

  [B] Clinical X-ray examples:

  1. Type I;

  2. Type II; and

  3. Type III.

Note. X-rays 1-3 are taken of the same patient at 15°, 5°, and 25°, respectively, showing that posture or slight angle variations can change projection, decreasing the reliability of this classification scheme.

with accuracy varying from 40% to 98%. With this test, the shoulder can be evaluated through a range of motion, and this may be a significant advantage in assessing rotator cuff tears if the interpreter is meticulous; assessment of labral pathology is poor.

In the patient who has expressed fear of dye-injection testing, ultrasound may be a good screening technique for rotator cuff pathology. To an experienced and interested radiographer, partial-thickness erosion into the rotator cuff (Figure 4.21), full-thickness tear without retraction (Figure 4.22, a and b), or full-thickness tear with retraction (Figure

4.23, a and b) may be demonstrated to almost the same accuracy as a CT-arthrogram, thus decreasing the cost of diagnostic testing.

Ultrasound can also help determine whether or not surgery, if necessary, can be scheduled as an inpatient or outpatient case: Erosion may be treated by outpatient subacromial decompression; minimally displaced tearing by outpatient decompression with miniarthrotomy repair; and major disruption by more formal inpatient repair or arthroscopic, rather than open salvage debridement procedures.

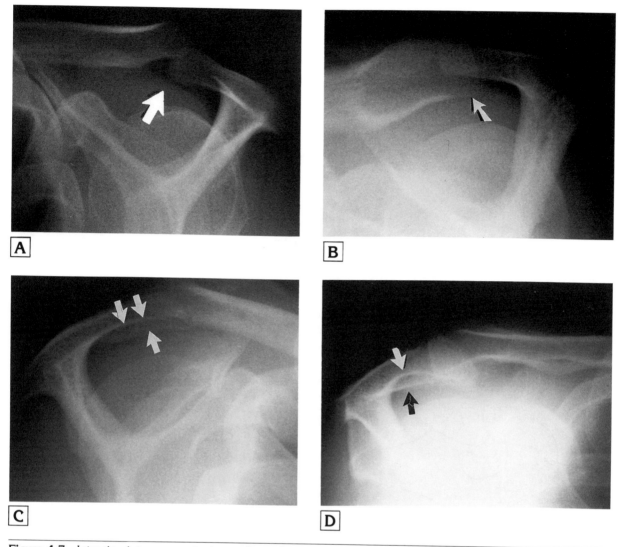

Figure 4.7 Intrusion into supraspinatus outlet and rotator cuff.

[A] Acromial impingement into the soft tissue shadow of the supraspinatus demonstrated on the office X-ray.

[B] Impingement due to inferior clavicular projection into the supraspinatus outlet.

[C] A Type II curve (two arrows) may fill in and build up due to periosteal irritation, converting to a Type I curve (one arrow).

[D] A Type III hook converting to a Type II curve may eventually develop into a Type I configuration by further periosteal build-up, decreasing reliability of the classification system.

Magnetic Resonance Imaging

Magnetic resonance imaging (MRI) is a noninvasive technique without radiation that measures the density of mobile protons in the tissue examined. The signal is produced by magnetized protons excited by radio waves. Echoes that depend on the density of the protons in the examined substance are picked up. Dense tissue such as cortical bone, tendon, and ligament produces no signal and appears as a black region on the MRI. Water-containing tissue such as muscle produces a medium-intensity signal, and fat produces the highest intensity signal and appears white on the MRI. Areas of bone necrosis are easily defined.

The main advantage of MRI is in assessment of rotator cuff tears. Full-thickness tears (Figure 4.24) or partial-thickness tears (Figure 4.25) can be easily demonstrated. One problem is that MRIs are often overread. A report stating, for instance, that "findings are consistent with impingement; rule out clinically" is redundant and decreases the usefulness of this test in a clinical setting. Also, an MRI does not well define labral pathology. Patients

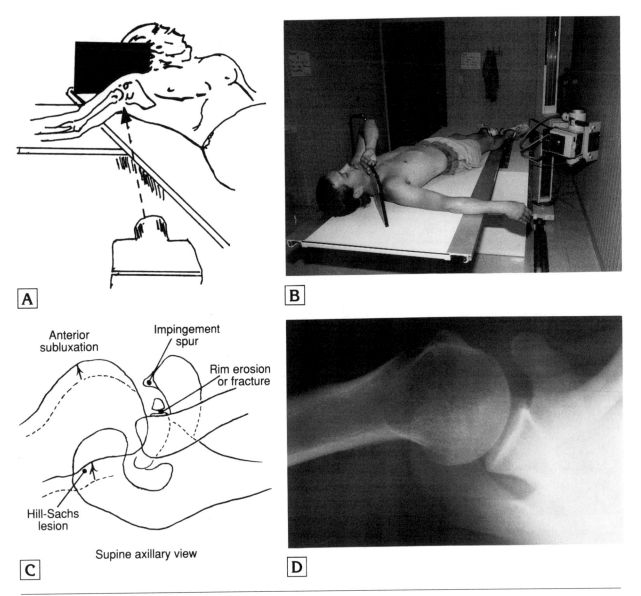

Figure 4.8 Modified Lawrence axillary view.

[A] Position drawing.

[B] Clinical positioning.

[C] X-ray drawing.

[D] Clinical X-ray.

weighing over 250 lb (113 kg) may not fit well into the gantry unless an oversized machine is available. The advanced surface coils are not generally available, and many insurance programs do not include MRIs as covered benefits. For this reason, newer generations of the device may not be available in a community, and therefore the sharper images that they reportedly produce—demonstrating subacromial bursitis, supraspinatus tendinitis, rotator cuff tearing, labral pathology, and so on—also may not be available. Testing is done in one position; motion MRIs are investigational.

At the present time, the CT-arthrogram remains the "gold standard." This is not to say that the MRI is not useful, as it has already changed the way we look at many clinical entities. Osteonecrosis may be picked up early, impingement wear into the rotator cuff by early A/C joint disease has been identified (Figure 4.26), pathologic entities such as suprascapular neuromas have been identified (Figure 4.27), and early arthritic changes, such as subchondral ossification and posterior osteophyte formation at the A/C joint (Figure 4.28), have been demonstrated through the use of MRI.

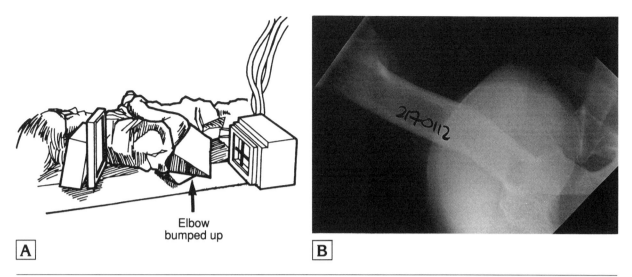

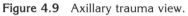

Figure 4.9 Axillary trauma view.

[A] Axillary view can be obtained even with the arm in a sling by merely propping the elbow forward.

[B] Posterior glenohumeral dislocation, taken in Velpeau immobilizer.

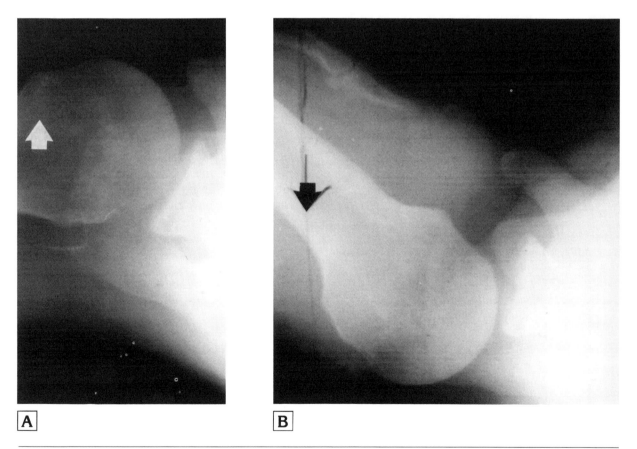

Figure 4.10 Stress axillary X-ray.

[A] Anterior push.

[B] Posterior stress. Axillary in external rotation commonly shows increased posterior motion with superior capsular mechanism disruption, SLAP lesion, or strict posterior laxity.

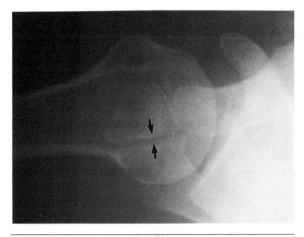

Figure 4.11 Mesoacromial nonunion or fibrous union not identified well on AP view can be seen on axillary view.

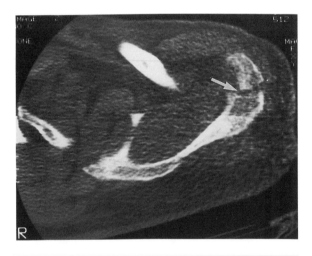

Figure 4.12 CT of acromial fracture.

Decreasing costs and the future ability to do real-time MRI, contrast studies, color enhancement, and so on may make this a more routine diagnostic tool. There may even come a day when the MRI is used to identify pathology in conjunction with a laser focused below the skin in order to do surgery without incisions.

Again, most clinicians presently rely more on CT-arthrogram and ultrasound than on the MRI to aid in diagnosis, but this varies among localities. The MRI is not to be done as a screening test; that is, a patient should not be referred to the orthopedist with a negative MRI, never having had a routine X-ray, although this is not unusual in the "gatekeeper" approach of many managed care programs. A CT-arthrogram in most situations is recommended as the most cost-effective screening test, yielding the most information.

Electromyography

The study of electrical activity associated with nerve conduction and muscular contraction yields useful diagnostic information in the care of the athlete's shoulder. One must try to identify a lesion before suggesting treatment if, in fact, treatment is feasible. A cervical root avulsion is not treatable, but a laceration to the brachial plexus or peripheral nerve may require immediate exploration and surgical repair for the best results. A neural stretch or contusion injury is expected to recover without surgical intervention. Electrical assessment can give evidence of recovery or lack thereof, rate of recovery, and subsequent need for surgical exploration or muscle transfer techniques. Understanding the terms involved helps to make such clinical tests useful.

Measuring Neuromuscular Activity

Electromyography concerns the methods of studying electrical activity of muscle. Graphic representation of such electrical currents produces an electromyogram (EMG). Neural transmission and myocontraction are achieved through transfer of electrically charged particles and associated depolarization and repolarization along cell membranes. Such electrical activity can be measured. By inserting an electrode into a muscle or by stimulating the nerve that supplies the muscle, muscular response can be recorded, yielding information on the integrity of the nerve and associated muscle fibers or motor units.

Although electrical recordings are no substitute for a history and physical examination, an EMG can augment the clinical assessment, help to find the actual pathology, and yield prognostic data. The status of the nerve, whether there has been segmental compression, or evidence of regeneration helps to establish the course of therapy. The maximal power of the muscle can be recorded to help establish the stage of rehabilitation and expected ability of the muscle to recover.

Surface recording of muscle electrical activity is very important in motion analysis and sports research (Nuber, Jobe, Perry, Moynes, & Antonelli, 1986). This can yield a rough estimation of muscular integration in the analysis of specific sport activity. Muscle electrical activity can help to establish what muscles are used, what muscles should be trained, and the percentages of muscular strength to integrate to achieve maximal performance and neuromuscular balance. This has

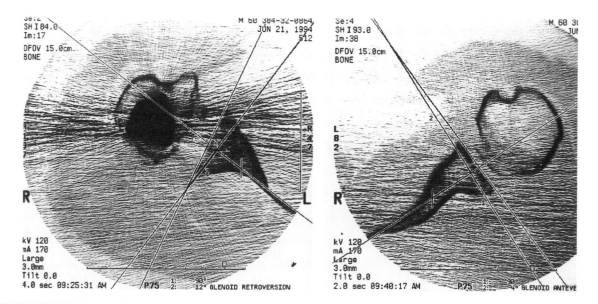

Figure 4.13 CT of glenoid: right shoulder with 12° retroversion, left shoulder with 4° anteversion.

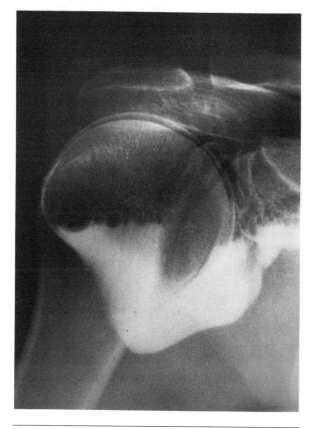

Figure 4.14 Normal arthrogram. Dye stays within confines of glenohumeral joint capsule.

prognostic implications for how to train to avoid injury or how to rehabilitate if injured.

Abnormal Electrical Patterns

When a *needle electric exam* (NEE) is done, a needle electrode is inserted or moved within a muscle,

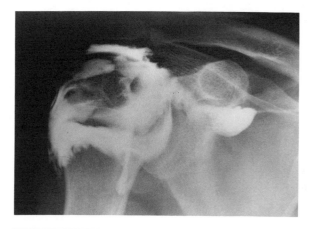

Figure 4.15 Abnormal arthrogram in which dye extravasates from the joint capsule into the sub-acromial, subdeltoid, subscapular, and subclavicular bursae (potential spaces) through a hole in the cuff; the size of the cuff tear is not well defined.

where it can detect a short burst of electrical activity that can be heard over a loudspeaker or recorded on an oscilloscope. *Insertional activity*, due to stimulation or injury to the muscle, normally stops 2 to 3 s after ceasing motion and twisting the electrode.

Much is learned from the *spontaneous activity* of muscle at insertion of an examining needle. Prolonged activity that leads to repetitive discharging *fibrillation potentials, fasciculations,* and *positive sharp waves* yields evidence of pathology. Insertional activity is eliminated when there is no functional muscle tissue available.

Positive Sharp Waves. A positive sharp wave is an initial positive deflection of rapid onset

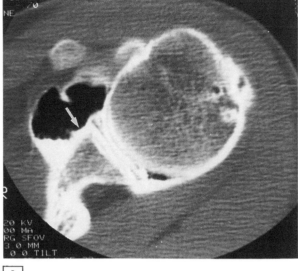

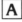

A

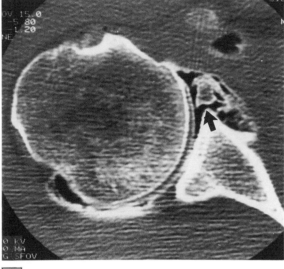

B

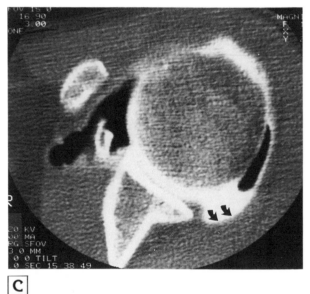

C

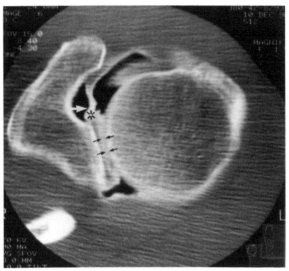

D

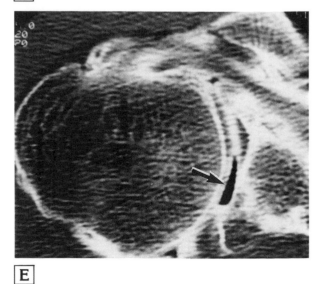

E

Figure 4.16 CT-arthrogram best defines capsulo-labral pathology.

[A] Anterior capsular stripping.

[B] Bankart lesion: anterior labral detachment.

[C] Posterior capsular redundancy.

[D] Detachment of coracoglenoid soft tissue at base of glenoid (* = pivot point), associated with thin superior glenohumeral ligament (white arrow). Note extravasation of dye within the superior labrum itself, identifying an associated SLAP lesion (black arrows).

[E] Air filling hole in central glenoid articular carti-lage loss.

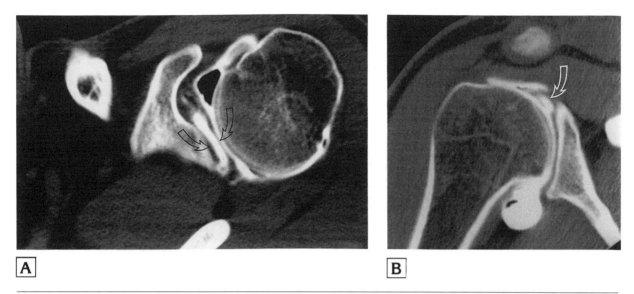

Figure 4.17 CT-arthrogram.

[A] Axillary reconstruction. Contrast filling defect with soft tissue glenoid labrum demonstrates SLAP lesion.

[B] AP reconstruction. Contrast filling defect in superior labrum where avulsed from glenoid (SLAP lesion).

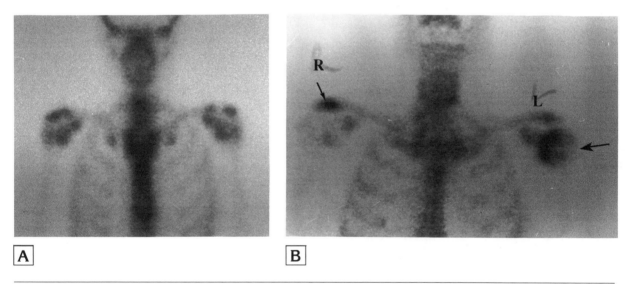

Figure 4.18 Bone scan.

[A] Normal.

[B] Areas of increased uptake indicate acromioclavicular joint arthritis in right shoulder and glenohumeral arthritis in left shoulder.

followed by a slower negative potential change that is prolonged. Positive sharp waves have a discharge frequency of 5 to 10 per s. Positive sharp waves occur spontaneously in denervated muscle and are a sign of injury or reinnervation.

Fibrillation. Within 100 hr of a crush or stretch injury, nerve fibers lose excitability distal to that injury, producing a prolonged discharge with a repetitive wave pattern. This produces electrical patterns called fibrillation potentials that are not associated with visible contracture of peripheral muscle and that are usually biphasic or triphasic in configuration with a discharge rate between 2 and 20 per s. They must be found in three separate areas within a single muscle to be considered present. They are found in denervated muscle, but disappear when reinnervation occurs or after the denervated muscle has atrophied so that no viable tissue remains. The absence of fibrillation potentials

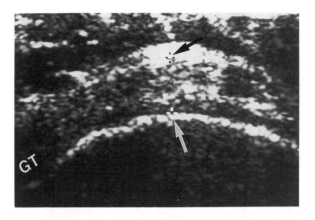

Figure 4.19 Normal ultrasound. Note markers used to estimate thickness of tendon to compare the opposite side (GT = greater tuberosity).

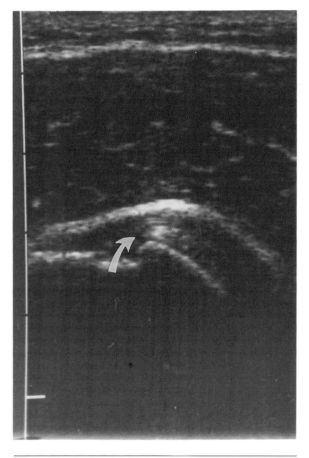

Figure 4.20 Ultrasound: biceps subluxated out of groove.

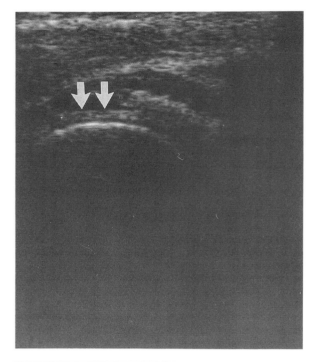

Figure 4.21 Ultrasound: partial-thickness rotator cuff tear.

may indicate recovery but may also indicate the inability to recover. Clinical correlation is mandatory. Fibrillation potential activity is related to injury to the muscle and to saponification of the fatty external layer of nerve necessary for saltatory conduction and will be registered in short nerves earlier than in long nerves. A short facial nerve may register such changes immediately, whereas long nerves to the shoulder and peripheral appendages may take 4 to 6 weeks to register abnormal activity.

Fasciculation. Fasciculations, or visible, rapid bursts of muscle activity in small ribbon-like areas, may be normal but can also indicate pathology, due to collateral reinnervation with instability occurring at the newly denervated and cross-innervated endplates. They are associated with exercising a muscle that is not warmed up, are increased in a cold environment, and may be enhanced by percussion. They produce a uniform and repetitive wave form that repeats from 1 to 50 per min. Fasciculation can be attributed to ischemia and electrolyte imbalance and therefore may be related to drug therapy, hydrational state, cramps, or metabolic disturbances, including hypokalemia.

Occasional spontaneous electrical discharge is recorded as a single fasciculation potential. Groupings of spontaneous discharges yield brief repetitive patterns. On physical examination, this correlates with the brief muscle twitch in a small area of muscle, random in distribution and electrical discharge pattern. These random twitches are related to new patterns of collateral reinnervation

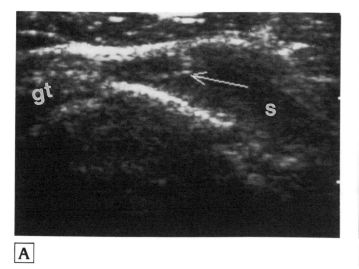
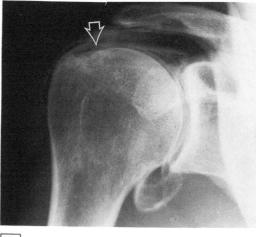

Figure 4.22 Nondisplaced full-thickness rotator cuff tear.

[A] Ultrasound (gt = greater tuberosity, s = supraspinatus).

[B] CT-arthrogram, same patient as in [A].

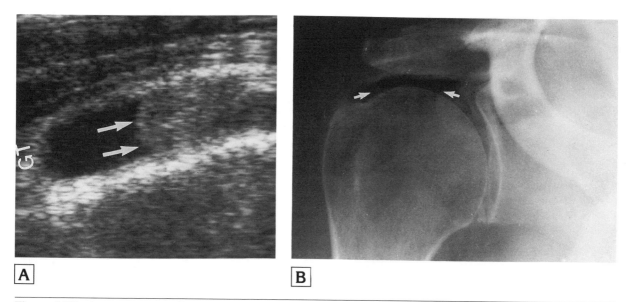

Figure 4.23 Large rotator cuff tear with significant detachment.

[A] Ultrasound (GT = greater tuberosity).

[B] CT-arthrogram, same patient as in [A].

by randomly scattered axonal twigs to the motor endplate.

Amplitude of Electrical Response

Electrical stimulation of a certain neurologic or somatic area can elicit a recorded response. There is a limit to this response because stimulation is limited by neurotransmission, the number of nerves involved, the nerve and muscle *motor units* involved, or the amount of muscle mass itself. Increasing the amount of electrical stimulation will increase myocontractility only up to a point. This point is called *supramaximal stimulation*, which records the electrical response of motor nerves to repetitive stimuli and gives useful information as to the status of the injury. Changes in the size of the *evoked response* can yield data on disorders of transmission at the neuromuscular junction. The size of the supramaximal stimulation will help

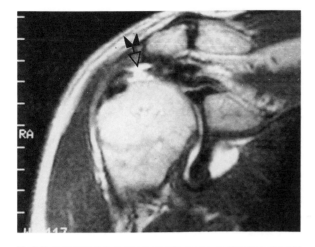

Figure 4.24   MRI: full-thickness rotator cuff tear.

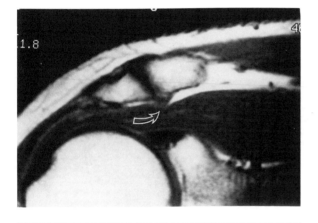

Figure 4.25   MRI: partial-thickness bursal-side rotator cuff erosion or tear.

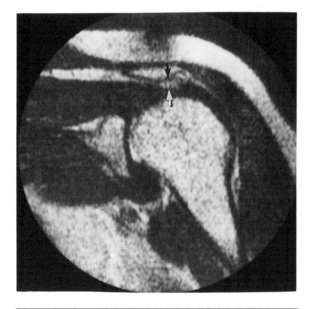

Figure 4.26   MRI: arthritis and swelling at A/C joint impinging into rotator cuff and causing tendon wear.

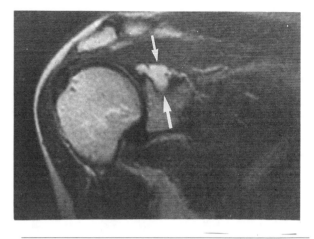

Figure 4.27   MRI: suprascapular neuroma eroding into superior glenoid notch.

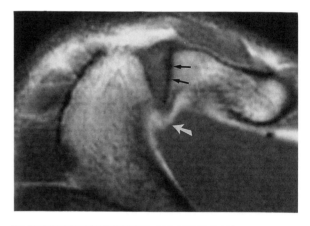

Figure 4.28   MRI: end-plate calcification (black arrows) and posterior osteophytes (white arrow), indicating early arthritis at the A/C joint.

determine recovery following crush or stretch of a nerve. Size changes necessitate serial analysis of the same area by the same examiner using the same diagnostic recording equipment for the most adequate interpretation.

Rather than the normal, small recorded range of depolarization and repolarization of a certain motor unit, occasionally after injury a number of phases overlap. This results in multiple units, or variable nerves in various stages of repair, demonstrating at least five components in the recorded response to an electrical stimulus. The average number of muscle fibers per unit may pathologically increase following denervation of muscle, because reinnervation by collateral branches of surviving neurons may lead to a scatter effect on the endplates of the motor units, so that the electrical charge may be dispersed over a wider area than usual. This is called *polyphasic* or *p-wave activity* and yields evidence of early regeneration, which decreases as normal nerve activity recovers.

Conduction Velocity

Conduction velocity can be measured, and decreases in velocity demonstrate specific areas of compression neuropathy or crush injury due to segmental demyelinization. Such slow-down, or *latency*, can determine the area requiring surgical decompression or conservative treatment such as a resting splint. Much information can be obtained through needle electrode analysis by stimulating *Erb's point*, the angle between the clavicle and the posterior border of the sternocleidomastoid, and recording distally. Compressive neuropathy such as a crutch palsy can be documented, although clinical presentation should be self-evident. Electrical assessment of radial nerve injury due to compression or humeral fracture near the spiral groove will show sparing of the proximally supplied triceps muscle but distal electrical abnormalities. Suprascapular nerve entrapment at the superior scapula, which decreases athletic performance and leads to imbalance and improper mechanics in activities like throwing or to difficulty in rehabilitation following rotator cuff repair, is best assessed by conduction velocity analysis. Ulnar nerve compression at the elbow, radial nerve entrapment due to humeral fracture, or carpal tunnel syndrome associated with a double crush phenomenon are also assessed by this technique.

Radiculopathy

Nerve root compression may limit electrical signals to muscles about the shoulder. This must be ruled out in differential diagnosis before treatment of intrinsic shoulder pathology that leads to decreased functional activity. *Cervical root compression*, due to disorders of bones and supporting structures around the spinal cord, can decrease the electrical impulses of exiting nerves and therefore decrease stimulus to their corresponding muscles. Such pathology may limit the expected response to surgery or greatly prolong rehabilitation due to interference with muscle balance, impeding the recovery of motor patterns needed for normal shoulder motion. *Radiculopathy* is defined as irritation of the spinal nerve root, leading to pain and paresthesia often accompanied by numbness and weakness. The most common C5 and C6 radiculopathies are hard to distinguish from each other, because the two nerve roots, due to plexus crossover, jointly innervate the shoulder muscles, including the supraspinatus, infraspinatus, deltoid,

biceps, and brachial radialis. C5 may potentially innervate the rhomboids more than C6 does, and the flexor carpi radialis may be more affected by C6, so that differentiation may be possible by EMG. C7, affecting the triceps, may also affect the anconeus with electrical changes picked up on the EMG.

Electrical Differential Diagnosis

EMG can help determine a root problem from a plexus problem, and electrical testing of sensory nerves, *somatosensory evoked potential* (SEP), is useful. Only the anterior primary rami contribute to the plexes, so that proximal radiculopathy can be distinguished from a plexus lesion by EMG sampling of muscles supplied by the posterior primary rami. If denervation, fibrillation, or other electrical disturbance is found in the paraspinal as well as limb muscles, this would indicate that the neurologic problem involves both the anterior and posterior rami and therefore is most likely a root lesion. Root lesions are not considered surgically treatable. Plexus and root lesions can also be distinguished by assessment of SEP. Sensory action potentials are lost if the lesion is beyond the posterior root ganglion, causing Wallerian degeneration of afferent fibers, but are preserved when the lesion is a proximal radiculopathy, in which peripheral sensory fibers do not degenerate. Thoracic outlet syndrome with chronic denervation of C8 and T1 can be documented by EMG as well. A true neuropathy exhibits thenar wasting, as opposed to a postural change or a *droopy shoulder syndrome* associated with a normal EMG.

Demyelinating disease and neuropathology discovered by EMG are beyond the scope of this discussion, because they do not primarily affect the athlete and because classification of the disease processes involved is usually made before *wheelchair* or *impaired athlete* status is achieved. If pathology is incidently identified, treatment and proper referral will be suggested by the EMG result.

A sudden jolt or a stinging and burning sensation throughout an outstretched arm, which may occur while trying to fend off a tackle or with point contact of the shoulder, may be associated with weakness lasting several minutes. This is commonly called a "stinger" or "burner" injury. These symptoms have been attributed to stretch of the upper trunk of the brachial plexus; however, symptoms are more commonly related to shoulder subluxation or a *dead arm syndrome*. When symptoms last more than a few hours or when the mechanism of injury suggests neurologic stretch, EMG characteristically demonstrates fibrillation potentials and positive sharp waves in the upper trunk muscles but not in paraspinal muscles. Paraspinal fibrillation would indicate a radiculopathy instead. EMG of the neck and periscapular muscles can help define a neurologic injury to the serratus anterior or trapezius muscle as distinguished from pseudowinging, which exhibits no electrical disturbance.

Summary

Plain radiographic, enhanced roentgenographic, nuclear magnetic, and electrical testing can assist in diagnostic accuracy. Such studies are not a substitute for clinical examination but must be used in conjunction with the exam to increase accuracy and suggest proper management. As has been demonstrated, the most expensive test is not necessarily the best. Each of these tests has a specific clinical setting in which it becomes relevant. At the present stage of technology, an MRI should not be the first diagnostic test ordered; as much information can be obtained from a plain X-ray, and more specific information may be obtained from a test such as a CT-arthrogram. In many cases, it is the clinical exam and the X-ray, rather than the MRI, bone scan, or arthrogram, that determines possible surgical intervention. Test results such as an arthrogram indicating an adhesive capsulitis or an EMG implicating neuromuscular dysfunction might predict a poor response to either surgery or physical therapy. Because no patients are the same, examination together with diagnostic studies as presented in this chapter are individualized to determine proper management and expectations for treatment of the athlete's shoulder problem.

5

Arthroscopy: Diagnostic and Surgical Tool

The shoulder ranks only behind the knee as the joint most commonly assessed arthroscopically. Shoulder arthroscopy is no longer just a diagnostic tool, because both sides of the rotator cuff can be evaluated and treated surgically by this technique—the subacromial space endoscopically and the glenohumeral joint arthroscopically. Many procedures that have been done through open surgical technique in the past can now also be done arthroscopically if the orthopedist is familiar with triangulation technique developed in knee arthroscopy and has the tools to arthroscopically deal with the shoulder. Many bony and soft tissue debridement procedures are commonly done arthroscopically. Arthroscopic repair of tissue is becoming more common as implants, tools, and techniques are developed.

The purpose of this chapter is to present arthroscopy as a diagnostic and surgical tool. In the early phases of clinical practice a clinician may do much diagnostic arthroscopy to confirm clinical impressions. As clinical experience progresses and diagnoses have been confirmed time after time, the clinician tends to depend more on the clinical examination for diagnosis and to reserve arthroscopy for surgical debridement, repair, and possibly helping to define the role of open reconstruction. This chapter is meant to familiarize the therapist and trainer with what can be done arthroscopically. It also presents variations of technique that have been found useful in over 5,000 shoulder arthroscopic procedures in one practice, some of which may be of use to the arthroscopist of the sports medicine team in dealing with his or her athlete's shoulder.

Patient Preparation

If the patient is referred for consideration of arthroscopic assessment or surgery, he or she should understand that this is not at the present time generally done in the office at the initial orthopedic assessment. Most offices are not set up for this; the procedure is usually done in an operating room under general anesthesia or regional block. History and physical examination, as well as adequate X-rays, are mandatory prior to arthroscopy. One would not wish to spread a bone tumor or fracture through osteopenic or displaced bone when positioning the patient for an arthroscopic procedure. Shoulder arthroscopy can reliably demonstrate an accurate diagnosis in most situations and is the most effective shoulder diagnostic method, if done in a routine manner and with a defined pattern of exploration.

Older patients go through preadmission testing. There is a high incidence of cardiac problems and hypertension in such individuals suspected of rotator cuff pathology and a high incidence of diabetes in patients with subacromial bursal adhesions. Pretesting helps avoid delays in the surgical schedule. Preoperative medical clearance and specialty consultation might aid in avoiding cancellation on the date of surgery.

Evaluation Under Anesthesia

The patient is usually examined under general anesthesia, although a viable alternative is use of an interscalene or brachial plexus supraclavicular block, specifically if there is a cardiac or respiratory problem. Although a regional block does not give the same relaxation of general anesthesia, manipulation under anesthesia can be accomplished nevertheless. In fact, with a pulmonary history of severe asthma or significant smoking, a regional block may become the anesthesia of choice in an effort to avoid postoperative pneumothorax; preoperative X-rays in these cases may identify blebs on the lungs of such patients at risk.

The patient is examined in the holding area prior to anesthesia, and X-rays are displayed in the operating room so that there is no confusion about which shoulder is to be examined. Drawing an X on the affected shoulder not only avoids the risk of operating on the wrong extremity, but is in fact found reassuring by the patient. The patient is anesthetized and reexamined for range of motion to see whether there is an actual mechanical block to motion. If there is a block, the patient is examined for instability in a supine position with the arm at the side at 40° and at 80° of abduction, prior to manipulation. With the arm in a neutral position, the amount of humeral head displacement in anterior-posterior translation, inferior translation, and superoposterior-to-superoanterior motion are assessed. This gives an indication of unidirectional instability, multidirectional instability, or superior suspension laxity (Figure 5.1, a and b).

Clicking and grinding should be noted, because with external rotation, a Hill-Sachs lesion or posterior labral pathology might be implicated; with

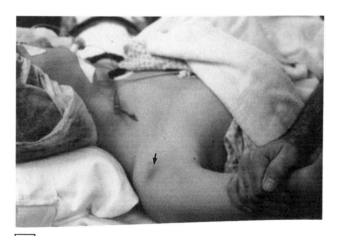

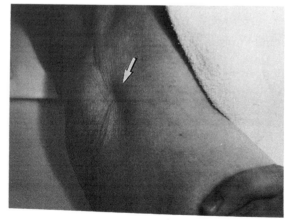
B

Figure 5.1

[A] Examination under anesthesia at 40° and 80° of abduction can help determine anterior, posterior, or multidirectional instability; a large anterior dimple with posterior pressure implicates superior laxity or a SLAP lesion. (Isolated posterior subluxation is best assessed with the arm in horizontal flexion, slight adduction, and posterior push.) Here it is present without a sulcus sign.

[B] Close-up of anterior dimple, indicating superior laxity or SLAP lesion, in examination under anesthesia.

internal rotation, grinding may indicate anterior labral material caught within the glenohumeral joint or a reverse Hill-Sachs lesion at the front of the humeral head. At this point, anterior-posterior stability of the A/C joint is also assessed; it may otherwise be easy to overlook. If there is full range of motion, the instability tests can be done. If range of motion is limited, assessment of instability is followed by manipulation and then a repeat instability exam to see if the laxity pattern has changed due to the reestablishment of the original injury by the manipulation. Manipulation of secondary adhesive capsulitis may reestablish the primary instability pattern, unmasking the original problem. If there is any question of fracture, an image intensifier or portable X-ray should be available to assess the shoulder.

Manipulation Under Anesthesia

The function of the shoulder is to position the hand through space. When that function is hampered, the hand may not be used, the upper extremity may be held close to the body, and the shoulder may gel. This is particularly true when there has been some erosion of the rotator cuff and the healing phase has caused too much scarring. Certain medical conditions in athletes—including disuse associated with cardiac disease, breast lesions or biopsies, and especially diabetes—commonly lead to fibrosis. These conditions may allow development of scar tissue between the deltoid muscle, rotator cuff, and acromion and thus inhibit the normal sliding of the rotator cuff under the acromion, capturing the central shoulder.

The small-vessel and neurologic loss associated with diabetes may lead to a loss of a "fidget factor," that is, loss of the micromotion normally found in sleep and daily activity. The minor bursal bands that may occur in the healing of rotator cuff tendinitis are not broken in this disease, leading to progressive bursal fibrosis that finally becomes symptomatic. Manipulation under anesthesia is an important part of the arthroscopic procedure for these diseases. Opening tissue planes may allow easier access to the pathologic areas and provide tissue stubs after manipulation that can be debrided to help prevent recurrence of adhesions.

Four-Step Technique

Manipulation under anesthesia should be done in a well-defined manner, whether it is done in conjunction with fluid injection to break adhesions in the office setting or in the operating room. This is a four-step technique. First, elevate the arm in forward flexion to break inferior capsular adhesions. Abduction in external rotation should not be the first maneuver, because torquing against a very scarred capsule can break the humeral head or cause spiral fracture of the humerus, particularly if there is significant osteopenia from disuse. The second step is to loosen the shoulder in horizontal flexion, because many fine posterior bursal and deltoid/rotator cuff adhesions will still need to be broken even after elevation in forward flexion. The third step is abduction in external rotation, which may freshen a preexisting Bankart lesion or anterior labral detachment. At this point the shoulder may redislocate; this is not due to the manipulation but to the preexisting injury, which is identified by the exam under anesthesia and unmasked by the manipulation. Internal rotation with the arm at 90° of abduction, or preferably behind the back, is done fourth in an attempt to regain full motion. Comparison should be made with the other shoulder. Breaking minor nonsymptomatic adhesions might in fact lessen the need for subsequent surgery in the presently nonsymptomatic side.

Postmobilization Care

Most often the adhesions are very fine and break very easily, and there is no evidence of concurrent subluxation, especially after cardiac problems, breast biopsy, or short-term disuse. In such cases, the shoulder is injected with 20 cc of 0.75 Marcaine with 1/200,000 epinephrine (except with unstable cardiomyopathy), using 10 cc in the subacromial space and 10 cc in the glenohumeral joint to diminish bleeding and for pain relief, with 2 cc of morphine in the mixture. The patient is transferred to the recovery room with the arm above the head, held in place with a loosely wrapped gauze roll. An ice bag or a circulating cold-water cuff is applied to the shoulder and utilized postoperatively (Figure 5.2). The patient is not placed in a sling until after he or she realizes the shoulder can be moved overhead.

Manipulation is usually considered an outpatient technique. The patient is sent to physical therapy five times a week for 2 weeks, then three times a week as necessary for immediate full passive range of motion, advancing to active motion, and then strengthening, in order to help prevent recurrence of adhesions. The same protocol is followed whether or not arthroscopic debridement is associated. The patient advances to a home program when able to exercise on his or her own.

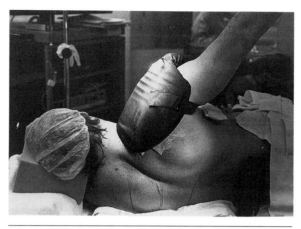

Figure 5.2 *Cryotherapy.* Circulating ice water following manipulation or shoulder surgery helps to allow such techniques to be done on an outpatient basis (IsoComforter, Nu Tech Medical, Inc., Grand Rapids, MI).

Further Intervention

If fine adhesions are easy to break through manipulation and there is no evidence of subluxation, arthroscopy is not necessary unless clinical evidence of internal derangement is apparent and is the probable cause of secondary stiffness. When manipulation is somewhat difficult, as in diabetic capsulitis, arthroscopic assessment and debridement are recommended, primarily to resect the ends of the broken scar (usually subdeltoid) so that they will not stick down again.

Except after artificial joint replacement in a stiff shoulder, the role of a continuous passive motion machine in treatment of adhesive capsulitis is limited. In most cases, active range of motion should be reestablished before considering open reconstructive surgery, because operating on a stiff shoulder usually results in a stiffer shoulder. Manipulation, arthroscopic debridement, and strengthening may eliminate the need for open surgery or help improve its likelihood of success.

Arthroscopy, Bursoscopy, and Endoscopy

The shoulder consists of three joints and two sliding mechanisms. Each of these can be addressed independently; however, they work in combination to provide shoulder function. The arthroscope lends itself to examining each of these areas without having to take down muscles, which may lead to temporary dysfunction or imbalance in the recuperative phase. Assessing the glenohumeral joint,

acromioclavicular joint, or sternoclavicular joint can be formally considered as arthroscopy. Examining the two sliding mechanisms, however, is not technically arthroscopic, because they are not within a joint; assessment of these mechanisms can be labeled more properly as an endoscopic or bursoscopic procedure.

Prior to the mid-1980s, shoulder arthroscopy was limited to the glenohumeral joint. Since then, endoscopic assessment and debridement of the subacromial space has become more popular as it is recognized that the glenohumeral joint does not work by itself. Nevertheless, glenohumeral arthroscopy and subacromial endoscopy are not the same procedure. Subacromial endoscopic technique is generally considered much more difficult than glenohumeral arthroscopic technique, because landmarks are fewer and both visualization and orientation are much more difficult. Although considered one technique by many insurance companies, these two distinct techniques address entirely different anatomic structures, each a discrete surgical area in itself. In addition, arthroscopic assessment and debridement of the acromioclavicular joint, subscapular endoscopy, and sternoclavicular arthroscopy are even more difficult technically but can also be accomplished with the arthroscope.

Glenohumeral Arthroscopy

Placing the arthroscope within the glenohumeral joint is the second most common arthroscopic surgical procedure; only knee arthroscopy is more common. The shoulder is one of the most complex joints and demands meticulous assessment to find primary pathology or amplifying factors that might contribute to or increase pathology in one of the other compartments that are associated with shoulder motion. A suggested method of assessment follows.

Patient Positioning. Two methods of visualizing the glenohumeral joint are possible: either with the patient in a sitting position, as recommended by Skyhar, Altcheck, and Warren (1988), or in the lateral decubital position, as popularized by Andrews, Zarins, Carson, Nemeth, and Ciullo (1983). The author has used both but reserves the supine "beach chair" position for very obese patients, because the lateral decubital position is more efficient (Figure 5.3).

In the lateral position it is important to tilt the patient back 15° to avoid surgical draping and thus get better clearance for anterior instrument passage. The arm is abducted 45° and forward flexed

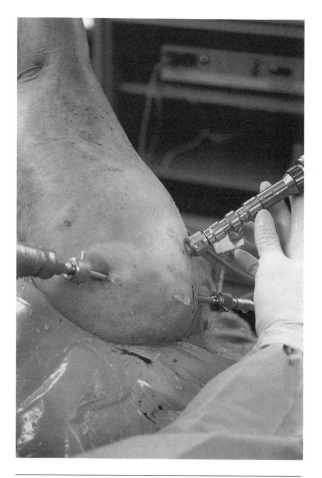

Figure 5.3 The lateral decubital position allows easy access to the front and back of the shoulder.

about 20°, placing it in the position of functional abduction, in which the anterior and posterior muscles are allowed to balance the joint. A sulcus with 5- to 15-lb (2.25- to 6.75-kg) balancing weight indicates significant laxity and multidirectional instability that is clinically underdiagnosed. With only 5-lb (2.25-kg) balancing traction while in the lateral decubital position, a *lateral laxity test* is done to test stability and is compared to that done previously in a supine position (Figure 5.4, a and b). It is interesting that multidirectional subluxation (increased motion circumferentially around the glenoid rim) is easier to define in this position than it is in the supine position.

Portal Placement. An additional 10-lb (4.5-kg) weight is attached, and the patient is sterilely prepared and draped (Betadine spray is sufficient). A needle is placed in the A/C joint for marking purposes. Using the posterior portal 1 cm medial the posterolateral point of the acromion, aiming through the marking needle toward the coracoid process, distend the joint with 40 cc of lactated ringers to provide a larger target. A small jab incision into the joint in line with deltoid fibers is made, following the entry angle of the previous needle. The arthroscope is introduced, usually in the "safe area" anteriorly between the humeral head and glenoid, aimed toward the interval between the superior glenohumeral ligament and the subscapularis tendon (Figure 5.5). A passing rod is passed through the arthroscope cannula into the safe area then angled slightly upward, tenting the skin on the outside; a small skin incision is made in this area. A larger cannula is then placed retrograde over the exposed tip of the rod. The rod is

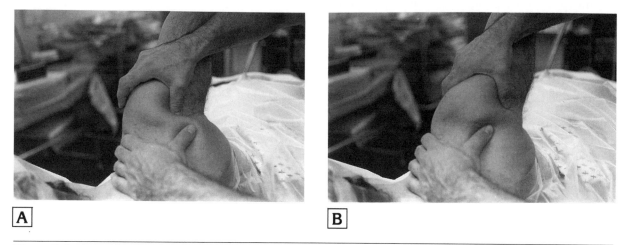

Figure 5.4 Lateral laxity test. In the lateral decubital position with 0- to 5-lb (0- to 2.25-kg) balancing weight on the arm, the humeral head can be easily pushed out [A] anteriorly or [B] posteriorly in an extremely loose shoulder. Inferior or multidirectional translational laxity is also easily assessed.

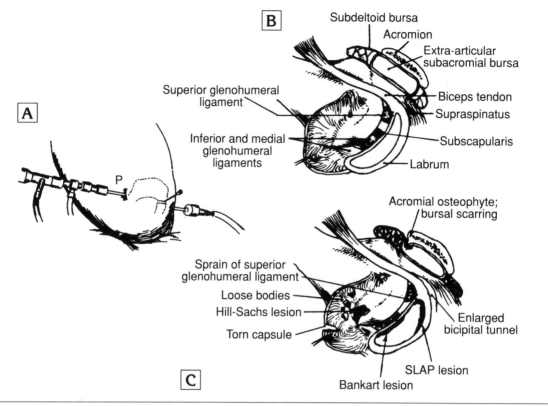

Figure 5.5 Glenohumeral arthroscopy.

[A] Anterior or posterior portals can be switched for visualization or operative purposes.

[B] Normal arthroscopic anatomy as viewed from the posterior portal (* = pivot point at attachment of superior glenohumeral ligament and coracoglenoid tissue).

[C] Pathologic anatomy identified arthroscopically.

removed, cannulas separated, and the arthroscope introduced. A third portal can be made in the notch between the clavicle and scapular spine if greater water inflow is necessary, but with the new high-inflow cannulas or a pressure pump set at 60 mmHg, this third portal is rarely needed; it risks injury to the suprascapular nerve. The shoulder is assessed first from the posterior portal and then from the anterior portal, with the opposite portal used for inflow, irrigation, or instrumentation.

Laxity Assessment. The balancing weight is then reduced to 5 lb (2.25 kg) or removed, and an assistant helps hold the arm in place to allow an *arthroscopic laxity assessment*. Remember that the non-pathologic anterior capsule is tightened in external rotation and the posterior capsule tightened in internal rotation. The arm is turned into external rotation and assessment is made of how far the shoulder can be moved out of the socket superoanteriorly, inferoanteriorly, and directly inferiorly. Forty percent displacement anteriorly and inferiorly is normal. Thirty percent displacement of the humeral head out of the glenoid socket inferiorly

or inferoposteriorly is normal. Any further displacement is considered abnormal and is usually associated with glenoid labral pathology, wearing, or notching of the humeral articular surface.

By moving the arm into internal rotation to tighten the posterior structures, inferoposterior and superoposterior subluxation is assessed. Note whether the humeral head is sitting out of the joint with or without weight in an inferoanterior direction. In patients with no significant glenohumeral laxity, such as those with diabetic stiffness or primary subacromial bursal adhesions, the humeral head will sit directly in the glenoid socket in spite of a 15-lb (6.75-kg) balancing weight (Figure 5.6a). In the majority of patients who undergo arthroscopic analysis, inferoanterior perching is not normal but is a factor of patient selection (i.e., elective arthroscopy usually is done in symptomatic patients), and some overlay of physiologic laxity or capsular stretching may be due to obesity (Figure 5.6b).

Posterior Portal Examination Sequence. The 15-lb (6.75-kg) weight is reapplied. From the posterior portal, tissue avulsion off the lesser tuberosity

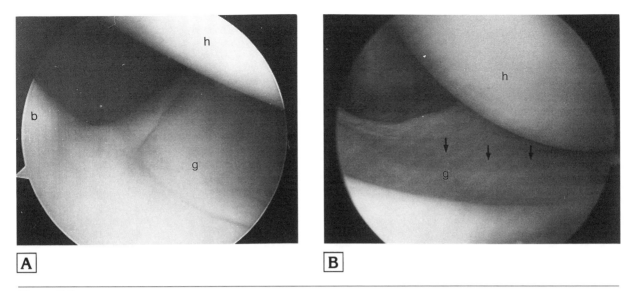

Figure 5.6

[A] Humeral head well centered in the glenoid socket, seen in "normal," or nonphysiologic, lax shoulder or in adhesive capsulitis.

[B] Humeral head perched on anterior inferior rim, seen with physiologic laxity, pathologic laxity, and obesity; note thin cartilage near glenoid rim (arrows) (b = biceps, g = glenoid, h = humerus).

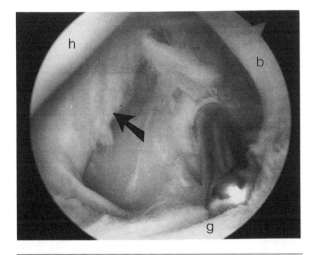

Figure 5.7 Subscapularis strain near attachment into lesser tuberosity (b = biceps, g = glenoid, h = humerus).

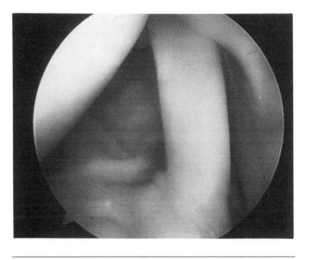

Figure 5.8 Normal biceps tendon tunnel opening, viewed from posterior portal.

and fraying of the subscapularis can be seen (Figure 5.7). Stretching or synovitis of the superior glenohumeral ligament and enlargement of the interval between the subscapularis and superoglenohumeral ligament is also assessed.

The biceps is then followed upward to the bicipital tunnel (Figure 5.8), pulled into the joint to check for vascular changes of tendinitis (Figure 5.9), and then followed downward; the supraspinatus is also visualized in the process. Fraying or full-thickness tearing of the rotator cuff in this area may be seen.

The posterior recess is then assessed to see if there is a significant synovitis, early arthritis, or hypertrophy of the labrum (Figure 5.10). In the process the superoposterior aspect of the labrum near the bicipital attachment can be assessed also, primarily to see whether a SLAP lesion exists (Snyder, 1989; Figure 5.11). Rule out loose bodies anteriorly, superiorly, posteriorly, and inferiorly, and then assess the inferior attachment of the rotator cuff to the humeral head.

There is usually a bare area of metaphysis between the rotator cuff capsular insertion and the

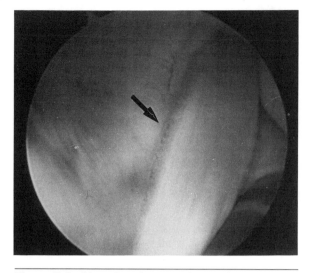

Figure 5.9 Vascular plexus on bicipital tendon retrieved from tunnel, showing tendinitis.

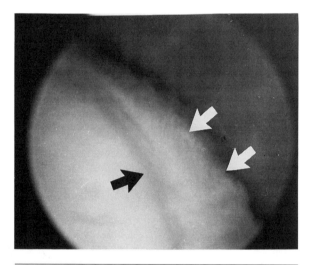

Figure 5.10 Posterior-rim, early-arthritic spur (black arrow) and labral hypertrophy (white arrows), seen through anterior portal.

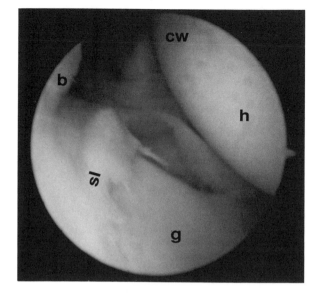

Figure 5.11 Superior labral anterior-to-posterior detachment (SLAP lesion) at biceps tendon base (g = glenoid, h = humerus, b = biceps, sl = detached superior labrum, cw = early superior chondral wear).

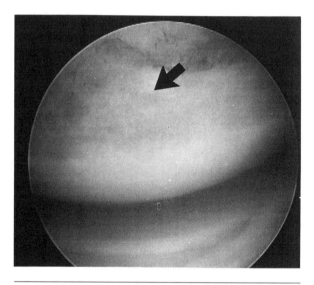

Figure 5.12 Normal intra-articular metaphyseal area at posterior lateral humeral head.

articular cartilage of the humeral head (Figure 5.12). This is normal, but fraying of the articular cartilage below this metaphyseal area correlates with subluxation. An actual notch or indentation of the bone, called a Hill-Sachs lesion (Figure 5.13), is pathognomonic of previous dislocation (Hill & Sachs, 1940).

The labrum is then reassessed by a *lift-off test*: If the arthroscope passes easily under the humeral head, there is enough capsular laxity to justify diagnosis of subluxation (Figure 5.14). In multi-directional or significant physiologic laxity the equal longitudinal pull of the arm weight may hide circumferential laxity, but this lift-off maneuver will remain positive.

SLAP lesions, posterior labral detachment (reverse Bankart lesion), anterior-to-posterior inferior labral detachment (APIL lesion), and infero-anterior labral detachment (Bankart lesion), with or without glenoid fracture, may be easily seen (Figure 5.15, a and b). Labral flap tearing, particularly in the superoposterior and superoanterior quadrants, will be evident. Synovitis in the superoposterior area where traction occurs, or anteriorly over a stretched superior glenohumeral ligament,

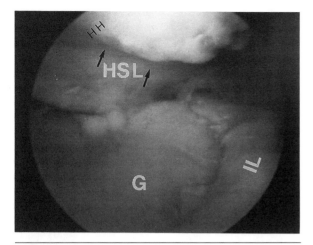

Figure 5.13 Posterior lateral humeral head compression from anterior glenoid rim, associated with anterior subluxation—a Hill-Sachs lesion (HH = humeral head, G = glenoid, IL = inferior labrum, HSL = Hill-Sachs lesion impaction fracture).

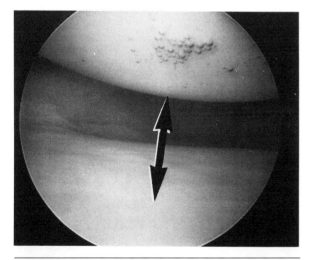

Figure 5.14 The ability to easily pass the arthroscope under the humeral head or to lift the head off the surface of the glenoid by 6 mm indicates glenohumeral laxity—a positive lift-off test.

can be seen, as well as fraying of or splitting into the biceps tendon.

Anterior Portal Exam. At this point, prior to any surgical procedure, the arthroscope is switched to the anterior portal, and instability reassessed. The significance of traction superoposterior rotator cuff fraying (Figure 5.16), other rotator cuff fraying, the possibility of such tears having a full-thickness component, the superior glenohumeral ligament (Figure 5.17), Bankart lesion, or capsular stripping are all best assessed from this anterior portal. The weight is released now, and the arm is brought

into adduction and slight internal rotation to see if the superior labrum and biceps tendon catch in the joint and cause a grinding phenomenon. If there is associated chondromalacia at the top of the humeral head, the SLAP lesion or stretched superior suspensory mechanism can be considered symptomatic, a condition labeled as *superior laxity* or *microinstability*.

Combined-Portal Surgical Consideration. When pathology is demonstrated, and especially with a SLAP lesion as previously noted, switching the arthroscope and debriding or repair tools back and forth between the anterior and posterior portals will lead to the most satisfactory result. If a frayed SLAP lesion is found, it is debrided; if a loose sleeve of tissue, it is repaired (Figure 5.18). The type of detachment correlates with bicipital firing at time of injury. If the arm was in a forward flexed position during injury, the SLAP lesion may proceed into the superoposterior glenoid quadrant. If the SLAP lesion developed in an abduction and external rotation injury, it tends to extend into a Bankart lesion segmentally, with a stretched inferior capsular counterpart, or to extend directly from the inferoanterior quadrant. Although SLAP lesions are highly correlated with instability and disruption, they can occasionally occur without instability, especially in throwing injury.

Labral tissue that catches in the joint can easily be debrided arthroscopically. Care must be taken in the superior region, because the biceps tendon usually inserts into the labrum and not into the superior glenoid tubercle. Arthroscopic repair by absorbable implants or suturing technique for the superoanterior quadrant is actually easier than repair through a larger, anterior, open arthrotomy incision. Arthroscopic tightening or shifting of the inferior capsule is not so easily accomplished, because the capsular tissue most commonly stretches before labral avulsion. Inferoanterior capsular tightening and more accurately balanced reattachment of the labrum is more easily achieved as an open procedure. After debridement of soft tissue, synovitis, frayed rotator cuff tissue, or torn labrum; removal of loose bodies; or chondroplastic smoothing of certain irregular articular surfaces at the glenohumeral interface, the joint is irrigated and all instruments are removed. Glenohumeral arthroscopy is complete.

Subacromial Bursoscopy

The same posterior portal used in glenohumeral arthroscopy is used to redirect the cannula above the rotator cuff to the area of the anterior edge of

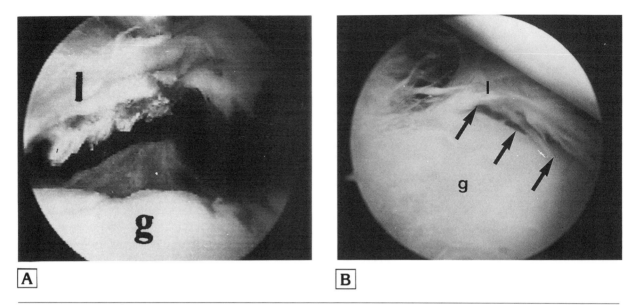

Figure 5.15 Inferoanterior labral separation—a Bankart lesion—seen through the posterior portal (g = glenoid, l = labral capsular anterior complex).

[A] Acute.

[B] Chronic.

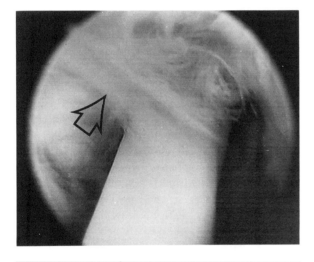

Figure 5.16 Partial-thickness superoposterior intra-articular rotator cuff "toggle" tearing demonstrated through the anterior portal.

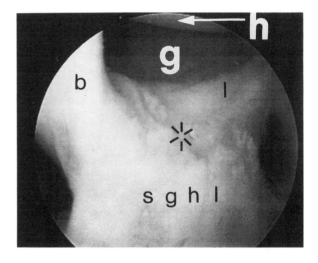

Figure 5.17 Superior glenohumeral ligament as visualized from the anterior portal (sghl = superior glenohumeral ligament, b = biceps, l = labrum, g = glenoid, h = humerus, * = pivot point).

the acromion for endoscopic or bursal assessment. The supraspinatus sliding mechanism is not actually within a joint, therefore its examination is an endoscopic, not arthroscopic, procedure. The switching rod is used to position the anterior cannula through the same anterior portal, but above the rotator cuff, to provide inflow or a working portal to this area. A third anterolateral portal is made 3 to 4 cm from the anterior edge of the

acromion if surgical subacromial or A/C joint debridement is to be considered (Figure 5.19).

If thick subacromial bursal adhesions are encountered in the process, first the posterior cannula with its obturator is used to break them; otherwise visualization is markedly restricted. If no thick adhesions are encountered between the deltoid and rotator cuff, the normal thin bursal cross-striations are left alone, and the soft clear spot under the

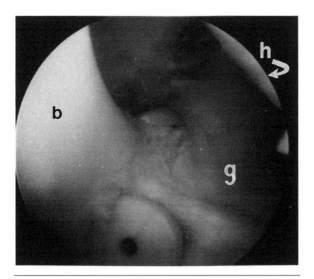

Figure 5.18 SLAP lesion repaired with absorbable Suretac rivets (Acufex, Smith & Nephew Endoscopy, Mansfield, MA) (b = biceps, h = humeral head, g = glenoid).

anterior edge of the acromion, almost universally seen after age 20, is sought. Thickened subacromial bursal walls or thick bands within the bursa (Figure 5.20, a and b), if clinically significant, should be resected; remove the subdeltoid–to–rotator cuff peripheral adhesions, as well as adhesions to the scapular spine, to aid in postoperative motion and restore the supraspinatus outlet gliding plane.

There may be a thickened, meniscoid rim in the front of the acromion and calcification within the coracoacromial ligament origin, particularly with subluxation (Figure 5.21). This may progressively wear into the greater tuberosity area of the supraspinatus insertion and the area over the biceps tendon, a process called *impingement*. The weight is removed at this point, and the arm is placed through a range of motion and rotated in functional elevation at about 90°. If there is erosion into the rotator cuff, even without a full-thickness tear, and a corresponding "crab meat" appearance of

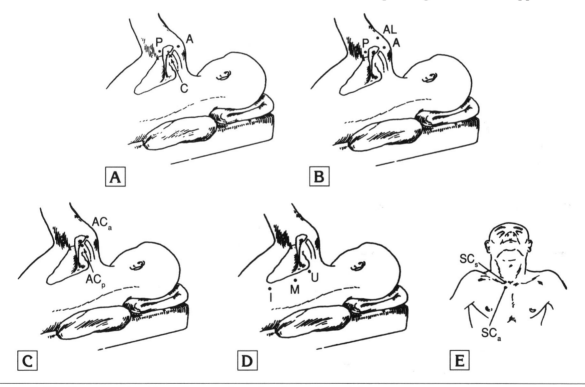

Figure 5.19 Common shoulder arthroscopic and endoscopic portals.

[A] Glenohumeral arthroscopy: (P) posterior, (A) anterior, and (C) rarely used central portals.

[B] Subacromial endoscopy, or bursoscopy: (P) posterior, (AL) anterolateral, and (A) redirected anterior portal, which may be of use for the A/C joint.

[C] A/C joint arthroscopy: (AC$_a$) A/C anterior and (AC$_p$) A/C posterior direct portals may be of use but are rarely necessary, because subacromial endoscopic portals are more useful and can preserve the posterior A/C ligament.

[D] Subscapular endoscopy: (I) inferior, (M) middle, and (U) upper portals, 2 to 3 cm medial to scapular edge.

[E] Supraclavicular arthroscopy: (SC$_s$) sternoclavicular superior and (SC$_a$) sternoclavicular anterior portals.

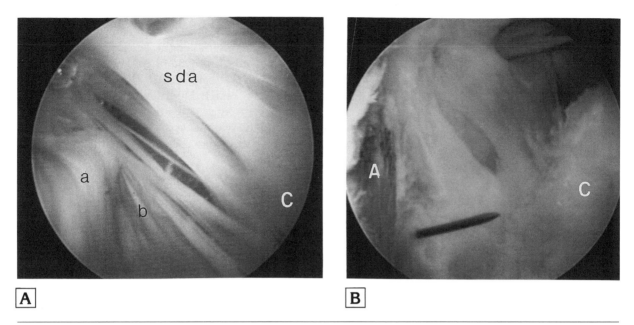

A

B

Figure 5.20 Thick bands may remain after fine cross-striations and bursal walls erode or after trauma.

[A] Prior to resection (a = acromion, b = bursal bands, c = rotator cuff/supraspinatus, sda = subdeltoid adhesions).

[B] Following resection and acromioplasty (note A/C marking needle).

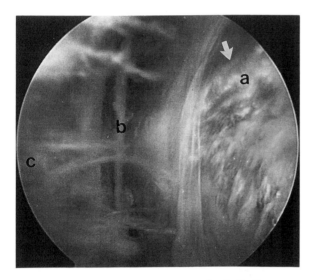

Figure 5.21 Pressure against soft tissue in the sub-acromial space leads to periosteal build-up at the front of the acromion, a meniscoid-type change that may progress to a bone hook and is responsible for further impingement (a = acromial edge, b = bursal band, c = frayed, eroded rotator cuff).

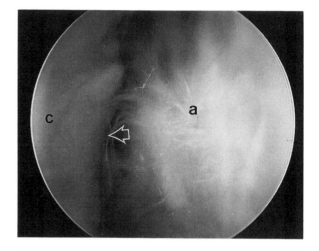

Figure 5.22 Acromial wear into rotator cuff, called impingement (a = acromion, c = rotator cuff).

the undersurface of the acromion (Figure 5.22), then impingement is occurring. The 15-lb (6.75-kg) weight is replaced and subacromial decompression can be done endoscopically (Figure 5.23), which may in fact be more effective than an open acromioplasty, because the deltoid is not taken

down and postoperative immobilization stiffness is minimized.

If there is no wear into the rotator cuff and no irregularity or wear of the acromial undersurface, then acromioplasty is not warranted. It is not unusual that, when testing with the weight off in this position, manually centering the humeral head back into the socket completely eliminates early impingement. In this case a minimal debridement of the rough acromial-surface fibrous build-up, which has not yet ossified, is all that is necessary to allow the patient to return to physical therapy.

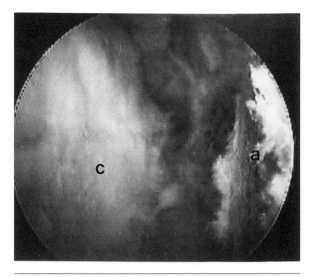

Figure 5.23 Impingement relieved following inferior acromioplasty (a = acromion, c = rotator cuff; same patient as in Figure 5.21).

Pain is completely relieved, and work on internal rotation strengthening and humeral head depression can better position the head in the socket (Ciullo, 1989b). With combined instability and impingement, isolated acromioplasty is not indicated because the acromion may have adapted to contain the humeral head. Removing this braking mechanism anteriorly can increase instability considerably, and the hook may quickly reform. With minimal instability, acromioplasty followed by humeral head depression exercises may control symptoms. Capsular stabilization may be necessary if the exercises are not sufficient.

In major instability, particularly capsular avulsion such as a Bankart lesion or SLAP lesion, the endoscopic subacromial decompression may decrease the extent of the open procedure. The open surgery may be limited to the glenohumeral joint, or the combined endoscopic decompression may limit the size of the skin incision and avoid the need to take down the deltoid muscle. Underlying subluxation is the main cause of failed acromioplasty; treating the primary problem is the only means of effecting a cure. Isolated impingement without subluxation does occur and usually responds well to endoscopic subacromial decompression if there has not been too much wear into the rotator cuff. With continued aching pain in the area where the impinging surfaces wear into the cuff, open imbrication may be necessary to restore a smooth supraspinatus component to this outlet sliding mechanism.

Dome decompression or distal clavicular resection at the A/C joint can be accomplished as

long as the surgeon has experience with arthroscopic cautery or familiarity with a pressure pump set at 80 to 100 mmHg. The A/C joint, lateral acromion, and mesoacromial apophyseal lines are best seen from the anterolateral subacromial portal (Figure 5.24).

Subacromial decompression, resection of peripheral scarring, and debridement of the rough surfaces of a torn rotator cuff can be done in massive cuff tearing; the amount of motion recovered with or without functional strength increase may be remarkable. The pain relief following endoscopic subacromial decompression may be so significant that the patient elects not to proceed with further open surgery to repair the rotator cuff; this has been a common experience in the last 8 years of the author's practice. The patient is made to understand that there might be some loss of motion as a trade-off for strength in attempting to surgically repair a large cuff tear. Rather than electing surgical repair, the patient usually asks to have the other shoulder scheduled for endoscopic debridement, being satisfied with debridement alone.

Prior to 1990, most arthroscopists believed that resection of small fragments of anterior acromial bone or soft tissue was sufficient to remove symptoms. It was obvious that resection of too much bone could lead to increased symptoms, because the humeral head was not well contained and instability might worsen. There was obviously a correlation between subluxation and impingement. Finding where the rotator cuff rubbed against the acromion by removing and then replacing the weight during arthroscopy gave clearance for surgery; removing the weight again could demonstrate whether enough bone and soft tissue had been removed. Since then, acromioplastic technique has become more accurate by using the scapular spine as a stable base to provide a more accurate and often more generous acromioplasty, as well as to allow debridement across the A/C joint to remove inferior clavicular spurs responsible for impingement.

Acromioplasty followed by rehabilitative exercises that emphasize supraspinatus and infraspinatus function to depress the humeral head are often successful in avoiding the need for an open capsular reconstruction. When therapy is not successful, a delayed capsular repair might be considered. With a large cuff tear, debridement of adhesions could allow recovery of full active or passive motion. A two-stage rotator cuff repair can be considered—first removal of the adhesions and then physical therapy in order to regain passive and,

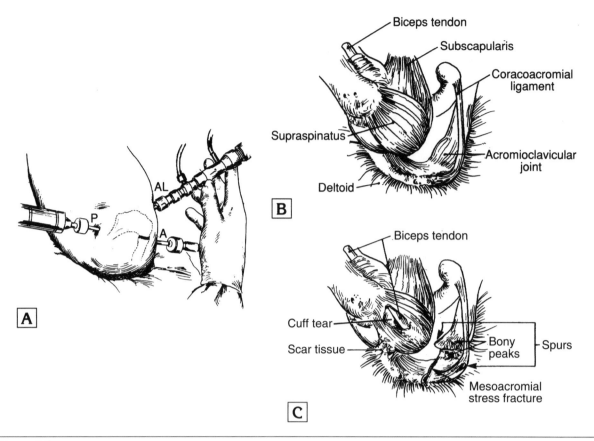

Figure 5.24

[A] Portal placement (A = anterior, P = posterior, AL = anterolateral).

[B] Normal subacromial anatomy, best assessed through the anterolateral portal.

[C] Pathologic subacromial changes.

possibly, active motion. If strength is still decreased but stiffness is no longer a problem, then a capsular or cuff repair is more successful.

With the newer pump techniques, arthroscopic surgical time has been minimized. Therefore, proceeding with an open repair at the same time is feasible in the absence of a significant amount of preoperative stiffness and excessive arthroscopic fluid extravasation. A large open reconstruction on a stiff shoulder often results in more stiffness. Mobilizing the tissue at the time of arthroscopy and releasing the adhesions that occur between the rotator cuff, acromion, and deltoid often permits a primary tendon repair rather than a tendon-slide or transfer procedure. Many so-called "impossible" cuff tears, when manipulated, debrided arthroscopically, and subsequently repaired in a staged manner with the open repair delayed by at least 3 weeks, are found repairable. This treatment allows repair of less friable and more mobile tissue, which can be pulled for a repair in a more anatomic direction. If substantive, the released tissue may be repaired concurrently with the arthroscopic release.

Subacromial spurs wear into the cuff by the A/C joint and respond well to endoscopic subacromial decompression by resting the sleeve of the debriding blade on the scapular spine, starting at the back of the A/C joint and swooping forward, thus eliminating impingement on both sides of the A/C joint (Figure 5.25). If pain persists, open imbrication of the cuff over the biceps tendon sleeve may be necessary to help eliminate pain by reestablishing a smoother supraspinatus surface to ride under the superior acromial arch.

Acromioclavicular Arthroscopy

Acromioclavicular joint assessment, debridement, or resection has traditionally been done as an open technique. It can be accomplished arthroscopically. This is not technically part of a glenohumeral arthroscopy but is a separate technique that can be mastered using the same equipment and most often under the same anesthesia. Pathologic changes within the glenohumeral joint can functionally subluxate the humeral head, jamming it

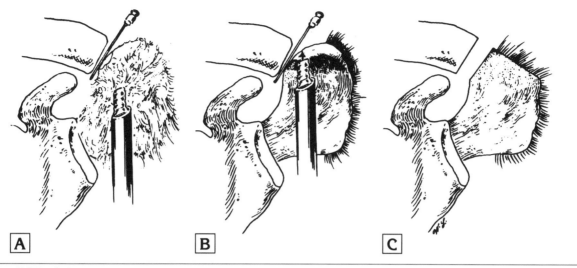

Figure 5.25 Subacromial decompression.

[A] Resection of subacromial scar and soft tissue may expose bony spurs at the front of the acromion.

[B] Endoscopic resection of bony spurs.

[C] With limited motion at the A/C joint or arthritic changes, the distal clavicle can be resected. Note marking needle for orientation in the A/C joint.

upward to cause secondary A/C joint symptoms. The importance of concurrent arthroscopic glenohumeral and A/C joint assessment cannot be over-emphasized if surgical failure is to be avoided.

Portal Placement. The A/C joint can be assessed through direct portals in front of and behind the joint, using a 2.7-mm arthroscope, or through the same portals used for subacromial bursoscopy (see Figure 5.19, b and c, on p. 71). The latter is preferred for two reasons: First, avoiding the direct portal approach helps preserve the posterior stabilizing A/C joint ligament. Second, A/C joint pain is often related to other shoulder pathology, that is, A/C joint overuse that compensates for glenohumeral laxity or stiffness, snapping transmitted by a SLAP lesion, or triad degeneration.

Combined Sequence Techniques. Glenohumeral arthroscopy is done first; if a pump is used, 60 mmHg of pressure is used intra-articularly. The pump is turned up to 100 mmHg for the A/C joint arthroscopy to minimize bleeding if necessary. A short 18-gauge needle placed through the A/C joint at the beginning of the procedure aids in proper placement of the portals used for the initial glenohumeral arthroscopy and then for the subsequent subacromial endoscopic and acromioclavicular arthroscopic procedures.

Dome Decompression. With A/C joint resection, concurrent subacromial decompression is most often necessary. It is best to resect infra-acromial and infraclavicular spurs on both sides of the A/C joint. Releasing these spurs, a *dome decompression*, may be all that is necessary to unlock the A/C joint (Figure 5.26).

Lateral Clavicectomy. If inferior osteophyte resection alone does not unlock the A/C joint so that there is at least 2 mm of play in the anterior-posterior and superior-inferior directions, or if there is significant pathology, the absence of a disk, irregularity of the articular endplates, cystic changes, or obvious arthritis, resection of the distal 1 cm of bone becomes necessary. The posterior portal is used to best visualize the anterior aspect of the A/C joint (Figure 5.27, a and b), usually with the anterolateral portal used for initial debridement.

The arthroscopic cannula is then switched to the anterolateral portal and inflow to the posterior portal or through the scope, with the anterior portal used to debride the back of the joint (Figure 5.28, a and b). Bare-ended arthroscopic cutters are most appropriate for this. When a pump is used, the posterior portal is available to remove large fragments of soft tissue, because the cutting tools often clog. Cauterization is usually not necessary but may be helpful near the back of the joint and for resection of fatty bursal tissue. Effort is made to preserve the superior periosteum and the posterior A/C joint ligament to preserve stability. Because it is not necessary to reflect the deltoid muscle, as is done in an open operation, arthroscopic debridement usually allows motion and activity out of the

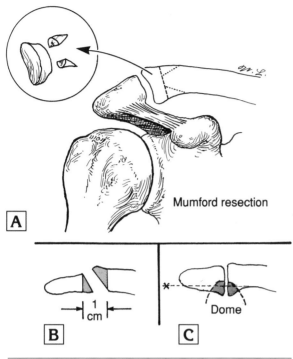

Figure 5.26 Unlocking the A/C joint or relieving arthritic symptoms can be accomplished by an open procedure or arthroscopically. The result should be a mobile joint, produced by a 1-cm parallel gap that fills in with scar tissue to act as a buffer.

[A] Lateral clavicectomy: *Mumford or GURD procedure.*

[B] *Modified Mumford*: resection of angled joint.

[C] *Dome decompression*: Unlocking the joint by removal of inferior osteophytes may restore motion.

sling the day following surgery, even with associated subacromial decompression and peripheral scar resection, unless concurrent glenohumeral repair procedures have been done.

Subscapular Bursoscopy

Evaluating the undersurface of the scapula for snapping due to partially torn muscle tissue (myonodular necrosis), bursal bands (adhesions), or protruding corners (bone spurs) is an advanced endoscopic technique. There is usually no true bursa under the scapula, but rather fine, wispy cross-striations of tissue that exist as a tissue plane. Once irregular erosion occurs due to overuse or perhaps postural change, the cross-striations may dissolve and allow the creation of a bursa. After trauma, superomedial subscapular periosteal tissue may wear down or hypertrophy, which leads to eburnation or bony changes. Erosive or traumatic involvement of muscle attachment leads to myonodular necrosis. Posttraumatic bands of scar can also cause snapping. MRI or CT assessment of the undersurface of the scapula is nonproductive.

Patient Positioning. If routine shoulder arthroscopy has been done previously, assessment of the subscapular space is best done in a prone position (Figure 5.29, a and b). Because there is a high correlation of glenohumeral pathology leading to scapulothoracic overuse and subsequently to subscapular pathology, in most cases glenohumeral arthroscopy and subscapular bursoscopy should be done first. Merely leaning the patient forward after routine arthroscopy will allow assessment of the undersurface of the scapula under the same anesthesia (Figure 5.30).

Portal Placement. With either a prone position or the lateral decubital position, the arm, placed in a stockinette, is positioned behind the back in order to elevate the medial scapular edge for clearance between the scapula and rib cage. Three portals have been found useful at the superior, medial, and inferior edges of the scapula, 2 to 3 cm medial to the medial edge (Figure 5.31), thus avoiding important neurovascular structures (Figure 5.32). A nick is made in this extremely thick dorsal skin with a knife, a hemostat is used to longitudinally spread soft tissue, and a large 5.5-mm cannula is positioned toward the scapula, inserted with a blunt obturator.

Debridement. Most often, in spite of grinding or snapping under the scapula, normal tissue planes are demonstrated, no bursa has formed, and there is no pathology. Nevertheless, due to direct trauma or progressive overuse, tissue can break down, and bursal bands, myonodular tissue, or periosteal erosion are seen. These can be easily debrided arthroscopically through a two-portal technique using adjacent portals. Large bone hooks at the top or the bottom of the scapula can be debrided, a process similar to inferior acromioplasty.

Sternoclavicular Arthroscopy

Pain or popping at the sternoclavicular joint may be due to a ruptured disk, fracture into the joint, arthritis, or chondromalacia. With an approach to this joint similar to that of other joints, debridement of the disk, chondroplasty of the articular cartilage, or removal of bone fragments is theoretically possible.

Sternoclavicular arthroscopy is another advanced technique. Preoperative X-rays to determine the slope of the joint are important. Familiarity with anatomy and extreme caution for posterior

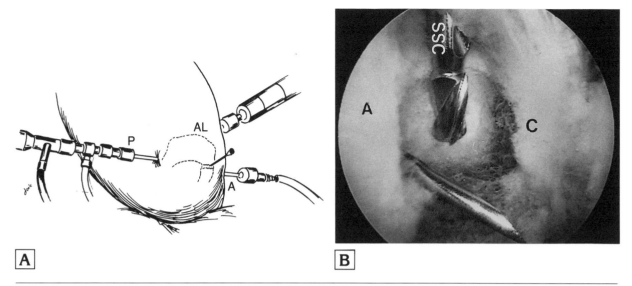

Figure 5.27

[A] Visualized through the posterior portal, the anterior A/C joint can be resected anteriorly (P = posterior, A = anterior, AL = anterolateral).

[B] Resecting the anterior aspect of the A/C joint (A = acromion, C = clavicle, SSC = Short Sheath clavicular resector, Dyonics, Smith & Nephew Endoscopy, Andover, MA).

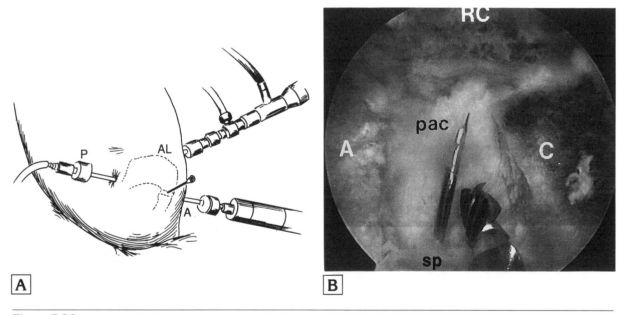

Figure 5.28

[A] Visualizing through the anterolateral portal allows posterior resection of the A/C joint through the anterior portal in order to establish a parallel gap.

[B] Endoscopic A/C joint resection leaves the posterior A/C ligament (pac) and the superior periosteum (sp) intact. After debridement of the acromion (A) and the undersurface of the clavicle (C), the remaining wear to the rotator cuff (RC) remains, but can heal or become nonsymptomatic. (Note the A/C marking needle.)

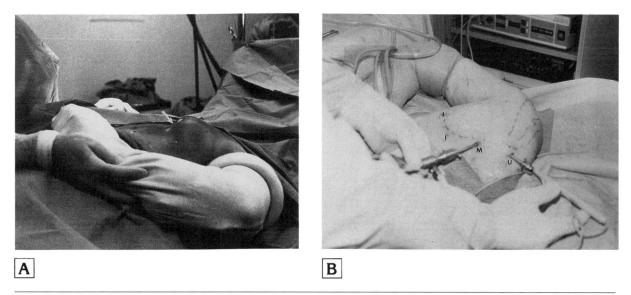

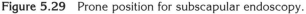

Figure 5.29 Prone position for subscapular endoscopy.

[A] Elevation of the medial scapula in the "chicken wing" position in the right shoulder.

[B] This position allows safe introduction of the arthroscope, cautery, or debriding tools, shown in left shoulder (U = upper portal, M = middle portal, I = inferior portal, L = accessory lateral portal).

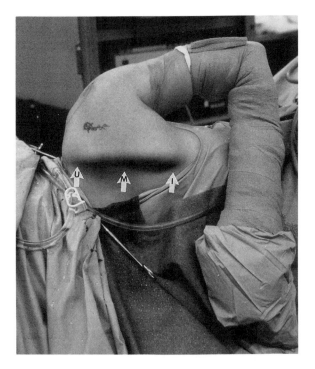

Figure 5.30 Lateral decubital position for subscapular endoscopy may follow normal glenohumeral arthroscopy and subacromial endoscopy by merely placing the arm in the "chicken wing" position, which avoids injury to neurovascular structures (U = upper portal, M = middle portal, I = inferior portal).

structures are mandatory. A neurologic head holder, extending the neck and turning the head to the opposite side, makes the approach feasible. This technique is best done with the patient in a seated position, which also allows concurrent arthroscopic assessment of the glenohumeral joint if necessary. Two portals, one directly anterior through the anterior sternoclavicular ligament and one superior through the interclavicular ligament, can be used (Figure 5.33). A 1.7-mm arthroscope passed through a cannula is necessary; the cannulas allow switching from one portal to the other. The largest tools that usually can be considered in this joint are 1.9-mm debriding tools or the 2.0-mm basket forceps, which are best passed through cannulas to minimize extravasation of fluid into the soft tissue.

In the last 10 years the author has found pathology in this joint responding to arthroscopic debridement on only three occasions: once to remove a loose body, once to debride a ruptured disk and associated chondromalacia, and once to debride arthritic changes. On one other occasion, no pathology was found; pain was considered to be due to overuse to protect from changes at the other end of the clavicle. In eight cadaveric arthroscopic explorations, no pathology was found. Arthroscopic or open sternoclavicular joint surgery is rarely done and rarely indicated. Definite contraindications to arthroscopy are an open physis, active ability to subluxate the sternoclavicular joint,

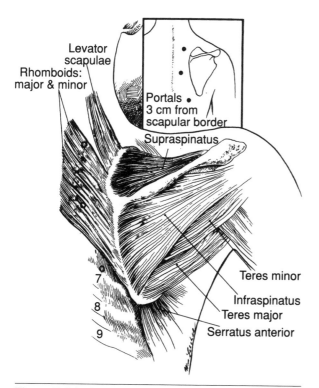

Figure 5.31 Portal placement for subscapular endoscopy.

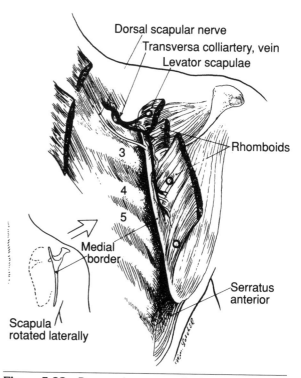

Figure 5.32 Proper placement of subscapular endoscopic portals and elevation of the medial edge of the scapula to avoid injury to neurovascular structures.

and clearly defined pathology at the glenohumeral joint, most likely leading to secondary sterno-clavicular overuse and pain.

Summary

Arthroscopy is a powerful tool both to assess pathology and to help deal with it. Each of the five mechanisms of shoulder motion can be assessed with the arthroscope, with concurrent assessment of more than one area often desirable. There is less need for diagnostic assessment as the clinician becomes more experienced and more secure in the meaning of his or her examination. With rapidly

evolving technology, arthroscopic assessment and surgical intervention become an alternative to open procedures done through larger incisions. Nevertheless, it is important to remember that the arthroscope is not a substitute for taking a good history, clinical examination, and diagnostic studies. It is more properly used as an adjunct when conservative therapy fails to restore sliding mechanisms, smoother motion, or more normal function within joints, so that flexibility training and muscular restrengthening can be effective. Arthroscopy thus becomes a major tool to help address certain specific pathologic conditions about the shoulder, which will be discussed in the next section.

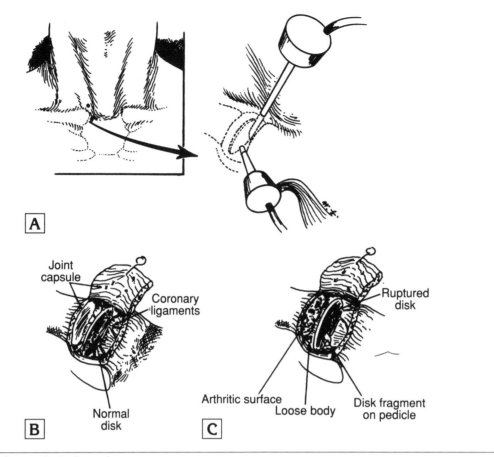

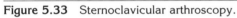

Figure 5.33 Sternoclavicular arthroscopy.

[A] Portal placement.

[B] Normal arthroscopic anatomy.

[C] Pathologic arthroscopic findings.

Part II

Shoulder Injuries

$\mathbf{B}$y coupling a knowledge of anatomy with the patient's complaint and his or her clinical examination, a diagnosis can usually be made. Further definition of the problem can be achieved through radiographic, nuclear, magnetic, and electrical testing. Arthroscopy can help diagnose or assess and treat the athlete's shoulder. These topics were presented in Part I.

Part II deals with assessment and treatment of specific structural problems. Sprains and strains are the most common athletic injuries of the shoulder and therefore deserve detailed analysis. Sprains and strains are presented in chapters 6 and 7, respectively, which are the longest chapters of this book. Although the subsequent chapters of this part deal with conditions that are less common, understanding the subject matter is equally important in an effort to assess and treat the athlete's shoulder.

Most injury patterns due to use and overuse have an acute phase and a chronic phase. It is best to assess the problems early, before they develop into long-term disabilities. The earlier an injury is assessed and treated, the less chance that muscle imbalance, improper mechanics, and structural damage will interfere with rehabilitation.

Many injuries that can be treated when acute are often ignored by the patient until tissue damage interferes with performance. The patient may have adopted the "no pain, no gain" philosophy, which the treating physician must discourage both in the athlete and in his or her coach. An initial overuse problem may become an abuse problem, ultimately leading to a less satisfactory result. Nevertheless, as will be seen in the following chapters, there may be means to diminish pain and increase performance even with chronic injury. If treatment is delayed, muscle imbalance, incoordination, and structural deficit tend to increase. With chronic or severe injury, salvage rather than return to competition becomes the goal. Ideally, an injury is identified early, treatment is initiated, and return to function is more complete.

The following chapters in Part II deal with assessment and treatment of specific shoulder injuries.

6

Sprains

Sprain injuries of the shoulder are very common in sports. Capsular ligaments and their extensions hold the bones of the shoulder together to afford stability while allowing motion. Injury to these capsular structures results in instability, which seriously hampers athletic performance. This chapter deals specifically with identification, management, complications, and prevention of sprain injury of the shoulder.

Glenohumeral Capsulolabral Sprain

When an athlete complains that his or her shoulder moves out of joint, the underlying problem is generally a sprain of the joint capsule. Laxity due to stretch or detachment of the capsule will allow the joint to move apart partially (subluxation) or totally (dislocation). The athlete may feel as if the arm has "gone dead." On the playing field, this sensation has also been described as a "zinger," "stinger," or "burner" and is generally attributed to stretch of the cervical roots or brachial plexus but in fact is more commonly associated with shoulder subluxation.

Chronic laxity has been labeled instability, subluxation, recurrent dislocation, shoulder laxity, and "dead arm" syndrome. All of these names have been applied to the condition in which the glenohumeral joint is no longer stable throughout its range of motion. A *chronic dislocation*, a condition in which the joint is out of socket for longer than 48 hours, is uncommon but sometimes seen in the athletic population.

Epidemiology

A sprain of the glenohumeral joint, or shoulder laxity allowing the humerus to be pried out of the joint, is one of the most common problems encountered in the athlete. It occurs in practically every sport activity but is most common in activities where momentum of the arm changes rapidly, as in throwing or pitching, and in activities where forward momentum can be forcibly stopped, as in a fall while playing football, rugby, soccer, or basketball. Force can be transmitted down the arm, leading to laxity at the shoulder, as in racquetball, tennis, karate, volleyball, and handball. Even pushing off the wall in the attempt to reverse forward momentum in swimming can lead to symptoms of shoulder instability. Congenital or physiologic laxity may make an athlete more injury prone to microtrauma, leading to clinical symptoms.

Because of the inherent instability of the shoulder, which allows the universal motion necessary in sports, acute subluxation or dislocation is the most common traumatic athletic shoulder injury. Ninety percent of dislocations in athletes less than 30 years of age will become persistent or lifetime problems. After age 35, dislocation is commonly associated with postinjury stiffness with or without a fracture of the greater tuberosity, which may limit resultant clinical instability so that the recur-

rence rate of symptoms decreases to 40%. Willingness to decrease activity with age, natural decrease in flexibility, and increase in arthritis may limit motion and symptoms.

Pathogenesis

There are two main mechanisms of acute traumatic injury, modified by the athlete's natural laxity or a tense biceps tendon during the injury. The first mechanism is an abducted external rotation injury, which stresses the normal corkscrew arrangement of the shoulder capsule and stretches the inferior glenohumeral ligament component, leaving it loose and unable to absorb energy well. It may heal redundantly and be unable to keep the shoulder stable (Figure 6.1a), which usually results in *multidirectional instability*. A straight posterior push

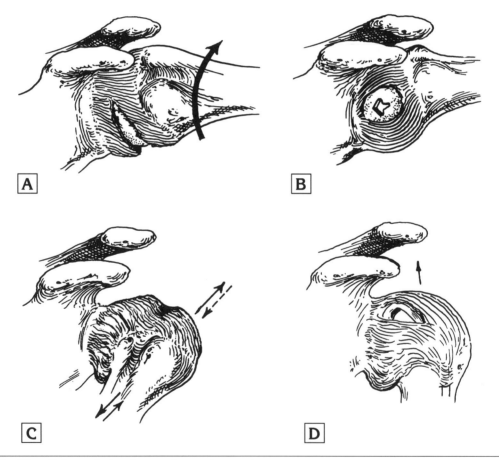

Figure 6.1 The etiology of glenohumeral capsular sprain.

[A] Abducted, externally rotated torque progressively tears the capsule, leading to multidirectional instability.

[B] A straight push may rupture the capsule and associated muscles anteriorly or posteriorly, or the capsule alone inferiorly.

[C] Adducted push or pull can generally stretch the capsule and lead to significant internal derangement.

[D] Superior push can enlarge the interval, lead to SLAP lesion, damage the rotator cuff, or produce an acromial fracture.

can lead to straight *anterior instability* by producing a hole in the capsule and subscapularis muscle (Figure 6.1b). Falling on an abducted, forward-flexed arm can jam the humeral head posteriorly through the thin joint capsule and infraspinatus muscle, leading to a straight *posterior instability*.

A straight push upward may result in injury to a tense biceps tendon during impact (Figure 6.1c). Falling onto a reverse extended straight arm or elbow or a contact pushing at the joint itself, thus prying the humeral head out of the socket, especially in an abducted position, may cause stretch of the superior glenohumeral ligament or supero-anterior labral detachment. A SLAP lesion may develop with or without enlargement of an interval defect. A fall occurring with the arm in forward flexion torquing toward external rotation can lead to a SLAP lesion that extends the anterior labral detachment, which propagates posteriorly. This prying mechanism may stretch the superior suspensory system of the shoulder (superior gleno-humeral, coracohumeral, or coracoglenoid ligaments) or may push the biceps depressor partially off the capsule superiorly or cause the humeral head to "buttonhole" through the superior capsule (Figure 6.1d).

Leverage against the abducted arm and a push downward on that extended arm can cause the humeral head to buttonhole through the relatively thin inferior capsule, which has no muscular protection, leading to *luxatio erecta* or a straight *inferior instability*. In a younger athlete, if laxity remains untreated, he or she will most likely have persistent subluxation or dislocation problems. In an older recreational athlete with stiffness and decreased activity levels, some of the capsular laxity can be compensated for.

Natural History

The etiology of chronic shoulder instability falls into three common groups related to capsular elongation or penetration or labral detachment; other causes are less common. The first common group is *atraumatic*; these problems tend to be bilateral and multidirectional. The second group occurs after *macrotrauma*, that is, a fall or a major traumatic event that translates the humeral head out of the shoulder socket and causes it to tear through the capsule, leading to a unidirectional and unilateral instability on one side. The third group, due to *microtrauma*, leads to gradual stretching of the entire joint capsule that may be bilateral or multidirectional, and is highly associated with secondary rotator cuff tendinitis or impingement.

Functional instability, or wedging the joint apart, will be discussed later. Other types of instability, such as *congenital* instability, exist that obviously are not due to athletic activity in itself but that set the patient up for a problem if he or she participates in athletic endeavors (Figure 6.2). *Neuromuscular* instability problems exist in the athletic population and are most commonly associated with conditions such as long thoracic or 11th cranial nerve palsy (winged scapula), which may alter scapular position so that the dynamic surrounding muscle stabilizers do not work in phase, and an altered glenoid version, which produces clinical instability.

Multiple instability patterns can be produced. The mechanism of injury, the trauma to tissue, and how that tissue heals determines which type of laxity develops (Figure 6.3). Abduction in external rotation produces a torque on the joint capsule that

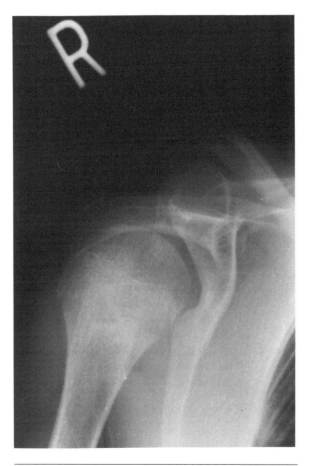

Figure 6.2 X-ray of congenital hypoplastic glenoid in a patient with osteogenesis imperfecta, who sustained 50 shoulder dislocations until a skateboard injury. The injury produced an inferior glenoid fracture and clavicular malunion, which contained the shoulder and which eliminated clinical subluxation and the need for surgical correction.

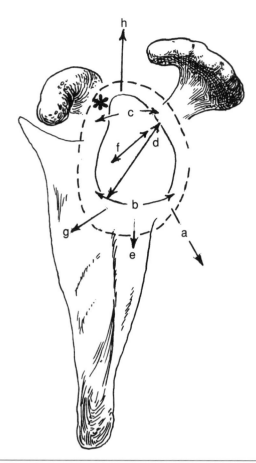

Figure 6.3 Instability patterns.

[A] Inferoposterior subluxation.

[B] Multidirectional instability.

[C] Microinstability/superior laxity (* = pivot point).

[D] Inferoanterior-to-superoposterior instability due to stretch or pull of the extremity.

[E] Inferior subluxation, or luxatio erecta.

[F] Superoposterior-to-anterior instability due to hole in rotator cuff superoposteriorly and to progressive stretching of the anterior capsule.

[G] Straight inferoanterior instability.

[H] Superior instability usually associated with SLAP lesion and occasionally with coracoid or acromial fracture.

can lead to multiple fiber failure and that commonly leads to a multidirectional instability pattern. Straight translational instability—that is, pushing the humeral head out of the socket while the arm is slightly abducted and either reverse extended or forward flexed—can lead to isolated fiber bundle rupture within the capsule and within external muscles and can lead to a clinical, unidirectional instability pattern.

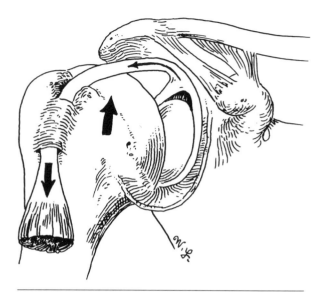

Figure 6.4 A SLAP lesion can be produced by pressure of the humeral head against an active biceps tendon and can lead to avulsion of the conjoined superior labrum and biceps long head origin.

An upward push of the humeral head against a tense long biceps tendon, as would occur in a fall, could detach the biceps base and superior labral attachment and cause a SLAP lesion to develop (Figure 6.4). Actually, there are many types of trauma from athletic or everyday activities that affect the recreational athlete and that can lead to superior labral detachment and interfere with subsequent athletic performance (Figure 6.5).

The SLAP lesion is a unique entity. Not only is a loose piece of labrum involved, but the attachment of the biceps tendon is compromised. When the biceps subsequently fires or is stretched, it may drag the labrum into the joint, causing functional subluxation and pain propagating down the biceps tendon. The capsular laxity that occurs may progressively stretch the superior capsule and jam the rotator cuff into the undersurface of the acromion, causing impingement symptoms and possibly an acromial stress fracture. Depending on the forces involved, dissection of the labrum off the glenoid rim can propagate forward, backward, or both. Dissection can progress up into the biceps tendon as well, leading to lack of stabilization and progressive superior humeral articular cartilage wear due to microinstability (Figure 6.6), eventually wearing into both the rotator cuff and biceps tendon, and leading to various tissue disruption patterns. These patterns can be categorized by a system expanded from Snyder's (1989) original scheme (Figure 6.7).

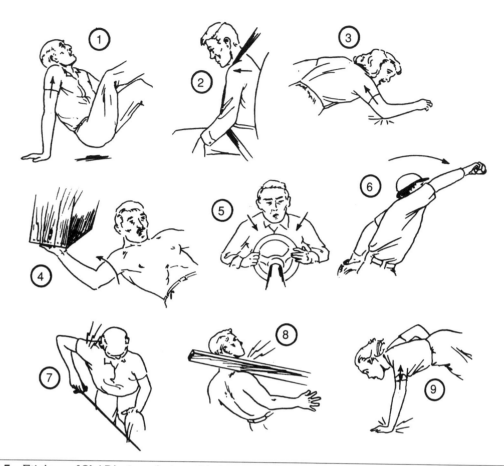

Figure 6.5 Etiology of SLAP lesions during athletic or everyday activity, limiting subsequent athletic performance.

(1) Fall onto an extended extremity, jamming the humeral head upward.

(2) Body momentum stopped, but humeral head continuing to move forward, as in pressure against shoulder harness.

(3) Fall onto elbow continuing force upward.

(4) Abducted external rotation injury while biceps is firing; Bankart and SLAP lesions can coexist. With slight adduction, the lesion will not progress posteriorly.

(5) Forward momentum stopped, but shoulders continuing to go forward, especially if the biceps is tense, as when holding onto a steering wheel.

(6) Stopping a forward throw allows the humeral head to work against a tense biceps tendon, avulsing the biceps origin.

(7) Pulling back without proper muscle balance may avulse the biceps origin.

(8) Tightening shoulder muscles, including the biceps, while colliding with an object such as a bat, a hockey stick, or a wall.

(9) Using an extended arm to try to stop an anterior fall may propagate labral detachment posteriorly.

A SLAP lesion is thus seen to be a very unusual entity in that it is both a sprain and a strain affecting the labrum and biceps tendon together. Although symptoms of tendinitis, pain along the biceps tendon, inflammation of the bicipital tendon sheath, and rotator cuff tendinitis are clinically evident, it is primarily the intermittent catching, snapping, and microinstability that lead to pathology. This is why this lesion is discussed primarily in this chapter but will also be discussed in chapter 7 as a strain.

With forceful trauma, the humeral head may skive against and partially avulse part of the glenoid labrum. The contact point will determine the area of labral detachment (Figure 6.8). With repetitive microtrauma, as may occur in swimming and throwing, the capsule tends to be circumferentially and progressively stretched, resulting in a

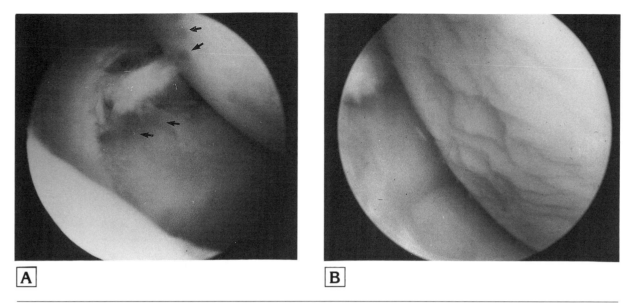

Figure 6.6 Microinstability related to stretching of the superior capsule, avulsion of the pivot point, or irritation caused by the loose labral fragment may lead to the following:

[A] Superior articular cartilage breakdown (arrows).

[B] Erosion of superior cartilage.

multidirectional instability. If the biceps fires during an attempt to stop forward momentum or during a backward fall that torques the shoulder in external rotation, the capsular tear may extend along the labrum, and a SLAP lesion may evolve that extends from an anterior or posterior labral detachment (Figure 6.9). Thus, superior labral detachment may be involved with concurrent multidirectional instability.

Disease Progression

If shoulder laxity remains untreated, outcomes are variable. Physiologic laxity varies from individual to individual. Even the clinical ability to pull the shoulder out of the socket may not be pathologic in an extremely loose-jointed individual. If laxity becomes painful, is associated with numbness and tingling in the fingers or the so-called "dead arm" syndrome, or leads to decrease in clinical performance or to secondary tendinitis of rotator cuff muscles, the underlying capsular laxity must be dealt with primarily. An extremely unstable shoulder cannot tolerate repetitive loading, and degenerative arthritis due to abnormal wear and tear may result. Osteophytic ridges around the periphery of the glenoid and humeral head can lead directly to erosion through the rotator cuff, particularly superoposteriorly, and to posterior capsular synovitis (Figure 6.10). Thinning of the articular cartilage will lead to a dysfunction of the shoulder

or to synovitis as chondral debris is generated by rough surfaces rubbing against each other. When it becomes too uncomfortable to move the glenohumeral joint, the scapulothoracic joint will be overloaded, and secondary muscles surrounding the scapula will be overused, leading to periscapular pain and muscle spasm.

If the instability occurs before age 20, there is an almost 100% chance of recurrent problems, decreasing to 90% at age 35. As tissue becomes less pliable with age, stiffness may develop after the dislocation, which may prevent recurrent problems; however, age is not an absolute safeguard against recurrent instability. It may be that the older nonathlete or "weekend warrior" may generally limit activity and restrict motion and thus avoid instability symptoms, but such self-restriction may not apply to the older athlete. Ideally, the problems of arthritis and recurrent dislocation can be avoided by prevention or adequate initial management. Repetitive episodes of either subluxation or dislocation have a greater need to be treated surgically.

The glenoid socket is buttressed superiorly by its outward curve and superoanteriorly by the biceps tendon, which originates from the superoposterior aspect of the joint and then moves over the humeral head and which works in conjunction with the acromion and the supraspinatus tendon as a spacing humeral head depressor. Although there is retroversion of the glenoid socket due to the

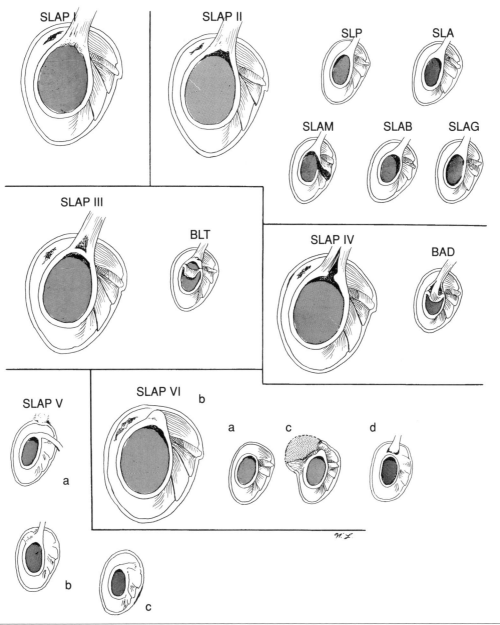

Figure 6.7 Expanded SLAP lesion calcification.

SLAP I: Fraying of the top of the joint without significant attachment, with or without rotator cuff damage, ranging from force-couple fraying to full-thickness tear.

SLAP II: Avulsion of biceps tendon origin extending posteriorly (SLP), extending anteriorly (SLA), detached with or into middle glenohumeral ligament (SLAM), extending into Bankart lesion (SLAB), and extending almost globally around glenoid rim (SLAG).

SLAP III: Erosion or hypertrophy of the biceps tendon base, BLT (bucket handle tear) in the joint, as well as superior detachment.

SLAP IV: Extension into biceps tendon, base advanced degeneration (BAD) extension into biceps tendon, and complex torn fragment that catches in joint.

SLAP V: Abnormal biceps [A] avulsed out of groove, [B] banded by adhesions to cuff, and [C] with congenital attachment to cuff, no bicipital tunnel.

SLAP VI: Biceps incongruity associated with SLAP lesion.
    [A] SLAP lesion with congenital absence of intra-articular biceps component.
    [B] SLAP lesion with residual stub.
    [C] SLAP lesions and biceps tendon stub with massive hole in rotator cuff.
    [D] Detached biceps tendon attached to cuff or superior tubercle but not to labrum.

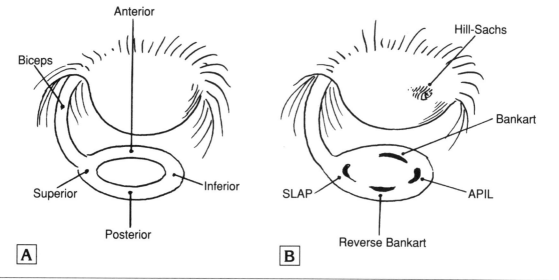

Figure 6.8

[A] Normal labral attachments.

[B] Labral detachment patterns: anterior detachment (Bankart lesion), superior detachment (superior labral anterior-to-posterior, or SLAP, lesion), posterior detachment (reverse Bankart lesion), and inferior detachment anterior-to-posterior inferior labrum, or APIL, lesion).

Note. Hill-Sachs humeral head impaction may be seen with anterior instability.

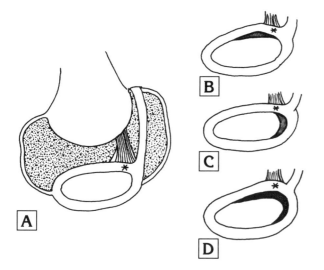

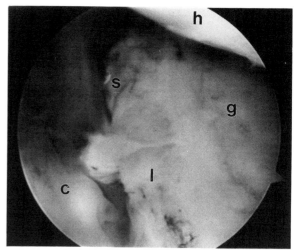

Figure 6.9

[A] The anchoring, or pivot, point may

[B] be detached anteriorly, extending into a Bankart lesion,

[C] extend posteriorly, or

[D] extend in both directions leading to complex instability patterns by destroying a normal joint signature and rotatory stability (* = pivot point).

Figure 6.10 As shown in this arthroscopic image, instability can lead to labral partial avulsion or hypertrophy, associated synovitis, and spurring of the glenoid rim. This leads to progressive thinning and fraying of the juxtaposed rotator cuff and continues the cycle by increasing instability (h = humeral head, g = glenoid, s = synovitis, l = calcified and hypertrophic labrum, c = eroded capsule and cuff).

positioning of the scapula on the rib cage, the posterior glenoid works as a buttress as well.

The function of the biceps tendon to work as a "monorail" to guide humeral rotation while continuing to depress the humeral head is allowed through a suspension system that is anchored to the base of the coracoid and the superoanterior glenoid edge. As the athlete reaches forward, the humeral head rotates around this critical anchoring point, allowing the humeral head stability yet mobility in order to position the hand in space. Being anchored superiorly and swinging inferiorly leaves the inferoanterior edge of the glenoid unprotected, which is why most shoulder dislocations occur in this direction.

Abduction and external rotation stretches the inferoanterior capsule most and makes these fibers most susceptible to injury. With decreased restraint, recurrent subluxation symptoms occur in this direction. If force is sufficient, however, the capsule and possibly the rim of the glenoid socket itself are avulsed off, with or without the labrum, leading to a Bankart lesion. Inferoanterior joint injury and lack of capsular integrity allow the humeral head to swing back and forth through the capsular defect.

The humeral head works much like the pendulum of a clock, swinging from its *pivot point* (O.H. Burt, personal communication, March 1988), the anchoring point of the superior suspensory system that attaches the superior glenohumeral capsular ligament to the superoanterior glenoid. When the superior suspensory mechanism is not intact, the humeral head may swing excessively inferiorly and anteriorly when reaching overhead, and the proprioceptive function of this tissue is lost. This excess wobble or abnormal play leads to further thinning or erosion into the cuff structures and to transmission of forces across the acromion. Such forces in turn lead to breakdown of the A/C joint, overuse of the scapulothoracic joint, or a symptomatic mesoacromion.

Overuse of the scapulothoracic joint leads to spasm and fatigue of the secondary accessory muscles, particularly of the levator scapulae, rhomboid major and minor, and serratus anterior. This overuse has been labeled *fibromyalgia, trigger point phenomenon, fibromyositis,* and other names and may lead to breakdown of the subscapular tissue structures, resulting in subscapular pseudowinging, subscapular bursitis, "snapping scapula," or "washboard syndrome." An acromial stress fracture may leave a loose anterior fragment to further wear into the rotator cuff, which may need surgery.

Transmission of force through the A/C joint will lead to A/C joint arthritis through calcification or breakdown of the intra-articular disk, or to enchondral ossification of A/C articular cartilages. Underlying impingement on the brachial plexus results in traction of the preaxial structures to the phylogenetically late addition of the coracoid and its tethering structures about the anterior shoulder. This combination of symptoms may lead to ulnar nerve symptoms (i.e., numbness and tingling in the small and ring fingers) or to the development of a double crush phenomenon (impedance of the axonal flow of the medial nerve from compression of the nerve at the shoulder and vascular congestion of the extremity due to disuse, leading to carpal tunnel irritation at the wrist).

As the superior suspensory mechanism of the superior glenohumeral, coracohumeral, and coracoglenoid ligaments breaks down or as primary superior quadrant subluxation stretches the superior structures, the apprehension sign is not as accurate, because the humeral head no longer is tethered by the superior pivot point and proprioceptive function may be altered. In this case other subtle signs of complex subluxation must be looked for. These include palm-up abduction being more painful than palm-down and a positive impingement sign in forward flexion and internal rotation. A SLAP lesion test in horizontal flexion and internal rotation is also positive, whereas an apprehension sign in abduction and external rotation is negative except for posterior shoulder pain due to scar-induced stretching of the cuff and posterior capsule.

Whether injury to the structures of the superior suspensory system (including the biceps, coracohumeral ligaments, superoglenohumeral ligament, rotator cuff interval, and superior labrum) is primary or secondary makes no significant difference because the end result is the same. This superior microlaxity contributes to overall laxity of the shoulder and leads to multiple fiber breakdown, an element of rotational or multiaxial instability, further stretch of the superior suspension mechanism structures, and wear of the rotator cuff that leads to impingement symptoms. Superior microlaxity may also lead to hypertrophy of the anterior rim of the acromion and thickening of the subacromial bursa, the body's attempt to restrain the humeral head. Such thickening of superior tissue may work as a braking or retaining system with the arm at the side, but when reaching, impaction and pulling against swollen tissue may lead to infra-acromial symptoms and then to A/C joint pathology. Both primary and secondary structures involved may need to be dealt with surgically in an effort to allow the athlete to return to functional activity.

The anterior capsule is stretched on external rotation so that the humeral head can be forced through this tissue, leading to inferoanterior instability. The posterior capsule is stretched on internal rotation so that sustained force, as in falling forward on an internally rotated straight arm, can lead to a recurrent posterior instability pattern. Directly forcing the humeral head downward can lead to stretching of the capsule inferiorly, as well as traction and stretch of the superior suspensory mechanism; therefore, a luxatio erecta or complex instability pattern can develop (Basmajian & Basant, 1959).

If the biceps fires as the arm is forward flexed and internally rotated, forcibly abducted and externally rotated away from the body, or extended backward in an attempt to stop backward momentum, the capsular defect may extend superiorly around the top, often affecting tissue only in the anterosuperior quadrant. The extension of the capsular defect may disrupt the superior glenohumeral ligament and possibly avulse the labrum, either producing a SLAP lesion, bicipital instability due to laxity of the coracohumeral ligaments and transverse humeral ligament, or widening the interval defect between the subscapularis and the superior glenohumeral ligament. Again, disruption of the superior suspensory mechanism leads to complex shoulder instability patterns. The fact that injury of the shoulder capsule itself (Townley, 1950) and of the subscapularis muscle (Symeonides, 1972) can cause recurrent subluxation has been well established and further complicates clinical presentation.

Diagnosis

In acute injury, if the athlete states that his or her shoulder came out of its socket, it probably did. If emergency room treatment was necessary to reduce the shoulder, there is further proof of dislocation. Examining the patient on the playing field may demonstrate that he or she is unable to lift the arm or is exhibiting the "dead arm" syndrome (Rowe & Zarins, 1981). Nevertheless, bringing the arm to abduction and external rotation (Rowe's apprehension test) may cause the patient considerable discomfort.

When the superior suspensory mechanism is avulsed, trying to move the humeral head out of the socket with the arm at the side can cause considerable pain, but more laxity is seen on the affected side than on the unaffected side (Hawkins's test; Hawkins & Boker, 1990). Also, when adduction or superior instability injuries have occurred, there is usually pain with forward flexion, internal rotation, and slight adduction (SLAP or superior laxity test).

History. When an athlete states that his or her shoulder feels as if it is "going out of the socket," "falling out of the joint," "feeling unstable," or "going dead," one should have a high clinical suspicion of recurrent subluxation or dislocation phenomenon. If he or she states that the shoulder has gone out before and was difficult to reduce, leading to multiple trips to the emergency room for reduction, then the need for definitive treatment should be obvious. In the past, it was felt that shoulder dislocation was to be treated only if there was X-ray documentation of the shoulder being out. Many patients whose shoulders recurrently subluxate or dislocate have learned how to reduce their own shoulders, and for this reason X-ray verification has little use.

It is important to find out how the patient dislocated or subluxated the shoulder the first time, how it was reduced, and whether it has gotten easier to reduce with subsequent instability recurrences. The patient who states that he or she has sustained a "stinger," "zinger," or "burner" or that the "arm goes dead" is usually telling you that the shoulder has an instability problem. The athlete who states that a click was heard or felt in the shoulder following a fall onto a hyperextended arm most likely has a SLAP lesion.

Physical Examination. On physical examination the examiner's thumb and index finger can hold the humeral head and attempt to shift it out of the socket while the other hand holds the scapular spine and clavicle (Hawkins's *load and shift test*; Hawkins & Boker, 1990). Being able to shift the humeral head out of the socket by more than 50% demonstrates a clinically relevant instability pattern. Longitudinal pulling on the arm, with the arm down at the side, may cause an indentation under the acromion [Warren's (1983) *sulcus sign*]. One must compare the opposite shoulder to check for physiologic laxity.

The most important clinical sign in assessing instability is Rowe's *apprehension test* (Rowe & Zarins, 1981), discussed in chapter 3. Classically, abduction and external rotation causes pain anteriorly when subluxation exists. Pain posteriorly is a sign of adhesions or synovitis and can be found when superior laxity coexists, giving a complex laxity pattern. From the abducted externally rotated position, a click on internal rotation is associated with labral capsular or synovial interposition, or *functional subluxation*. A click or grinding felt on external rotation, even without pain, correlates with a subluxation as the humeral head slides out of the joint.

A *containment maneuver* is clinically relevant (Ciullo, 1989a, 1989b). Placing the patient in the supine position, trapping the scapula against the examining table, and abducting and externally rotating the arm at 90° of abduction leads to classical anterior shoulder pain. By pressing the humeral head backward, or essentially back in the socket, thus containing the head, the pain may go away, particularly if there is a relationship between underlying subluxation and secondary rotator cuff tendinitis or impingement. This is commonly the case when, during impingement testing, there appears to be more pain in palm-up abduction (when the greater tuberosity is cleared from the acromion) than there is in palm-down abduction (which classically should cause the impingement pain; Kessel & Watson, 1973). In such cases, tenderness over the A/C joint made worse by horizontal flexion and hyperabduction can implicate tertiary A/C joint irritation and breakdown of the A/C joint. *Triad degeneration* is set up: The A/C arthritis wears and thins the rotator cuff, leading to further instability of the glenohumeral joint.

Crossing the arm in front of the body with internal rotation may cause pain at the top of the joint. The shoulder may posteriorly dislocate, but this is uncommon. More likely, there is pain radiating down the biceps from the top of the joint backward. Superoanterior-to-posterior subluxation due to stretch or avulsion of superior structures is relatively common but poorly recognized. Injury to superior structures produces atypical clinical findings and symptoms due to associated rotator cuff tendinitis and glenohumeral instability components. A click felt while internally rotating the arm in this position is pathognomonic of a SLAP lesion. Pain radiating down the biceps can occur with a SLAP lesion or with any of the other factors associated with superior suspensory mechanism dysfunction, such as a widened rotator cuff interval, subluxation of the biceps tendon, incompetency of the transverse humeral ligament, or a stretch of the coracohumeral-superoglenohumeral anchoring complex (Ciullo, 1989a).

When the superior suspensory mechanism is compromised, the classic signs of shoulder subluxation may or may not be positive. In this regard, the examiner may need to use other signs, including a *lateral laxity test*, to document instability. The lateral laxity test is done while the patient is positioned for arthroscopy in the lateral decubital posi-

tion and the arm is suspended with 5 lb (2.25 kg) of balancing traction at about 40° of abduction. Superoanterior-to-posterior, straight, and rotational instability patterns are well defined in this manner, like the Hawkins load and shift test.

With the patient in a supine position just after anesthetization for surgery, testing for instability with the arm at the side at 40° of abduction and then at 80° of abduction yields extremely important clinical information. With the arm in neutral rotation there may be a normal subluxation of the shoulder in an anterior, posterior, or inferior direction up to 40% out of the joint, and this must be compared to the opposite side. Internally rotating, pulling anteriorly, and pushing posteriorly tightens the posterior capsule; posterior instability past 50% is pathologic. Likewise, testing the arm at the side at 45° and at 90° of abduction in external rotation should tighten the anterior capsule. Instability persisting in spite of this tightening is pathologic. Of particular interest is when posterior motion at 80° of abduction in internal and external rotation is significant enough to cause an anterior dimpling in the front of the shoulder. This is pathognomonic of injury to the superior suspensory mechanism.

Even when laxity equals that of the other shoulder when testing in any of these positions, if a click or grind is associated with subluxation or reduction, a pathologic condition exists within that shoulder that most likely needs to be dealt with surgically. If there is any further question, arthroscopy should be considered prior to, or concurrent with, an open capsular reconstruction.

Imaging. Radiograph showing notching of the back of the humeral head, bony glenoid or greater tuberosity fracture, or a loose body may demonstrate factors that contribute mechanically to the instability problem. The most important X-rays of the four-view office survey are the axillary and the 15°-downward-angled AP (modified Grashey) film. On the axillary view, look for persistent subluxation anteriorly or posteriorly, or for possible locking that identifies chronic dislocation (Figures 6.11, a and b, and 6.12, a and b).

Subluxation is primarily a soft tissue problem of the capsule and suspensory ligaments, and commonly the X-rays will look normal. However, subtle fracture signs, such as notching on the back of the humeral head—Hill-Sachs lesion (Figure 6.13, a-c) or anterior or posterior glenoid rim avulsion—or Bankart lesions (Figure 6.14, a and b) on the internal rotation AP or the external rotation axillary views, may occur.

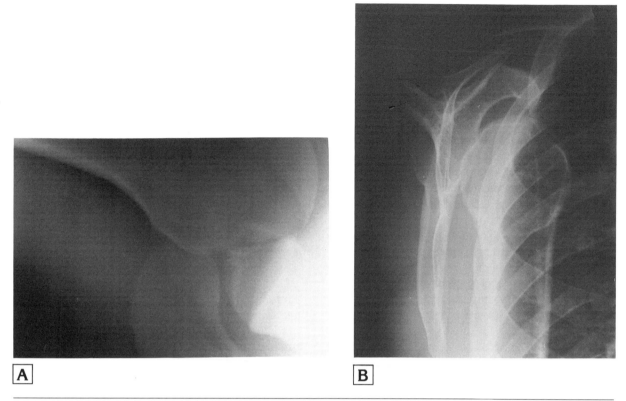

Figure 6.11 The importance of three-dimensional analysis: Chronic anterior dislocation looks relatively normal on the AP X-ray due to bone overlap.

[A] Dislocation locked into Hills-Sachs lesion on axillary film.

[B] Dislocation locked anteriorly to the glenoid rim of the scapular Y film.

A SLAP lesion may be associated with superior glenoid rim avulsion as well (Figure 6.15, a and b). Bony overlap may give a false impression of a normal joint on the AP film. The axillary and scapular Y views are useful in identification of acute anterior and posterior dislocations and help prevent the problem of missing an injury that might become chronic.

Utilization of the glenoid scapular spine angle on the axillary film can help identify excessive retroversion or anteversion occasionally associated with recurrent subluxation patterns (Ciullo et al., 1984; Figure 6.16). Calcification of the rim of the glenoid or calcification of the articular edge of the humerus demonstrates degenerative arthritis, which is found late in instability patterns. The angle-up AP view can show late involvement of the A/C joint in triad degeneration. Spurring or change of the anterior angle of the acromion on the lateral 15°-downward-angled supraspinatus inlet or scapular view helps define the changing acromial pattern related to glenohumeral instability. No other imaging is acutely necessary unless the humeral head is difficult to reduce or unless a

scout X-ray has found a split associated with fracture dislocation; a CT scan would then be useful, and open surgical reduction or repair indicated.

When X-rays appear normal and there is some question of coexistent rotator cuff tear overlapping with glenohumeral instability, then a CT-arthrogram should be done. Capsular stripping of the glenoid neck, labral damage, Bankart lesions, and articular cartilage defects, as well as injuries to the superior suspensory mechanism (if the radiologist is aware of such pathology) can be defined with these studies. Coexistent tears of the rotator cuff can occasionally be identified. However, if a large tear in the cuff exists, then dye extravasation may not allow for proper assessment of the glenohumeral structures, and arthroscopy would be the next step. Allergy to the iodine used in CT-arthrographic technique would lead to consideration of nonionic contrast or arthroscopy rather than routine arthrographic assessment of the shoulder.

If there is a break in Maloney's line on the AP X-ray—that is, if the inferior scapular neck and the inferior aspect of the humerus at the joint do not

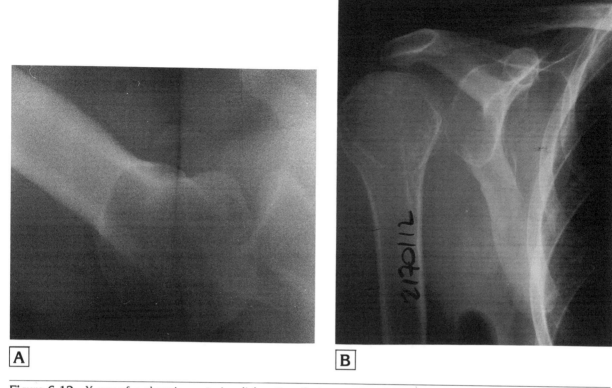

Figure 6.12 X-ray of a chronic posterior dislocation that was missed for 8 weeks and treated as rotator cuff tear. Three sets of anterior X-rays were read as normal.

[A] Dislocation locked posteriorly on the axillary film.

[B] Dislocation locked posteriorly on scapular Y film.

match up—then ultrasound is useful to check the integrity and thickness of the cuff. When there is a late involvement of the cuff and A/C joint symptoms are indicated, one must rely on clinical examination and plain X-ray assessment rather than bone scan to define the interrelated role of the A/C joint. MRI has comparatively little use in assessment of intra-articular glenohumeral structures, although fluid enhancement may yield better labral detail (Figure 6.17).

Grading the Injury. Much has been said about delineating instability patterns from unidirectional to multidirectional or combined categories. Rowe (1963) and Matsen (1988) have described post-traumatic unilateral and unidirectional instability and have compared this to atraumatic bilateral multidirectional instability patterns. Matsen has described two mechanisms of injury, which he labels traumatic, unidirectional Bankart detachment needing surgical repair (TUBS) and atraumatic, multidirectional, bilateral rehabilitation with rotational strengthening in 80% inferior capsular shift for failed PT (AMBRI). It is assumed that traumatic

injuries require a higher incidence of surgical reconstruction; atraumatic injuries, apparently with some underlying physiologic laxity, may have a less favorable surgical outcome.

Although classification schemes can give some guidelines, they are gross generalizations. In careful arthroscopic clinical examination, pathology is found to vary significantly. Treatment must be directed toward pathology. Not all unidirectional instability patterns present with Hill-Sachs lesions and Bankart lesions, nor do all generalized laxity patients present with capsular laxity without labral or bone pathology. One can find bony rim avulsions and other Bankart lesions without Hill-Sachs lesions, and one can find multidirectional instability with capsular laxity and Hill-Sachs lesions. These may or may not be combined with SLAP or APIL lesions.

Clinical examination, X-rays, and arthroscopic assessment are essential for identifying the actual pathology, defining proper management, and leading to the best clinical result. The type of initiating trauma is of minor importance to the risk of recurrence (Hovelius, 1982). Associated lesions,

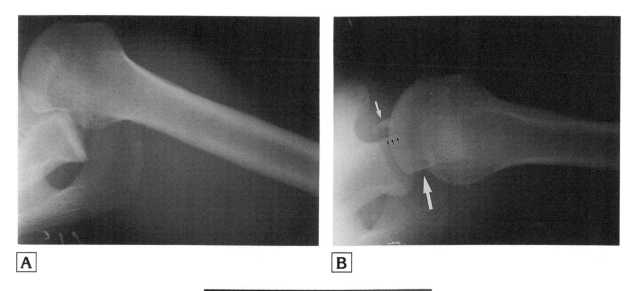

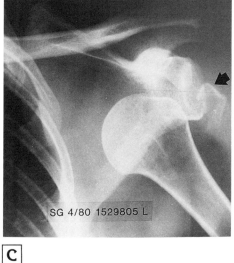

Figure 6.13 X-ray of an anterior dislocation.

[A] Prereduction: humeral head locked against anterior glenoid.

[B] Postreduction: residual posterior humeral head impaction fracture (Hill-Sachs lesion, large white arrow) and anterior glenoid rim fracture (Bankart lesion, small white arrow).

[C] Anterior humeral head dislocation with avulsion of greater tuberosity fracture fragment.

Note. Glenoid rim is smaller and the capsule may need to be attached to the edge of the shortened rim (small black arrows in [B]).

such as clavicular fracture, coracoid fracture, triad degeneration, or A/C joint separation, must be noted and may have to be dealt with if surgical management becomes necessary.

Differential Diagnosis

Correct management demands proper diagnosis. Differential diagnosis is important to rule out a *functional subluxation* or an interposed-tissue torn labrum and to distinguish between a loose body

wedging the shoulder out of the socket (Figure 6.18) and a capsular laxity that no longer restrains the joint. With a history of the arm going dead, brachial plexus injury, thoracic outlet syndrome, or cervical radiculopathy, carpal tunnel syndrome as well as full-thickness rotator cuff tear must be ruled out, although this generally does not have to be done on an acute basis. In fact, EMG changes may not occur for 4 to 6 weeks.

Glenohumeral arthritis, subscapular bursitis, snapping scapula, or rotator cuff impingement

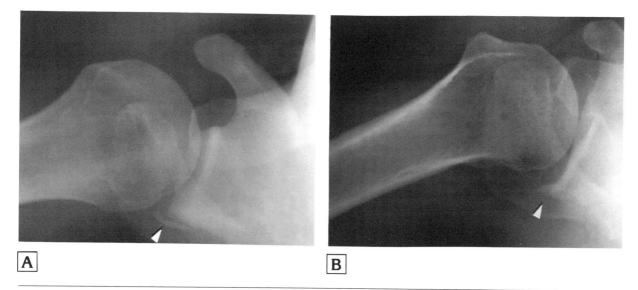

Figure 6.14 Posterior subluxation or capsular avulsion can lead to bone change.

[A] Acute avulsion fracture of posterior glenoid rim.

[B] Healing forms posterior osteophyte or "baseballer's exostosis" evident 2 yr later in the same patient as in [A].

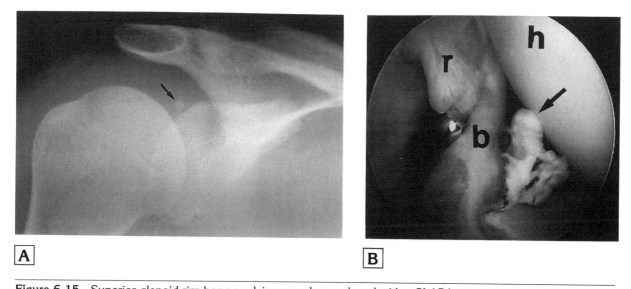

Figure 6.15 Superior glenoid rim bone avulsion may be produced with a SLAP lesion, a common skiing injury.

[A] X-ray appearance.

[B] Arthroscopic equivalent. Note associated rotator cuff tear and synovial pannus of posterior labrum biceps complex (b = biceps, r = rotator cuff tear, h = humerus, arrow = bony avulsion associated with SLAP lesion production).

may give findings that mimic instability. Careful history taking, examination, and X-ray studies must be augmented by repeat examination in an effort to arrive at the proper diagnosis. If there is any question regarding the results of the tests outlined in this section, CT-arthrography and ultrasound should be followed by evaluation under anesthesia (with or without the use of an image intensifier) and shoulder arthroscopy.

Management

If first-time subluxation is suspected or a dislocation has occurred, the primary treatment, regardless of etiology, is sling immobilization for 4 weeks.

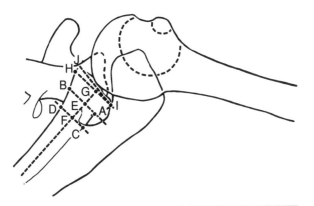

Figure 6.16 Glenoid version can be measured on axillary film by drawing a line (IGH) perpendicular to a central orienting line (FEG) of the distal scapula. The incident *glenoid angle* (IJ) measures version (Ciullo et al., 1984); this has been modified in CT scan analysis, demonstrated in Figure 4.13 in chapter 4.

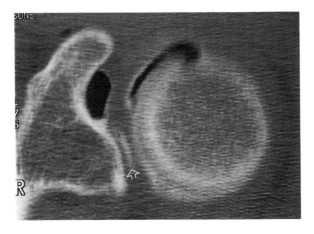

Figure 6.17 MRI identification of a SLAP lesion highlighted by contrast fluid in a soft tissue defect.

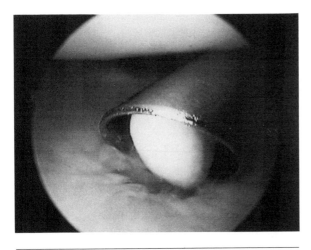

Figure 6.18 Arthroscopy reveals the capture of an intra-articular loose body.

The arm is held in internal rotation in front of the body in a sling that can be removed for bathing (Figure 6.19a); the sling is necessary even for sleeping so that the anterior capsular fibers mend tightly, not in a stretched position that could potentially lead to chronic instability. The exception is posterior dislocation for which the sling is turned sideways; here the elbow is kept behind the body in order to keep the posterior capsular fibers shortened to allow healing and minimize pain (Figure 6.19b).

In many younger athletes and in most athletes older than 35, enough fibrosis occurs that laxity may not remain a clinical problem. If conservative management is effective, 4 weeks of immobilization must be followed by adequate strengthening prior to returning to athletic activity in an attempt to avoid recurrence. After a short period of immobilization full motion must be sought; a strengthening program is then initiated (Table 6.1). Immobilization in an effort to prevent recurrence is not as effective for multidirectional or superior subluxation.

Anti-inflammatory medications are usually not necessary and may in fact be counterproductive, because inflammation is part of the healing process. Pain medication may be useful for the first week, especially for sleeping. The player should avoid contact activity for 4 weeks and then start using the arm in a forward plane, avoiding abduction and external rotation. When full motion has been regained he or she can start weight training or weighted activity. Emphasizing internal and external rotator strengthening at that point allows the subscapularis and infraspinatus to depress the humeral head and contain the shoulder.

When weighted activity does not cause discomfort, the athlete can return to full activity without restriction, which is usually after a minimum of 6 weeks and more likely 3 months. At least 80% of normal strength must be regained prior to returning to full training activity, or 90% before return to competition. Prior to returning to contact sports it is important for the athlete to work on internal and external rotation strengthening to hold the shoulder in the socket and to help prevent recurrence of injury. Returning to activity prematurely can risk reinjury and a more complicated subluxation pattern.

Whether the athlete complains of repetitive dislocation or subluxation, the arm "going dead," or the arm being pulled out of the socket when throwing a ball, the treatment is the same and tends toward surgical management. The underlying pathology must be identified and treated appropriately to obtain a satisfactory clinical result.

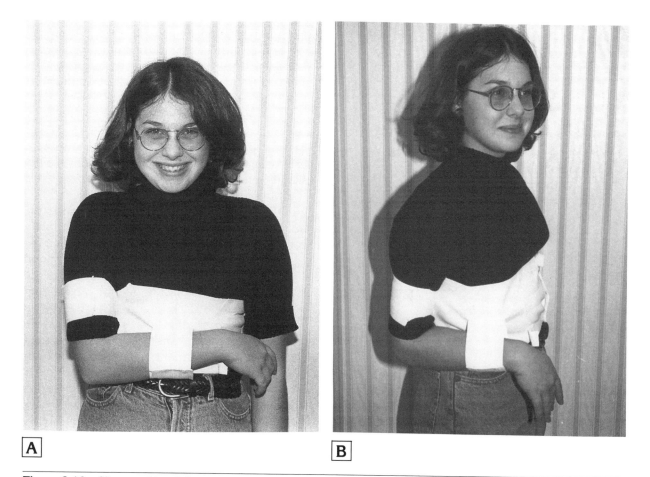

Figure 6.19 Sling position following injury or surgical repair.

[A] Anterior position decreases tension on the anterior capsule.

[B] Lateral position decreases tension on the posterior capsule.

The athlete is seeking the ability not only to do everyday activities, but also in most cases to return to competitive activity.

About half of recurrent subluxators will respond to a conservative program of anti-inflammatory medication and physical therapy geared toward their pathology. Treatment would be as described in Table 6.1, without initial immobilization. Immobilization in the management of recurrent laxity probably serves no purpose. It may be counterproductive by causing more atrophy of the secondary stabilizers and therefore more instability.

In *unidirectional* straight instability patterns, internal rotation strengthening can tighten the subscapularis in anterior subluxators and help to contain the shoulder until the isolated area of redundant capsule scars down to the hypertrophied subscapularis; either this cures the pathologic situation, or the capsular defect can be compensated for as long as the subscapularis remains hypertrophied. Once exercise stops, the instability

may return. In posterior subluxation the response is less predictable because of the common coexistence of superior suspension injury. Regardless, external rotation strengthening in isolated posterior instability may work if maintained for a long period of time.

Overall, for *multidirectional* instability and *superior laxity* lesions, conservative management tends to be less successful, and surgical stabilization is more often needed. Both of these entities are underdiagnosed clinically. When conservative management fails, surgery must be considered for the athlete.

Proper surgical management directly depends on addressing underlying pathology. Unidirectional instability can occur after the humeral head has ''buttonholed'' directly through the capsule and subscapularis anteriorly, without a Bankart lesion. This problem is approached by capsular repair and subscapularis imbrication over the defect. Where a Bankart lesion exists, even in

Table 6.1 Conservative Rehabilitation Program for Acute Glenohumeral Capsular Sprain

---

Stage 1   Weeks 0-4

Immobilize affected arm in sling for 4 weeks

Anterior capsular sprain: forearm in front of body to close anterior capsule and allow healing.

Posterior capsular sprain: forearm at side with elbow behind body (sling turned sideways) to allow posterior capsular healing.

Dependent pendulum exercises q.i.d. start immediately; sling removed for exercise or showering only.

Stage 2   Weeks 4-6

Internal or external rotation exercises with elbow at side.

Anterior capsular sprain: internal rotation strengthening for anterior laxity.

Posterior capsular sprain: external rotation strengthening for posterior instability.

Stage 3   Weeks 6-8

Balancing humeral head depressors (subscapularis and infraspinatus) to contain shoulder in socket. The same amount of exercise in each direction.

Stage 4   Return to sport, usually by Weeks 6-8

Motion is returned to normal.

Flexibility is returned to normal.

Muscles are balanced, strength normal.

Return to training.

---

multidirectional instability, a Bankart repair by exposure of a fish-mouth opening and retraction of the subscapularis, shortening and directly anchoring avulsed tissue by drilling holes to the freshened glenoid rim, and "pants-over-vest" imbrication of the remaining medial capsule is needed to give a stable repair (Figure 6.20). If a large inferior pouch exists, this must be taken up as well, and often the Bankart reconstruction is modified to incorporate capsular shift of the inferior capsule. The Bankart

lesion can occasionally be reattached arthroscopically with transglenoid suture or absorbable rivet technique (Figure 6.21). However, significant residual capsular stretch may still require tightening.

With an extremely large notch in the back of the humeral head, infraspinatus transfer into the bony defect is occasionally necessary as a soft tissue spacer to provide stability (Figure 6.22). Subscapularis avulsion, when part of the anterior instability picture, must also be repaired either through open or arthroscopic technique (Figure 6.23, a and b).

In the absence of a Bankart lesion, a tear in the anterior capsular ligaments, avulsion of the anterior capsule, or a fracture of the glenoid rim, the capsule can be shifted superiorly and medially and reattached through direct exposure over the rim to avoid redundancy of the inferior capsule and to incorporate the slack (Figure 6.24). Because in most of these cases the interval defect between the subscapularis and superior capsule-coracohumeral ligament complex has been widened, this upward capsular shift allows closure. Of course, in such cases there is no medial flap to imbricate over the lateral flap, and anchorage is either through bone or directly to the remaining labrum and capsule on the anterior glenoid. Just closing the interval defect, imbricating the infero-anterior pouch, or superolateral capsular transposition can be effective when there is no Bankart avulsion of the capsule off the glenoid rim.

Where a SLAP lesion coexists with an enlarged interval defect, these defects should be repaired concurrently so that the superior suspensory mechanism is reestablished to allow the biceps to track properly within its groove and remain a humeral head stabilizer and to avoid abnormal instability patterns that can lead to progressive degeneration of the surgical repair (Figures 6.25, a-c, and 6.26).

If there has been a concurrent rotator cuff problem, subacromial decompression to repair the worn rotator cuff or bursal sheath over the cuff (with or without acromioplasty to resect the thickened bursa under the acromion) should be done concurrently. If the A/C joint has broken down, then a Mumford procedure should be considered in addition to the preceding. These can be done concurrently through the same saber incision (Ciullo, 1989a; Figure 6.27). A Bankart lesion can occasionally be repaired arthroscopically with suture or rivet technique.

Reanchoring a stretched superoglenohumeral ligament and tightening the extra-articular component of the coracohumeral ligament, if stretched,

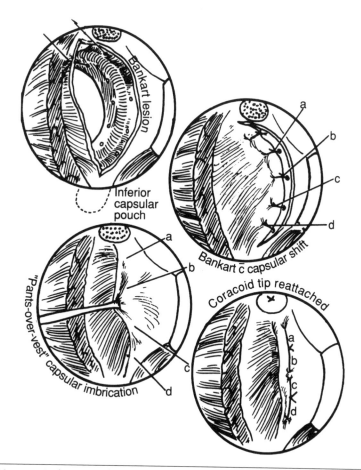

Figure 6.20 Bankart type anterior capsule repair. Redundant capsule is shortened, or avulsed capsule is reattached to drill holes in glenoid rim. (Note additional surgery: reattached superior labrum.) Note the suture placement anterior to the glenoid rim for associated Bankart repair.

are mandatory to ensure long-term beneficial results. These are done most easily at the present time with open exposure, which most often includes coracoid osteotomy and occasional use of a nonabsorbable anchor (Figure 6.28). An absorbable rivet can alternatively be used to attach a firm tissue sleeve to the base of the coracoid (Figure 6.29). Arthroscopic absorbable implants can also effectively accomplish the same results without technically difficult open exposure (Figure 6.30).

Posterior instability can be handled by external rotation strengthening advancing toward balancing external and internal rotation strength. Balancing the periscapular musculature is mandatory. If symptoms persist, posterior saber incision and elevation of the infraspinatus can allow tightening or imbrication of a redundant posterior capsule. A large reverse Hill-Sachs lesion contributing to the instability can be treated with subscapularis implantation into the anterior humeral head defect. If a lesion is too large, however, hemiarthroplasty is occasionally considered.

Postsurgical rehabilitation after reanchoring a straight instability consists of at least 2 weeks of immobilization, progressive motion with wall-climbing exercises, and gentle self-assisted motion for the next 6 weeks (Table 6.2). If full motion has not been regained after 8 to 10 weeks, then physical therapy should be started, first for mobilization and then for strengthening. After repairs of the superior suspensory mechanism or combined repairs (including rotator cuff repair, subacromial decompression, or Mumford procedure) to correct multidirectional instability, immobilization is for at least 4 to 6 weeks to allow adequate scarring and healing of the glenohumeral capsular and deltoid attaching fibers. Self-regulated pendulum exercises, gravity assisted only with no actively induced muscular motion, are started 2 days postoperatively. At 4 to 6 weeks, wall-climbing exercises and active assisted motion are encouraged, avoiding reverse extension and abducted external rotation so that the capsule is not jeopardized. When full motion has been reestablished,

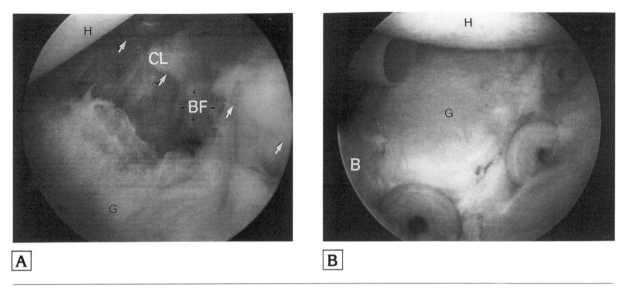

Figure 6.21 Arthroscopic Bankart repair.

[A] Avulsed capsulolabral tissue and bony rim fracture at the anterior glenoid, as seen through the posterior arthroscopic portal.

[B] Reattachment using Suretac II absorbable rivets following freshening of the glenoid rim, as seen through the anterior arthroscopic portal (Acufex, Smith & Nephew Endoscopy, Mansfield, MA) (H = humerus, G = glenoid, B = biceps, CL = capsulolabral tissue, BF = bony fragment). Shortening of reattached capsule may also be needed.

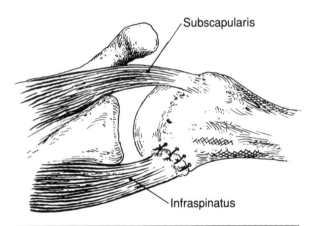

Figure 6.22 Infraspinatus transfer into Hill-Sachs lesion acts as a soft tissue block. A slight amount of external rotation is sacrificed to eliminate the mechanical cause of subluxation (Connolly procedure).

and definitely by 3 months, strengthening exercises are initiated. When the recreational athlete has about 80% normal strength measured isokinetically or the competitive athlete 90%, he or she can return to training. This can be as early as after 2 to 4 months. If at 3 months motion is not full, physical therapy is initiated, first to regain motion and then progressing toward strengthening. Again, when isokinetic testing demonstrates that there is less than 20% deficit, commonly at 6 months, return to training can occur, although with combined rotator cuff surgery, especially if a Mumford procedure was done concurrently, rehabilitation is commonly prolonged by about 2 months.

The patient does not return to athletic training until full internal rotation, external rotation to within 10° of normal, and full clinical strength (less than 20% deficit measured isokinetically in the recreational athlete or 10% in the competitive athlete) have returned. Premature athletic activity or physical therapy can lead to surgical failure.

Of course, surgical reconstruction does not make the athlete immune to further injury. The same trauma can recur and reinitiate the instability. The best prevention is proper strengthening for anterior subluxation; external rotation strengthening for posterior subluxation; and combined anterior and posterior strengthening to keep the humeral head depressed for secondary impingement, A/C joint symptoms, or superior suspensory mechanism problems. It is reasonable for the athlete to undergo a short period of physical therapy prior to surgical consideration, either to avoid surgery or to teach him or her the exercises that will be necessary in rehabilitation and for long-term avoidance of recurrence.

Complications

Complications that occur with acute injury are significant capsular laxity, which leads to future repetitive subluxation or recurrent dislocation, and

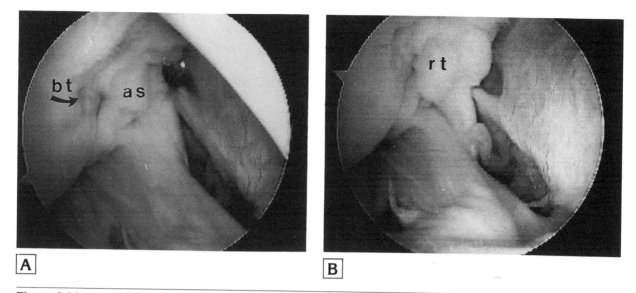

Figure 6.23 Arthroscopic repair of avulsed subscapularis tendon and humeral avulsed glenoid ligaments (HAGL lesion) from lesser tuberosity.

[A] Avulsed subscapularis (as; bt = bare lesser tuberosity) and capsule.

[B] Reattachment of combined tendinous strain and capsular sprain with absorbable rivet (rt = reattached tendon).

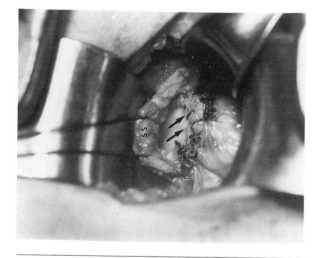

Figure 6.24 Capsular shift. The glenohumeral capsule is shifted to remove inferior and anterior redundancy. The subscapularis (ss) is elevated for exposure then reattached. Here a capsule is shifted superolaterally (arrows), but it could be shifted superomedially or plicated centrally to achieve a similar effect.

fracture of the humeral head or glenoid rim, which leads to loose body formation, catching in the joint, and a mechanical instability. Rotator cuff tearing can occur, specifically in older athletes with less pliable tissue, and axillary nerve stretching can lead to deltoid atrophy, which rarely becomes permanent but prolongs recovery. More than 4 weeks in a sling can lead to significant fibrosis or adhesive capsulitis in the older individual. Immobilization is not necessary after recurrent dislocation, because

the capsule is already stretched or detached and instability will continue regardless.

One must not initially be too aggressive surgically. Frayed tissue is hard to sew together. Waiting 4 weeks will yield more tissue to work with, especially if the capsule heals in a stretched or lengthened position. Avulsion of the labrum from the glenoid rim should not degenerate in that time interval and should still be repairable.

Long-term problems are related to chronic instability, development of more complex laxity patterns, and loose fragments of bone within the joint. Acceleration of degeneration may occur from fracture, interposition of loose bodies, avulsed labrum or soft tissue caught within the joint that leads to lack of cartilage nutrition and subsequent breakdown, or abnormal wear of the joint surfaces secondary to instability and lack of containment. Recurrent dislocation can progressively notch the back of the humeral head and the glenoid rim, and degenerative spurs within the joint may lead to erosion through surrounding soft tissue such as the capsule and rotator cuff.

Multiple dislocation or subluxation phenomena lead to progressive stretch of the rotator cuff, capsular tissue, and superior suspensory mechanism, such that an initial unidirectional instability may turn into a multidirectional, global, or even more complex instability pattern. With secondary impingement and A/C joint arthritis wearing through the rotator cuff, the supraspinatus breaks down and fails to contain the humeral head. A hole

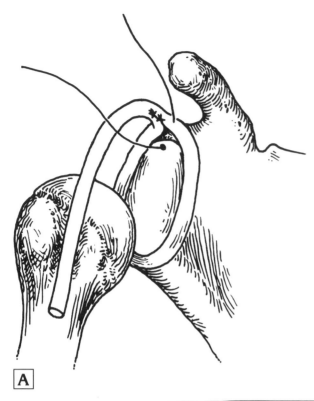

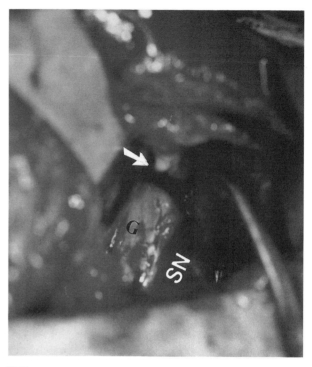

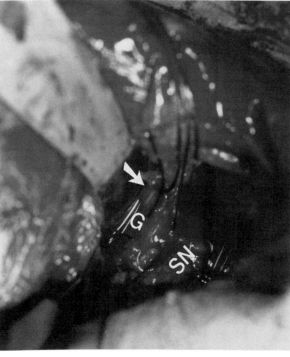

Figure 6.25

[A] Open repair of a SLAP lesion usually necessitates coracoid tip osteotomy for exposure.

[B] Surgery on a detached superior labrum.

[C] Reattached superior labrum. Note the absorbable sutures on the anterior rim for associated Bankart repair (G = glenoid, SN = scapular neck).

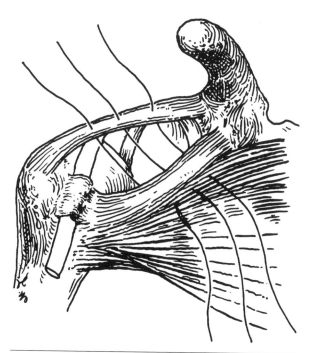

Figure 6.26 Interval defect repair.

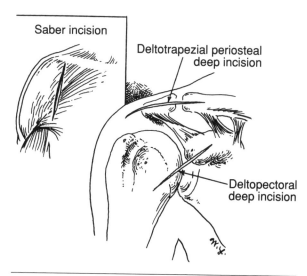

Figure 6.27 Saber incision of skin allows deep deltotrapezial periosteal exposure of the rotator cuff or A/C joint and deltopectoral exposure of the anterior joint capsule and humeral head.

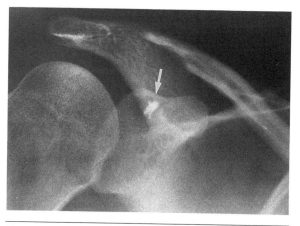

Figure 6.28 Reattachment of coracoglenoid soft tissue at the base of the coracoid with a GII Anchor subcortical metallic rivet (Mitek, Norwood, MA).

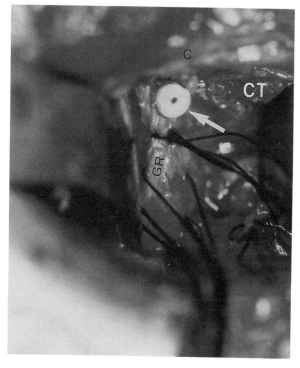

Figure 6.29 Reattachment of a firm soft tissue sleeve at the coracoid base with a Suretac absorbable rivet (Acufex, Mansfield, MA) combined with multiple absorbable sutures along the glenoid rim for open Bankart repair (arrow = implant, C = coracoid, CT = retracted conjoint tendon, GR = anterior glenoid rim with absorbable sutures placed for Bankart capsular reattachment).

in the rotator cuff can lead to loss of hydrostatic pressure and further instability. With a buttonhole through the cuff, the humeral head may move in a superoposterior direction, irritating the biceps and placing traction on the inferoanterior capsule, thus stretching that capsule and leading to further instability. In treatment the patient may be sent to therapy prematurely, and breakdown of the surgical repair can occur.

Occasionally neurologic conditions develop in concurrence with the subluxation phenomenon or may lead to the subluxation phenomenon. Injury to the axillary nerve is the most common neurologic injury that occurs with subluxation, and it

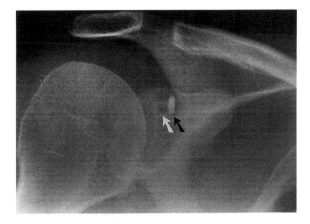

Figure 6.30 Either an absorbable implant placed arthroscopically (white arrow) or a nonabsorbable anchor placed during an open procedure (black arrow) can be used to reattach a soft tissue sleeve at the base of the coracoid, the pivot point.

occurs in at least 10% of cases. It is usually transitory but may take up to 1-1/2 years to resolve. Very rarely it remains, resulting in an inability of the deltoid to restrain or elevate the humeral head. Brachial plexopathy occurs with dislocation and generally has a more dismal outlook; however, it can spontaneously resolve entirely. Suprascapular nerve palsy, which rarely occurs, leads to loss of the supraspinatus and infraspinatus as mobilizers or stabilizers; this may result in progressive superior laxity and eventual stretching of the entire capsule, which persists even if the nerve recovers. Long thoracic nerve palsy can be related to recurrent posterior subluxation and anterior subluxation due to malpositioning of the scapula. It is a mistake to operate on the glenohumeral joint when long thoracic nerve palsy is present, because this condition usually resolves over the next 1-1/2 years. When it does resolve, the associated subluxation or dislocation usually disappears.

Glenohumeral capsular sprain injury is most judiciously managed to contain costs by adequately treating the original incident so that chronic instability and associated arthritis are limited. Once arthritis develops it may be too late. Tightening two worn surfaces together may increase friction and therefore increase symptoms. Although surgery is done to decelerate the possibility of arthritis, arthritis may progress nevertheless. Tightening or perhaps overtightening the anterior capsule in this situation may accelerate symptoms and muscle weakness due to disuse and may therefore accelerate arthritis (Figure 6.31, a and b).

Care must be taken when inserting hardware near a joint and nonabsorbable implants near the

Table 6.2 Postoperative Glenohumeral Capsular Reconstruction Therapy Plan

---

Preoperative education

Pendulum, Codman, internal rotation towel stretch behind back, external rotation cane stretch with elbow at side.

Internal and external rotation strengthening with elastic tubing and weights.

Postoperative immobilization   Weeks 0-6

Anterior capsular repair: sling with forearm in front of body, 4 weeks for Bankart, 6 weeks for capsular shift.

Posterior capsular repair: sling with forearm at side of body, elbow behind back for 6 weeks.

Pendulum exercise initiated at day 1 post-op: over-the-top inward rotation following anterior repair, over-the-top external rotation following posterior repair. The patient can shower at day 2, otherwise avoid heat for 72 hours.

Ice packs as needed for 72 hours; heat can be used after this time to minimize muscle spasm.

Postoperative early motion/flexibility, initiated when out of sling   Weeks 4-8

Externally rotated cane exercise stretching with elbow at side following anterior repair, internally rotated flexibility towel exercises behind back following posterior repair.

Wall climbing.

Active motion as tolerated below clavicular plane.

Strengthening   Weeks 6-20

Initiate internal rotation strengthening following anterior repair once motion has returned. Emphasize external rotation strengthening following return of motion after posterior capsular reconstruction.

Balance internal and external rotation strength.

Neuromuscular proprioception retraining (facilitation exercise), advance to open kinetic chain exercises; anticipate plyometrics of throwing sports by allowing stretching of capsule and then throwing.

Return to recreational sport or training activity as motion, strength, neuromuscular integration regained; emphasize home or training maintenance program to help prevent reinjury.

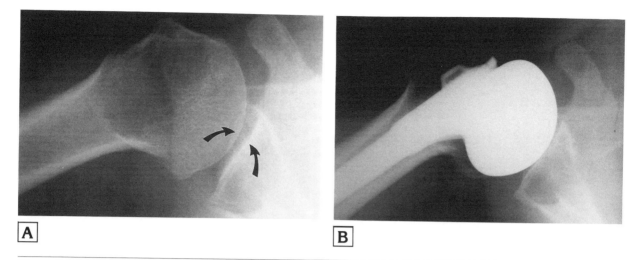

Figure 6.31 Arthritis may be initiated or accelerated by making the anterior capsular repair too tight.

[A] Failure of repair related to continued progression of degenerative arthritis.

[B] Hemiarthroplasty provides at least one smooth surface to relieve pain.

joint surface (Figure 6.32, a and b). Such placement should be avoided, because intra-articular intrusion causes wear and metal is unforgiving.

Instability persisting beyond implant fixation may lead to wear against implants and acceleration of the arthritis, so that artificial joint replacement may be the ultimate salvage procedure (Figure 6.33, a-d). Of course, even without hardware penetration, if surgery is not done early enough or is not found effective in decelerating the rate of arthritis, hemiarthroplasty or total shoulder arthroplasty remains as a salvage technique.

Prognosis

The minimum amount of time necessary prior to a return to sports after the initial instability episode is 4 to 6 weeks. After initial subluxation or dislocation, a short course of immobilization should be followed by mobilization and strengthening exercises. Surgical management of chronic instability, just like successful conservative management of initial instability, does not make the patient invincible. When subluxation or dislocation episodes have recurred and the patient wishes to avoid surgery (at least until the end of the season), then immobilization becomes less important, and the patient can return to athletic activity as soon as he or she is comfortable, as long as the patient understands that he or she is at risk of further injury or recurrence. A restraining brace may be of some use in this instance (Figure 6.34).

Nevertheless, with continued instability the long term prognosis is that the athlete may be apprehensive and may avoid full glenohumeral motion. This

not only decreases athletic performance, but may lead to overuse of secondary muscles, causing tenderness along the levator scapulae and rhomboids or secondary symptoms of subscapular bursitis. With recurrent dislocation, the process of triad degeneration may eventually lead to breakdown of the rotator cuff or A/C joint.

If the patient elects not to exercise postoperatively, the muscular atrophy from injury, surgery, and immobilization leads to decreased joint stability, and the capsule may again progressively stretch out. In the race against muscular atrophy, the patient must be committed to exercise both to protect the surgical repair and to avoid reinjury that would need future surgery. Preoperative physical therapy also has a role either in avoiding such surgery or in instructing the patient about postoperative exercises.

The immediate goal of joint stabilization through exercise or surgery is to allow the athlete to return to regular activity. The long-term goal is to avoid the stiffness and arthritis that jeopardizes athletic performance and that might eventually lead to artificial joint replacement as the athlete ages.

Patient Education

The physician must inform the athlete that he or she must be rehabilitated prior to returning to sport. The athlete must achieve a full range of motion without pain to protect the affected shoulder and must strengthen the other arm so that returning to the same activity does not cause a similar problem or overuse on that side. The athlete who has sustained a subluxation problem must

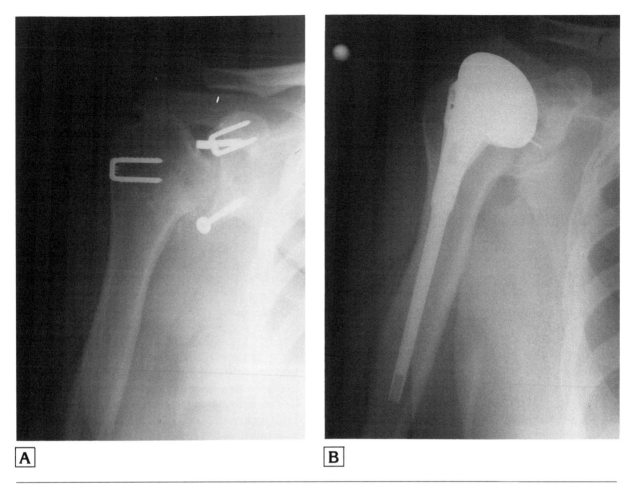

Figure 6.32 Metallic implants should not be placed close to articular surfaces. Degenerative arthritis may progress in spite of open repair.

   [A] Repair of anterior capsule and SLAP lesion with metal staples.

   [B] Total shoulder revision to relieve arthritic pain.

understand that he or she is at risk of further injury. Physical therapy or strengthening may markedly diminish initial symptoms, but strengthening must be maintained in an effort to prevent progressive increase in laxity. Nevertheless, even with exercise such increased laxity can occur, and surgery may become necessary.

Prevention

In many sport activities acute subluxation and dislocation may be preventable, for example, by learning proper falling techniques in the martial arts or by strengthening internal and external rotators and developing coordination through training so that the shoulder is more well contained and less easily caught off guard in sports such as football and wrestling.

Many young athletes, particularly swimmers or throwers, who have developed capsular laxity over time or who have underlying excess physiologic laxity may avoid symptoms if stroke mechanics are correct and muscle strengthening contains the humeral head on a persistent basis. Mobilization and flexibility are important to allow exercise of the muscles through their full range of motion and to gain maximum effects of conditioning. Nevertheless, he or she can still be caught off guard in any sport or daily activity, and injury can occur.

Glenoid Labrum Interposition

The term *functional subluxation* must be accredited to Pappas, Goss, and Cleinman (1983), who attributed clicking, catching, and locking sensations within the joint to labral interposition or wedging apart of the joint. The joint can be separated by tissue interposition, which is distinct from gleno-

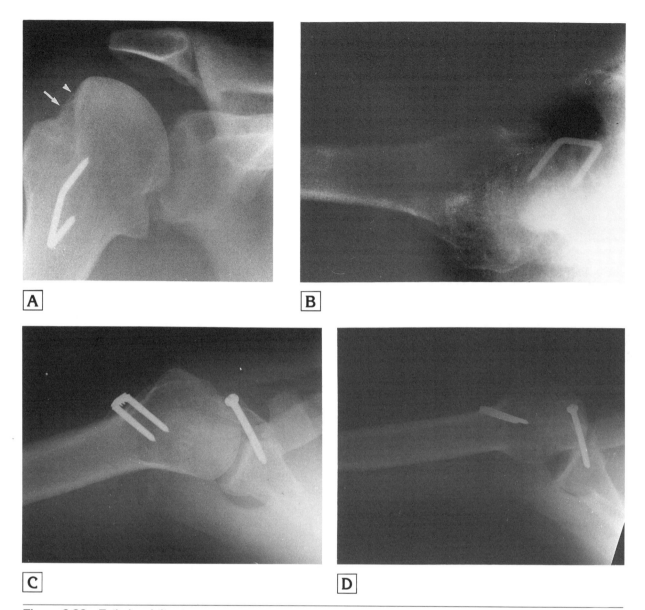

Figure 6.33 Failed stabilization attempt.

[A] Lateral transfer of subscapularis tendon with staple fixation (*Magnuson-Stack procedure*) may fail if mechanical symptoms persist. Note Hill-Sachs lesion.

[B] Subscapularis tendon may pull out with repeat dislocation, causing the staple to avulse into the joint and leading to progressive arthritis.

[C] Internal factors (Bankart lesion and Hill-Sachs lesion) are not compensated by extra-articular muscle transfer (staple) or bone block (screw) procedures.

[D] Dislocation into bony defect (Hill-Sachs lesion) occurs anyway, indicating persistent instability.

humeral laxity due to stretched or detached capsular restraints. Tissue interposition can also be labeled *microinstability* and leads to subluxation, amplification of instability symptoms, or eventually dislocation. In fact, any soft tissue loose in the joint, such as a torn capsule, torn superior glenohumeral or middle glenohumeral ligament, partial tear or stub of a biceps tendon, loose body, chondral flap, or partial tear of the rotator cuff can lead to such intermittent catching or locking within the joint.

Epidemiology

Wedging apart of the glenohumeral joint by soft tissue may follow trauma or become symptomatic in any sport but is most commonly associated with throwing or loaded hurling activity such as

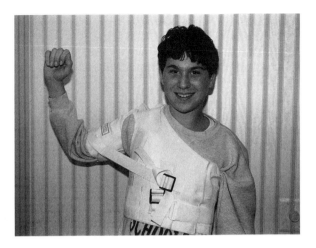

Figure 6.34 An abduction restraint brace may allow the athlete to return to activities such as football or hockey while avoiding surgery for at least the remainder of the season (Sawa Brace, Brace International, Scottsdale, AZ).

pitching, football throwing, handball, tennis, and boxing. McMaster (1986) has described this entity in swimmers as well. Interposition occurs most commonly in high school–age and college-age athletes but has also been found in younger and older individuals.

Pathogenesis

A single episode of subluxation, in which the dynamic stabilizers—such as the external muscles of the shoulder—are caught off guard, may lead to a situation in which the capsular stabilizers are caught and shear or are overcome while they are stretched in an energy-storing capacity. This can lead to wedging of soft tissue within the joint and associated symptoms. A small tear may propagate into a larger tear with repeated trauma in spite of a tight capsule. Even if the capsule is only partially torn and heals, a residual labral fragment may intermittently catch within the joint.

Natural History

If untreated, the athlete may remain extremely apprehensive and avoid positions that cause distress, thus decreasing his or her performance. The athlete may never know when this catching will occur, although certain activities—such as shaking the joint loose while stretching, feeling a snag either while or after throwing a ball, or placing the arm in a certain position—may reproduce a click within the shoulder and lead to a transient subluxation and even to a "dead arm" phenomenon. McMaster

(1986) notes that swimmers may complain of pain at hand entry and during the catch phase of swimming as the hand leads the arm into flexion and internal rotation.

The problem with soft tissue wedging that is either intermittent or locked within the joint is primarily twofold. First, soft tissue pressure against the articular cartilage may lead to localized arthritis or degeneration of chondral tissue, which may shed and cause secondary synovitis, leading to decreased motion and muscle atrophy. Second, recurrent wedging apart of the shoulder can stretch the surrounding capsular tissue so that capsular laxity and related rotator cuff impingement rather than functional instability become the major problem. The athlete's apprehension caused by not knowing when this clicking or catching will occur can seriously hamper athletic performance. With progressive capsular stretch, spurs peripheral to the articular surface can develop to take up the slack. This is counterproductive in that decreased motion and increased arthritic complaints are the consequence (Figure 6.35, a and b).

Diagnosis

The athlete will often tell you that he or she feels a click in the shoulder in certain positions; allow the athlete to demonstrate this. He or she may state that pain, including a snap or catch that is like "popping a knuckle," recurs while performing athletically or during the warm-up maneuvers. The athlete may state that the arm "goes dead" when this occurs, or that he or she has pain at rest or during glenohumeral motion immediately following or the day after athletic activity. The athlete may remember a single episode of subluxation or dislocation that led to this clicking or catching phenomenon.

During the physical examination an apprehension test may or may not be positive. Pain may be primarily posterior while doing this maneuver, but while turning the shoulder toward internal rotation from an abducted, externally rotated position, a click may be reproduced 60% to 80% of the time. The patient may confirm that this is the type of catching that he or she has experienced. With the patient's arm down at the side, utilizing Hawkins's load and shift maneuver while moving the humeral head back and forth in the glenoid socket, the examiner may feel a grinding that, again, implicates labral pathology, although a loose body or other interpositional tissue can cause the same sort of findings. The patient may experience tenderness along the anterior glenoid labrum, and there may

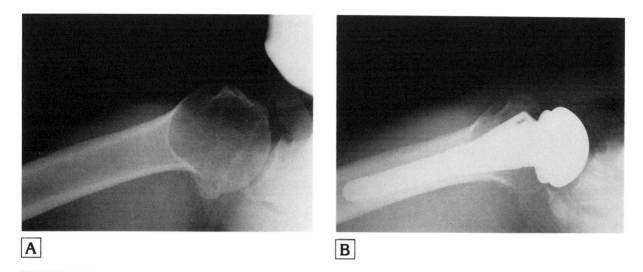

Figure 6.35 Instability may lead to arthritis.

    [A] Instability associated with baseball pitching has led to development within 10 years of spurs that tighten the capsule but also lead to symptoms.

    [B] Relief of symptoms with total shoulder arthroplasty.

be no feeling of subluxation in early presentation. The examination of the shoulder must rule out recurrent subluxation or dislocation in which a soft-tissue interposition may be only a component. Of particular interest is the horizontal flexion–internal rotation test, which may cause a catching in the superoanterior quadrant, identifying a SLAP lesion. In these situations the patient may volunteer in his or her history that it hurts to turn a steering wheel or door handle.

Inferior labral detachment or bucket-handle tears are made worse with cross-flexion (starting from a palm-up position with the arm directly extended down at the side and then bringing the arm up toward the opposite shoulder). If a catch or pop is produced by this maneuver, an APIL injury is commonly found (Figure 6.36). This lesion can best be repaired arthroscopically by debridement and repair of the freshened glenoid rim (Figure 6.37).

Even with a negative apprehension test, a Bankart lesion may produce symptoms when the arm moves from the abducted, externally rotated position toward an internally rotated position. A reverse Bankart lesion or a posterior labral detachment can cause a posterior clicking or posterior shoulder pain when the arm moves toward the apprehension position of abducted external rotation. These are positions similar to the McMurray test for meniscal pathology in the knee that can catch torn tissue in the joint.

X-ray examination is important; however, this primarily soft tissue interposition will not be demonstrated on most plain films unless a loose body

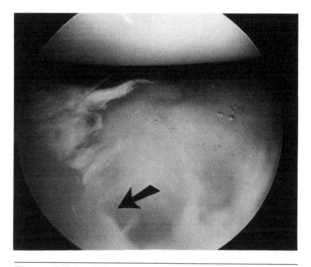

Figure 6.36 Arthrogram of APIL lesion, or avulsion of anterior-to-posterior inferior labrum.

or a Bankart-type lesion including a partial bony avulsion coexists. CT-arthrogram is extremely valuable in these situations to demonstrate a torn labrum even without capsular redundancy.

Differential Diagnosis

When the patient states that his or her shoulder "slips out," "hangs up," or is able to "slip back in place," one must include recurrent subluxation or dislocation in differential diagnosis. Catching can also be due to articular cartilage local impaction damage and initial glenohumeral arthritis,

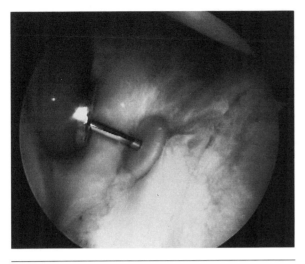

Figure 6.37 Arthroscopic repair of APIL lesion by debridement of frayed labral edge, abrasion of non-articular glenoid rim to bleeding bone, and reattachment with an absorbable rivet.

which can occur with diabetes or direct impact loading, causing central breakdown of cartilage within the glenohumeral joint. Synovitis, particularly along the posterior rim of the socket, can cause catching, but this is difficult to assess without arthroscopic differentiation.

With loss of distal clavicular cartilage at the A/C joint, bone-on-bone contact can cause grinding due to sliding of bone against bone at the A/C joint with horizontal flexion or circumduction. This is differentiated in that the arthritic pain is located strictly at the A/C joint, whereas the labral catching feels deep.

Management

Many symptomatic flap or bucket-handle tears of the labrum, or other soft tissue interpositions, can be managed with initial nonsteroidal anti-inflammatory medication and humeral head depressor or internal and external rotation strengthening exercises to contain the shoulder in the socket and leave less room for soft-tissue interposition. This may eliminate or markedly restrict the number of catching episodes that occur. A short period of rest along with anti-inflammatory medication, internal and external rotation exercises, and a graduated throwing program may be useful for return to pitching activity. If catching does not resolve with conservative management and interferes with athletic performance, then arthroscopic assessment is indicated.

If examination under anesthesia and arthroscopic analysis demonstrate no concurrent instabil-

ity problem, then resection of soft tissue—either torn labrum, loose body, biceps partial tear or stub within the joint, rotator cuff debris, or synovitis—should be done; repair of a SLAP lesion may be necessary (Figure 6.38, a-e).

Mobilization can start the next day following resection of Grade I fraying or at 4 weeks following repair of a more advanced superior labral detachment. After repair when motion is limited but relatively painless, an organized therapy program emphasizing first mobility and then strength should proceed (Table 6.3). Graduated throwing exercises leading to the ability to return to training is the goal. Internal and external rotation strengthening to depress the humeral head and prevent further subluxation or superior migration problems should be continued indefinitely. With concurrent instability, a superior labral repair most likely will not hold up by itself, and capsular tightening may be indicated. This is much like a meniscal repair that needs anterior cruciate reconstruction to protect that repair.

Complications

Labral flap tears or mechanical interposition may merely be components of a greater problem. A posterior or anterior bucket-handle tear, in spite of causing occasional clicking within the joint, may act as a buttress to provide considerable stability to that joint, and resection (although relieving the snapping) can lead to increased symptoms of instability. This resultant instability following labral debridement may necessitate an open reconstruction. Soft tissue against articular cartilage can lead to breakdown of that cartilage and to secondary synovitis, which in fact leads to atrophy of primary muscles and accessory muscle overuse. Periscapular spasm, trapezial muscle spasm, or scapulohumeral dysrhythm may result.

Prognosis

The athlete may return to full activity when he or she is asymptomatic. This means either that there has been response to conservative management using anti-inflammatories and strengthening or that the athlete has responded to arthroscopic or open resection of the labral tissue. One would hope that arthroscopic debridement would lead to faster recovery, but full motion and strength should be regained prior to return to athletic activity, whether debridement was done arthroscopically or as an open procedure. If the labral problem occurred in the superoanterior quadrant and is related to a stretch of the superior suspensory

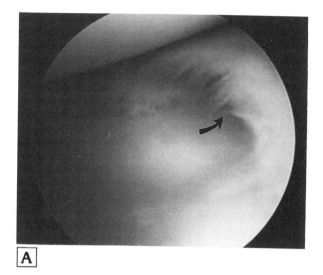

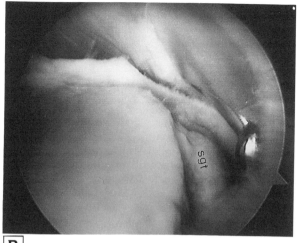

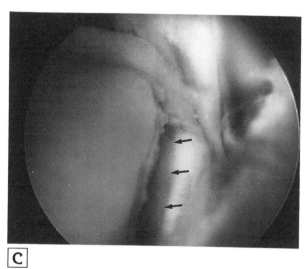

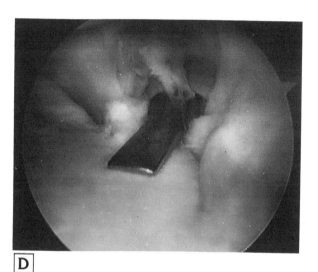

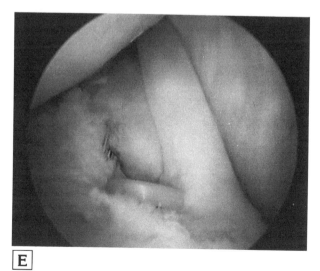

Figure 6.38 SLAP lesion repair.

[A] Labrum frayed by joint interposition must have shag debrided.

[B] Superior labrum and biceps tendon base detached from superior glenoid rim and superior glenoid tubercle (sgt).

[C] Abrasion of nonarticular rim to bleeding bone.

[D] Reapproximation and advancement of detached labrum–superior glenohumeral ligament complex (pivot point).

[E] Reattachment of labrum and biceps tendon base with absorbable rivets.

Table 6.3 Postoperative SLAP Lesion Repair Program

Preoperative

Internal and external rotation strengthening with elbow at side to decrease capsular volume, depress humeral head, compensate for instability, and with luck avoid surgery. Pendulum and Codman training, internally rotated stretching behind back, external rotation strengthening at the side with a cane, and horizontally flexed, hyper-abducted stretching of A/C joint and posterior capsule, with subdeltoid scar immobilization.

Postoperative immobilization following arthroscopic repair   Weeks 0-1

In sling for 4 weeks (but permit showering at day 1).

Pendulum exercises out of sling three times a day, then back in sling even during sleep.

If significant subdeltoid adhesions were resected, passive range of motion by the physical therapist, forward flexion and external rotation at the side once a week for 4 weeks, then back in sling.

Flexibility and motion   Weeks 4-8

Passive supine forward flexion in external rotation with the arm at the side trapping scapula, until full motion is regained. Emphasize posture and then advance to directed active range of motion.

When active range of motion (at least 90° of forward flexion or 80° of abduction, still emphasizing full passive motion by the therapist) balances internal and external rotation strength with the elbow at the side, gradually increase strength in abduction.

Weeks 8-16

With full passive and active range of motion and internal and external rotation strength with deficit less than 20%, initiate proprioceptive neuro-muscular recoordination, open kinetic chain exercises, and plyometrics with elbow at side stretching in external toward internal rotation, as well as abducted external rotation in a throwing motion. When accomplished, patient can return to training or recreational sport activity.

Note. Following open or arthroscopic SLAP lesion repair or superior mechanism reconstruction combined with open capsular repair, follow post-operative capsular repair program (Table 6.2). Use this program following arthroscopic SLAP lesion repair (with or without subacromial decompression or endoscopic Mumford procedure).

mechanism, both proprioception and stability will be affected. Symptoms may worsen over time and either superior laxity (microinstability) or progressive breakdown and synovitis of the entire joint capsule (combined multidirectional instability and superior laxity) may develop.

Patient Education

The physician must warn the athlete with a clicking shoulder that resection of that tissue may lead to greater instability. He or she must also warn the athlete that the labral or soft-tissue interposition itself (such as a loose body related to a Hill-Sachs or Bankart lesion) may not be the total problem and may be only a component of a much larger problem, such as capsular laxity, recurrent subluxation, or dislocation. It is mandatory that the athlete continues to emphasize internal and external rotation strengthening to contain the shoulder in an effort to avoid recurrence of symptoms that are resolved by conservative management.

Prevention

There is perhaps no way to adequately prevent interpositional injuries other than maintaining proper throwing or stroke mechanics and keeping the muscles strong to work as shock absorbers, thus minimizing the potential of being caught off guard and shearing tissue within the joint.

Acromioclavicular Sprain

The scapula is attached to the body essentially through the acromioclavicular joint capsule and the coracoclavicular ligaments. Injury to these ligamentous structures can lead to instability at this joint, particularly capsular ligament injury leading to anterior-to-posterior instability, capsular tearing combined with coracoclavicular ligament sprain producing superior-inferior instability, or direct pressure due to abnormal superoanterior glenohumeral motion. Injury to the acromioclavicular complex is quite common in sport activity and is frequently called *shoulder separation*. This results from a fall onto the point of the shoulder forcing the acromion inferiorly or from a direct lateral push, as in a football tackling injury. A fall on an outstretched arm with slight adduction can push against the acromion and separate the A/C joint. Tackling another individual with the point of the shoulder or hitting the shoulder into the boards while playing hockey can lead to the same injury.

Epidemiology

The sports in which A/C joint problems commonly occur are those associated with impact or a fall during play, such as football, rugby, wrestling, hockey, skiing, equestrian sports, basketball, soccer, and even falling over the handlebars in bicycling.

Pathogenesis

Separation or sprain of the A/C joint consists of injury to the joint capsule itself (acromioclavicular ligaments) or to the coracoclavicular coronoid and trapezoid ligaments (Figure 6.39). Injury commonly involves all of these structures because the ligaments work in concert to provide stability; however, isolated trauma or certain combinations can occur that lead to different clinical patterns.

Natural History

It has generally been felt that there is no significant consequence of untreated acromioclavicular sprain, other than forcing the athlete to throw a little more to the side or possible future arthritis needing resection of the distal end of the clavicle. There is growing concern that a step-off deformity at the A/C joint may lead to progressive wearing of the acromion into the rotator cuff in such a way that rotator cuff erosion may develop in time, and so perhaps an initial surgical stabilization may be justified.

Diagnosis

The athlete will usually state that trauma was sustained to the tip of the shoulder or in a fall with the arm outstretched either behind or in front of him or her. The athlete may indicate that it hurts at the top of the shoulder when attempting to lift the arm. Physical examination may reveal an associated contusion due to blunt trauma or a step-off deformity, which looks like a piano key. The end of the clavicle can usually be reduced manually down to the level of the acromion, but in some cases this deformity is fixed, in which case the need for surgical management may become more evident. Injury to the coracoclavicular ligaments is assumed with the ability to move the distal clavicle superiorly and inferiorly at the A/C joint. There may be a fixed separation with the clavicle posteriorly herniated through the trapezial fascia, in which case reduction is not possible. Pain in this area can also occur from isolated acromioclavicular joint capsular injury, in which superior-to-inferior subluxation may not be possible but anterior-to-posterior instability will be clinically evident.

X-rays are important to see whether there is increased widening at the A/C joint, which implicates acromioclavicular capsular sprain on the 15°-upward-angled AP film. In the athlete under age 18 a fracture of the distal end of the clavicle may occasionally occur and may be confused with a growth plate injury (Figure 6.40). These fractures usually heal and should be essentially immobilized in a sling for 3 to 4 weeks rather than risk nonunion (Figure 6.41).

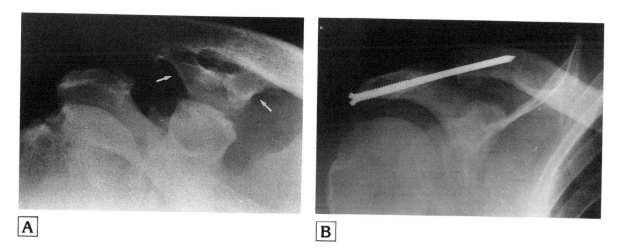

Figure 6.39

[A] X-ray of concurrent injury to the coracoclavicular ligaments and A/C joint capsule that allows separation of the clavicle from the acromion; calcification of avulsed ligaments can occur.

[B] Heterotopic bone excised and ligaments reconstructed; maintained repair with pin-screw fixation, removed at eight weeks (Pin-screw, Biomet, Warsaw, IN).

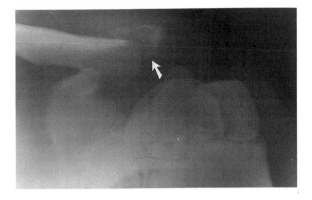

Figure 6.40 Acute injury of distal clavicle with A/C separation may be growth plate injury or capsular sprain equivalent. The X-ray shows pulling off a fleck of bone.

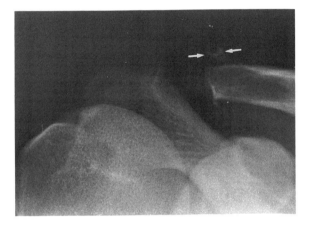

Figure 6.41 Twelve years following distal clavicle fracture and A/C joint capsular injury, an X-ray reveals that the bone fragment is still not healed and remains symptomatic; in spite of widening, there has been no surgical intervention.

In the past, weighted X-rays were done routinely (Figure 6.42), but these are not mandatory, and in fact clinical examination can give you most of the same information. There is no need to purposely subject acutely traumatized ligaments to further stress. Clinical grading of the injury, as developed by Rockwood (Rockwood & Green, 1984), helps to evaluate the need for conservative versus surgical management.

Rockwood and Green's classification of six types of injury is extremely useful but has been expanded to encompass most injuries at the A/C joint (Figure 6.43). Type 1A, sustained with depression at the top of the acromion, leads to capsular sprain injury with no considerable instability. Point tenderness at the A/C joint is made worse with horizontal flexion, hyperabduction, or reverse extension, and X-rays are in most cases normal.

Type 1B is usually due to an anterior push on the front of the acromion. Again, X-rays are normal, and the same clinical findings are produced except that the distal clavicle can be moved anteriorly to posteriorly with no significant step-off deformity demonstrated, showing that the capsular ligaments have been torn but the coracoclavicular ligaments may remain relatively intact. On X-ray, there may or may not be widening of the affected A/C joint compared to the opposite one, although a stress axillary X-ray will show the amount of possible displacement in an anterior-posterior direction (Figure 6.44, a and b; Ciullo, Koniuch, Teitge, & May, 1982). There is less than 3 mm of step-off even on a weighted X-ray, and in most cases a weighted A/C joint film shows no difference.

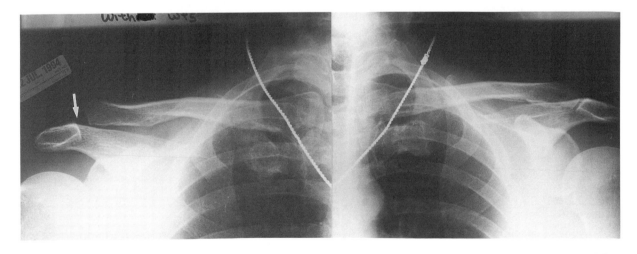

Figure 6.42 Comparison of affected and unaffected shoulders with 15-lb (6.75-kg) weight distraction demonstrates lack of ligament integrity; second degree sprain not obvious on plain, nonweighted X-ray view.

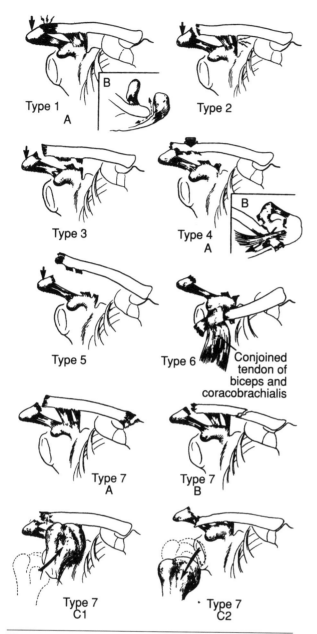

Figure 6.43 Expanded A/C joint sprain classification system.

In Type 4 A/C joint sprains, the coracoclavicular ligaments are completely disrupted, and the distal end of the clavicle buttonholes through the trapezius muscle. The AP X-ray may give the illusion of normal anatomy; however, an axillary X-ray will be the key to pathology, revealing that the distal clavicle is posteriorly displaced.

A Type 5 injury is sustained with much more trauma. The acromioclavicular and coracoclavicular ligaments are disrupted. The clavicular-coracoid interspace is at least 100% and possibly up to 300% that of the opposite shoulder. Deltoid and trapezial sleeves are detached from the distal clavicle, which may appear to tent the skin in a thin individual. Horizontal flexion or an attempted shoulder shrug may accentuate the displacement.

Type 6 injury is sustained when traction on the elevated arm is not released until after the A/C joint is disrupted. This causes the clavicle to slip under the acromion or even the coracoid, with a high concomitance of neurologic injury.

A seventh category has been found useful. In Type 7A, both the acromioclavicular joint and the sternoclavicular joint are separated. This usually implies significant rotational energy in etiology. In Type 7B injury, the acromioclavicular joint sprain occurs in conjunction with a clavicular fracture. Malunion of a midshaft fracture with A/C joint arthritis may lead to a high incidence of secondary subscapular bursitis when the normal function of the A/C joint is compromised by malalignment and stiffness. Distal clavicular fractures, either near or into the A/C joint, tend to remain symptomatic for a prolonged time, even years.

A Type 7C injury occurs when the A/C joint is injured in conjunction with a glenohumeral subluxation or dislocation. Type 7C1 A/C joint injury occurs in conjunction with a superior push of the humeral head, for example, when a football player is pushing up from the ground and his shoulder is tackled from above (Figure 6.45). Many individuals with symptomatic mesoacromial findings that lead to impingement later in life have sustained this type of injury. Superior humeral subluxation can lead to a nonunion or loosening of an acromial apophysis; the mesoacromial deformity may, however, be a stress fracture. In Type 7C2 injury, an inferior pull on the humeral and scapular mechanism may disrupt the A/C joint. This is rare but may be seen in conjunction with weight-training exercises when the spotter suddenly releases the weight, catching the athlete's shoulder off guard.

Differential Diagnosis

The differential diagnosis includes acromioclavicular joint arthritis and overuse. Osteolysis of

A Type 2 injury may have a mild step-off at the A/C joint, because the coracoclavicular ligaments are partially torn along with the A/C joint capsule. Horizontal flexion, hyperabduction, and reverse extension are similarly painful, and the acromion will be depressed less than the width of the clavicle.

In a Type 3 injury, there is a clinical step-off at the A/C joint, and on X-ray the coracoclavicular interval is 25% to 100% greater than in the opposite, normal shoulder due to the acromioclavicular capsular ligaments and coracoclavicular ligaments both being disrupted.

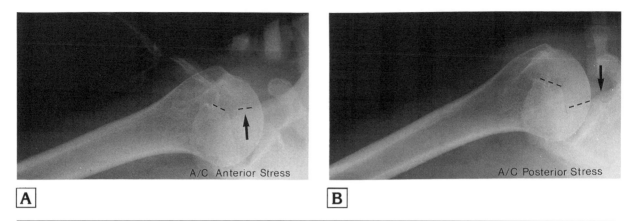

Figure 6.44 Stress X-ray assessment of A/C joint capsular disruption with coracoclavicular ligaments remaining intact.

[A] Examiner's fingertips around clavicle and skin can reduce the clavicular displacement with anterior pressure.

[B] Fingertip pressure displaces the clavicle backward. There is no displacement noted on the AP film or the 15-lb (6.75-kg) stress films.

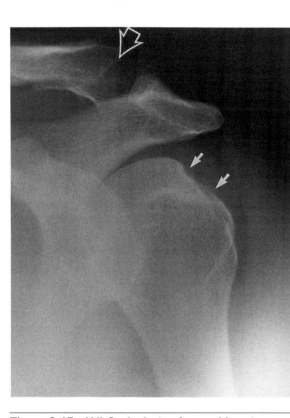

Figure 6.45 Hill-Sachs lesion from subluxation (small arrows) against superoanterior acromion and A/C joint separation and distal clavicle growth plate fracture with periosteal stripping (large arrow).

the distal clavicle is common in weight lifting, but may present as an acute A/C separation that is ruled out by X-ray. Although commonly considered a "male" injury, with women increasingly active in weight training, osteolysis is seen in either sex. In athletes septic arthritis is rare but can be seen with intravenous drug abuse and can be confused with an A/C joint sprain. Pain radiating into the A/C joint can occur with athletic trauma, rheumatoid arthritis, or bursal invagination into the joint. Rotator cuff pathology may lead to excess joint fluid irritating the A/C joint, and arthrography may be useful to define this situation. A primary cyst may occur in the A/C joint and be defined on X-ray; other pathology may not be involved. In an adolescent athlete, the clavicle may be pushed out of the periosteal sleeve, and if left alone, a double clavicular deformity may develop (see Figure 10.5 in chapter 10). If there is difficulty in reducing the clavicular portion, reossification may occur within the periosteal sleeve (Figure 6.46); the extruded fragment may need to be resected for cosmesis or due to tenting of the skin.

Management

Treatment of A/C joint sprains Types 1 through 3 is usually conservative. This means immobilization in a sling for up to 2 weeks until comfortable and then gradually regaining strength and activity as tolerated (Table 6.4).

The Type 1B sprain is the exception. If laxity persists in an anterior-posterior direction past 3 to 4 weeks, then operative repair is indicated. The author's preference is a Simmon's pin to help redevelop normal A/C joint motion (Figure 6.47). A Type 3 sprain in the dominant arm of a throwing athlete may warrant initial repair, again with a smooth-tipped, threaded-base screw. With chronic instability, transposition of the acromial portion of

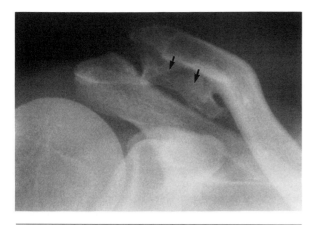

Figure 6.46 Periosteal avulsion from inferior clavicle and attachment of coracoclavicular ligament can lead to subperiosteal bone and heterotopic bony build-up.

the coracoacromial ligament, or tip of the coracoid, with the conjoined tendon may be necessary to reduce displacement.

Type 4 injury should have immediate reduction under anesthesia and then conservative management in a sling if this maintains position. If there is considerable anterior-posterior laxity, the use of a Kenny Howard splint can help stabilize this joint. A Type 5 injury warrants immediate operative reduction with repair of acromioclavicular ligaments and pin fixation of the A/C joint. A Type 6 injury necessitates open repair and exploration, because there is a high incidence of injury to the musculocutaneous nerve. Type 7A injuries require open reduction and internal fixation. The sternoclavicular joint may be reduced with a sandbag between the scapulae posteriorly; if the A/C joint remains subluxated, repair is indicated. In Type 7B injuries open reduction and internal fixation of the clavicle is indicated to help maintain normal scapulothoracic orientation when there is concurrent A/C joint sprain. In an older individual with concurrent A/C joint arthritis a Mumford procedure can be done, with the distal end of the clavicle used as bone graft for the clavicular fixation.

Type 7C is more difficult to manage, and is usually identified late (Figure 6.48). It is mandatory to listen to the patient's history, and if glenohumeral instability is suspected, it must be dealt with primarily. Testing the athlete's shoulder in a supine position at 20° of forward flexion, 40° of abduction, and neutral rotation on the forearm with posterior pressure on the upper arm may cause a dimple in the front of the shoulder. A dimple indicates disruption of the superior suspensory mechanism, which was injured prior to the continued superior

Table 6.4 Conservative Rehabilitation Program for Acute Acromioclavicular Joint Sprain

Stage 1   Weeks 0-3
Immobilization in sling until A/C joint not tender

Approximately 1 week for grade 1 sprain.
Approximately 2 weeks for grade 2 sprain.
Approximately 3 weeks for grade 3 sprain.
(Grades 4 and above are operated on.)

Stage 2   Weeks 1-3   Mobilization

With joint tenderness gone, initial range of motion exercises: gravity-dependent pendulum exercises, advancing to wall climbing (Figs. 12.3 and 12.5).
Active, functional, non-weight-bearing range of motion.

Stage 3   Weeks 3-6   Flexibility and strengthening

After healing of tissue, horizontal flexion and hyperabduction stretching (Figs. 12.6 and 12.7).
Internal and external rotation strengthening with elbow at side.
Upper-range and cross-pattern strengthening of periscapular, neck, chest, and shoulder muscles; postural training and muscle balancing.

Stage 4   Weeks 4-8   Return to sport

No tenderness and full range of motion.
Normal flexion and strength.
Neuromuscular coordination.
Return to training.

motion of the humerus that caused the A/C joint sprain. The 2 weeks in the sling primarily to rest the A/C joint should be followed by internal rotation strengthening exercises to contain the humeral head in the socket. This will diminish residual subluxation, which can cause impingement and further trauma to the already damaged A/C joint.

After initial management of the A/C joint injury, when there is no injury to other joints, the athlete may proceed with internal and external rotation, functional abduction, and forward flexion

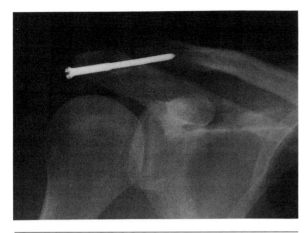

Figure 6.47 Reduction of A/C joint separation by a smooth-tipped, threaded-base pin-screw allows capsule and coracoclavicular ligaments to heal and reestablish normal rotation through this joint. This outpatient reduction was done percutaneously through a quarter-inch incision; the implant is removed at 6 to 8 weeks (Biomet, Warsaw, IN).

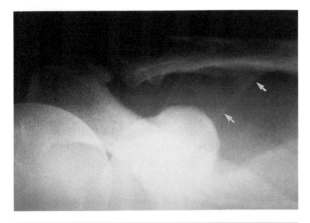

Figure 6.48 Superoanterior displacement of the humeral head can propagate force upward, leading to A/C capsular and coracoclavicular ligament injury. Note the avulsed inferior clavicular periosteum and slightly calcified coracoclavicular ligaments.

strengthening. When there is a full range of motion without pain and return of normal strength, the athlete can return to the coach for proper training in falling technique and to practice his or her sport activity. Returning to sport prematurely risks further injury or new injury to secondary structures that may be overused in compensation.

Complications

The main complications of nonoperative management of A/C joint injuries consist of stiffness due to wearing the sling, skin irritation due to the prominent distal clavicle or pressure of a sling, residual deformity, calcification of the coracoclavicular ligaments, pain with soft tissue interposition into the disrupted joint, and the fact that the athlete will throw more to the side if injury was to his or her dominant arm. Early muscle fatigue is seen in association with deltotrapezial disruption and step-off at the A/C joint.

Surgery is not without complication. There may be residual deformity, a scar instead of the bump, and a risk of hardware migration, as well as infection or osteomyelitis. Calcification of the coracoclavicular ligaments may follow surgical reduction of the joint. It usually takes much longer to rehabilitate and get back to sport activity following surgical repair.

Prognosis

In Types 1 through 3 injuries to the A/C joint it is not uncommon for the athlete to return to sport within 2 to 4 weeks following injury. Again, the athlete should have no tenderness, no pain with motion, a full range of motion, and full strength prior to returning to sport. If surgery is done on Types 3 through 7, a fixation pin may need to be removed at 8 weeks, and return to sport delayed from 3 to 6 months. If a plate or hardware is used for clavicular shaft fixation in Type 7 injury, the patient may be able to return to sport with the plate still in at about 8 weeks. In Type 7C injury, if glenohumeral stabilization is necessary, return to sport can be delayed by an additional 2 months when the A/C joint is involved.

The long-term problems associated with A/C joint injury consist of late arthritis, residual deformity, fatigue, and possible need for reconstructive surgery, which becomes more difficult when delayed. There may not be an effective means of cost containment other than early management of the injury so that repair rather than reconstruction can be done.

Patient Education

It is important for the physician to tell the patient that surgery may only trade a scar for a bump in Type 3 injury and that surgery is indicated in most Type 4 through 6 injuries. The athlete must know that if the injury is initially managed conservatively, there is still a chance of late arthritis development and the need for surgical reconstruction.

Prevention

There may be no effective way of preventing an A/C joint injury, which usually occurs when the athlete is caught off guard. Coordination drills and knowledge of the sport as well as practice in falling technique may perhaps limit occurrence of injury. It is important for the athlete not to return to sport activity until pain is gone, motion is full, and strength and agility have been recovered.

Sternoclavicular Sprain

The shoulder is attached to the body medially at the sternoclavicular joint. This joint is held together by a series of ligaments binding the clavicle to the sternum, a joint capsule, an intra-articular disk, supporting ligaments to the first rib, and a superior ligament over the top of the sternum to the opposite clavicle. Although the athlete rarely injures this joint, injury, when it does occur, is usually a sprain.

Epidemiology

Injury to the sternoclavicular complex is rare, and although motor vehicle accidents are the most common cause, sport activity ranks second. The athletes most prone to injury of this joint are those involved in auto racing, motorcycling, jogging or cycling (when hit by a motor vehicle), weight training, and football.

Pathogenesis

Disruption of the sternoclavicular joint can be caused by anterior and medial compression of the shoulder girdle complex pushing the proximal clavicle anteriorly or by posteromedial pressure on the shoulder girdle disrupting the clavicle at the sternoclavicular joint posteriorly. Direct pressure on the front of the clavicle, as in sustaining a kick in karate, also may cause posterior disruption of the clavicle at this joint.

The sternoclavicular joint is quite unstable. The majority of stability is provided by the intra-articular disk and extra-articular ligament structures. The epiphysis at the proximal clavicle is the last of the long bones to close, so many diagnosed fractures may in fact be injuries through the physeal plate. The proximal clavicle rests on top of the manubrium and first rib and is held in place by an intraclavicular ligament, an intervening soft-tissue disk, the sternoclavicular ligaments (anterior and posterior), and the costoclavicular rhomboid ligament. The pathologic entity in sternoclavicular sprain is injury to these ligaments or disk.

Natural History

If left untreated, a recurrent click may be felt due to a partially ruptured disk, and sternoclavicular arthritis may develop. Anterior or posterior subluxation has a higher incidence of arthritis than dislocation. An anterior dislocation can be left alone with little cause for concern. A posterior dislocation or clavicular separation through the physis may cause injury to the structures behind the sternum, including the common carotid artery, innominate artery, subclavian veins, subclavian artery, trachea, and esophagus.

Diagnosis

Because of the extent of motion that normally occurs at the sternoclavicular joint, any type of shoulder activity causes pain at this joint after injury. The patient frequently supports the affected arm across the front of the body with the opposite arm. The shoulder appears to be pushed forward, but this is actually an ipsilateral postural change. There will be swelling over the sternoclavicular joint with prominence of the end of the clavicle in an anterior subluxation, or depression with a posterior separation. A posterior subluxation is quite fixed, and an anterior injury may be fixed but most likely is quite mobile. Edema or skin mottling due to venous congestion may be prominent on the ipsilateral shoulder with posterior clavicular displacement. The patient with posterior subluxation may complain of an inability to swallow or may present with a pneumothorax. Because of swelling, however, it is often difficult to tell whether dislocation is anterior or posterior.

X-rays are generally not helpful. Routine X-rays are difficult to interpret. Because of overlapped tissue, lateral X-rays are also not useful. The best roentgenographic view is Rockwood's *serendipity view* (Figure 6.49), which was named for its chance discovery (Rockwood & Green, 1984). The patient is placed supine on the X-ray table with a film behind his or her back. The X-ray tube is angled down 40° cephalad, 45 in. from children and 60 in. from adult patients. The affected joint, when compared to the opposite joint, is found to be superiorly displaced with anterior dislocation and inferiorly displaced with posterior dislocation.

An *inspirational view* is also useful. Having the patient breathe while the X-ray is shot at a 45° angle in position will blur rib detail yet keep A/C joint detail. Tomograms are also useful for assessment of this joint, specifically if a fracture through the physis or near the proximal shaft must be differentiated. A late finding of arthritis at the

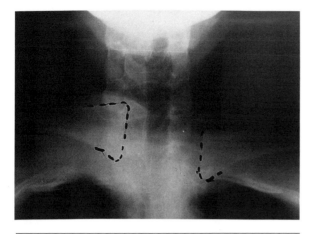

Figure 6.49 Serendipidity X-ray view is angled down 45° to show relative displacement of clavicle at the sternoclavicular joint.

sternoclavicular joint can also be defined by tomogram. A CT scan is the best method to assess the sternoclavicular joint. A bone scan is relatively useless in demonstrating acute inflammation or arthritis at this joint, because presentation is usually late; it is best to rely on a tomogram or MRI in clinical assessment, as will be discussed in chapter 11.

Injuries to the sternoclavicular joint are graded 1 through 4 (Figure 6.50). A Grade 1 injury is injury to the ligamentous, disk, or capsular structures without displacement. Grade 2 injury, either anterior or posterior, has displacement of less than 100%. Grade 3 injury is displacement of 100% or more at the joint, in either an anterior or posterior direction. Grade 4 sprain includes any type sprain plus a fracture at the S/C joint, which may be comminuted.

Differential Diagnosis

The most common entity to be confused with sternoclavicular sprain is posttraumatic hematoma; X-ray and CT scan are useful in differentiation. Spontaneous subluxation also occurs when anterior subluxation is noticed with overhead motion and weight training. It is frequently asymptomatic and reduces with lowering of the arm. Infection can cause swelling at the sternoclavicular joint, but is usually related to intravenous drug addiction. Other inflammatory conditions include osteoarthritis, which is usually unilateral and has a history of preceding trauma, and condensing osteitis, which is similar to osteitis pubis in that it occurs in women of about 40 years of age and bone scan may be positive. Rheumatoid arthritis or rheumatoid variants can cause swelling of the sternoclavicular joint, as can avascular necrosis, Tietze syndrome, and sternoclavicular hyperostosis. This latter condition occurs in women between 30 and 50 years of age, is usually bilateral,

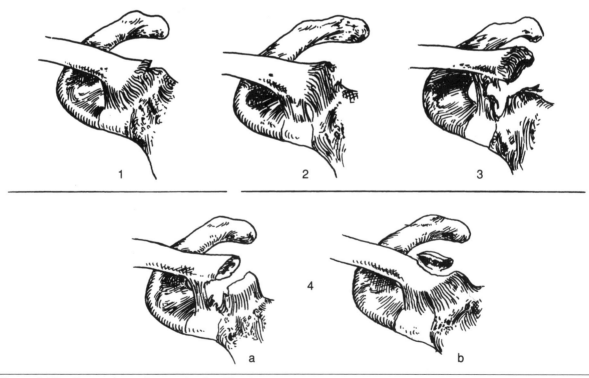

Figure 6.50 Sternoclavicular sprain classification system.

primarily involves the ligaments, and later involves the bones of the clavicle, sternum, and ribs (Sonozaki et al., 1979). Rickets, secondary hyperparathyroidism, syringomyelia, leprosy, gout, and metastatic disease can all rarely cause swelling in this area. Beware of concurrent voluntary glenohumeral subluxation and sternoclavicular subluxation. Some loose-jointed individuals, most frequently those involved in swimming, weight training, and basketball, are able to voluntarily subluxate both the sternoclavicular joint and the glenohumeral joint. This condition is usually painless—merely a parlor trick—and must be left alone.

Management

In Grade 1 injury, ice inside a plastic bag with water to avoid frostbite is applied for pain relief and to diminish swelling over the first 72 hr. Activity increases with more comfort over the next week. With Grade 2 subluxation, again, ice is useful. Keeping the shoulder back seems to provide the most comfort, and a clavicular strap is useful for this purpose. If pain in horizontal flexion persists past 4 weeks or if extension produces a pop or a grinding sensation, then joint exploration is warranted for the purpose of providing disk repair, partial disk or articular fragment removal, loose body excision, repairing ligaments that could provide stabilization, or identifying or repairing a bony fragment that may have been identified earlier on a CT scan. Joint exploration can be done as an open procedure or with an arthroscope smaller than 3 mm. If a dull, toothache-type pain with lifting develops later, it is most likely attributable to arthritis, and excision of the medial part of the clavicle, usually with a soft-tissue interpositional spacer, may be considered, as will be discussed in chapter 11.

One should attempt to reduce a Grade 3 sternoclavicular sprain or dislocation (Buckerfield & Castle, 1984). Anterior dislocation usually can be easily reduced, but the reduction is not maintained except for a Grade 4A injury—a fracture into the physis—which may snap back in place and stay there. An anterior dislocation that persists after an attempt at reduction can be left alone. There is usually no consequence other than a low incidence of secondary degenerative arthritis, which may respond to resection of the proximal clavicle (reverse Mumford procedure), anchoring of the residual clavicle to the first rib or sternum with ligament repair (anchovy procedure), and reconstruction by filling the defect with a coiled tendon, fascia lata, or umbilical tape ligament reconstruction.

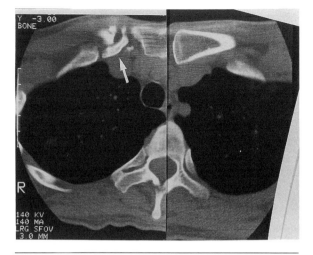

Figure 6.51 Proximal clavicular fracture associated with sprain injury, not appreciated on routine anterior X-ray, is easily identified on CT scan.

Grade 4B injury—fracture into the S/C joint—is more ominous. It is more highly associated with postinjury arthritis and pain (Figure 6.51). Conservative management with pain medication and activity as tolerated should nevertheless be attempted as healing progresses.

Painful arthritis may necessitate proximal clavicular resection; however, posterior bony fragments are often left behind, because there is a justifiable tendency by the surgeon to cautiously avoid important structures behind this joint. The fibrous tissue that forms within bone fragments or within the residual apophyseal plate will often give the surgeon the false impression that enough bone was resected. Fragments left behind may remain painful (Figure 6.52).

Complications

Because of poststernal anatomy, complications, which should be managed on an emergent basis, are more common with posterior dislocation (Buckerfield & Castle, 1984). If there is any question of vascular embarrassment, then aortography, contrast studies, and perhaps even MRI may be of some use to assess the poststernal structures. Open reduction is generally not necessary; stable reduction usually is accomplished by giving the patient mild sedation, placing a sandbag between the scapulae, and applying some traction in abduction of the arm. If this is not sufficient, fingertip pressure or a towel clip can be utilized to pull the medial clavicle back in place. Because sternoclavicular sprain is often a physeal injury, it reduces with a snap and is stable. When it is not stable a small

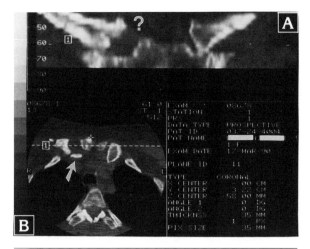

Figure 6.52 CT scan identifying a retained fragment following resection of the proximal clavicle for late arthritic pain associated with earlier fracture sprain injury. Retained fragment causing symptoms

[A] not seen on scout film but

[B] identified on sagittal film.

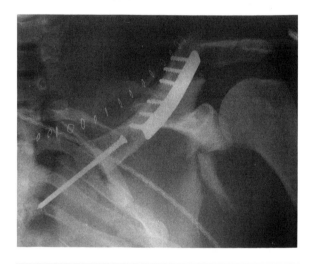

Figure 6.53 Repair of sternoclavicular capsular ligaments stabilized by smooth-tipped, threaded-base pin screw fixation. A jogger hit by a bus had the proximal clavicle resected to allow a vascular repair in a multitrauma situation, leading to a floating shoulder. The proximal clavicle was retrieved, sterilized, replaced, and attached with a plate distally. Capsular repair proximally was reinforced successfully with a temporary pin-screw device (no pain or arthritis at 12-year follow-up).

incision can be made, disk and ligamentous structures can be repaired, and internal fixation is usually not necessary.

Internal fixation is discouraged, primarily because motion at this joint risks hardware migration into the important structures behind the sternum. When forced to use internal fixation in an acute case with significant ligamentous disruption, the use of a smooth-tipped, threaded-base screw with a large head prevents migration. The pin screw is removed at 6 weeks. Internal fixation has been successful in one case in a 12-year follow-up (Figure 6.53).

The major complication of anterior displacement of the proximal clavicle is cosmesis. This is not life threatening, and even chronic dislocation does not lead to significant loss of motion. Late arthritis may be a problem. Posterior displacement of the proximal clavicle may be life threatening, however, particularly if postmediastinal structures are disrupted. The clavicle may enter the pulmonary artery, trachea, or esophagus or merely cause vascular venous compression. The use of a towel clip or surgical reduction may lead to infection or osteomyelitis, internal fixation or even the use of dacron tape may cause erosion through bone, and metal has a propensity to migrate. Fracture dislocation may lead to fibrous nonunion of the proximal clavicle; if bony resection is done, a fragment may be left behind inadvertently because exploration is hampered by the attempt not to injure postmediastinal soft tissue (see Figure 6.52). Many of these injuries are associated with the physis, and a significant incidence of remodelling occurs even in chronic unreduced dislocation. Even a posterior dislocation, if asymptomatic and not reducible by closed means, can be left alone. If difficulty breathing or claudicatory vascular changes are evident later, such dislocations can be reconstructed later. Other complications include reduction failure, infection, and late arthritis.

Prognosis

Prognosis of a displaced sternoclavicular sprain is generally good, because most are physeal injuries and will snap back into place; anterior displacement that does not easily reduce is not generally symptomatic. The athlete can return to activity when he or she is comfortable. Because the athlete is initially treated in a figure-8 splint for the first 4 to 6 weeks until soft tissue heals, mobility must be reestablished, and it may take 6 to 12 weeks postinjury to return to full activity. After surgical intervention, recovery time may be prolonged, from 3 to 6 months for the rehabilitation process.

The long-term problem is essentially cosmetic or the development of arthritis. Because these injuries are rare, there is no significant method of cost containment other than avoiding unnecessary X-rays.

If injury is suspected, a serendipity or inspirational view X-ray is justified, but one should proceed to a CT scan to better define the injury, that is, to differentiate a sprain versus a fracture dislocation.

Patient Education and Prevention

The physician should tell the patient that this is an unusual injury and that it will be mandatory to use a figure-8 splint for 6 to 8 weeks postinjury to allow soft tissue to heal. The patient should also be warned that arthritis is a late complication and that as this is a rare injury, there is perhaps no good way to prevent it.

Summary

Stability and guarded motion about the shoulder is provided by a series of capsular ligaments and their extensions. Sprain injury to these structures can jeopardize athletic performance. Early intervention is necessary to help prevent propagation of fiber damage, which leads to further instability, disuse, muscle weakness, and ultimately arthritis. Keeping the muscles strong as a second layer of defense will allow the muscles to work as shock absorbers, serving a protective function in rehabilitation and in prevention of future injury.

The separate capsular structures about the glenohumeral, acromioclavicular, and sternoclavicular joints help provide orientation so that the muscular sliding mechanism of the supraspinatus outlet and scapulothoracic mechanism can work effectively. Disruption of the capsular stabilizers seriously hampers the overall athletic performance of the shoulder.

There is a complex relationship between sprain injury and strain injury, because stability and strength must work in concert. This will be further explored in the next chapter.

7

Strains

Strain is the injury pattern involving tissue disruption of the muscles, tendons, and their bony insertions. In most areas of the body, muscle dysfunction would lead to imbalance, further tissue disruption of the injured area, or secondary concentric muscular overuse trauma. In the shoulder there are further considerations.

Lack of a deep bony socket and the amount of motion needed within the joint capsule itself to allow shoulder function means that the muscles are also forced into the role of stabilizing the joint. The muscles not only move the joint by contraction, but allow movement due to sliding mechanisms within the supraspinatus outlet and under the scapula.

In this chapter, injury to muscular tissue affecting shoulder performance will be explored. The most common injuries will be presented first, followed by less common but also important injuries that must be considered in analyzing the athlete's shoulder performance. The interrelationship of impingement and instability will be further explored. It will be seen that the complex role of the shoulder musculature in directly moving the joint, in allowing motion of the joint, and in assisting in the joint's stabilization must be taken into consideration by the treatment team. In no other joint of the body is the concept of triad degeneration more important.

Rotator Cuff Strain

The muscles that depress and contain the humeral head and that attach to the lesser and greater tuberosities are called the rotator cuff. Due to surrounding structures or imbalance of muscular strength, the supraspinatus tendon is the shoulder structure most commonly injured in athletic performance. In fact, the supraspinatus is the most commonly strained tendon overall in the human body. Tendinitis or inflammation of the rotator cuff and primarily of the supraspinatus has been labeled as bursitis, supraspinatus syndrome, baseballer's bursitis, swimmer's shoulder, bicipital tendinitis, calcific tendinitis, and rotator cuff disease. The newest buzz word is "impingement," which unfortunately is a wastebasket term like "internal derangement" of the shoulder or "chondromalacia" of the knee. There is considerable clinical overlap of structural problems about the shoulder, and there are many underlying causes of what clinically presents as rotator cuff tendinitis. Again, this is the most common shoulder problem seen in clinical orthopedic practice. However, many athletes choose to ignore early symptoms, and the opportunity of successful early management may be lost.

Epidemiology

The athletes most prone to acute supraspinatus tendinitis are swimmers, pitchers, weight lifters, and throwers. We have seen 8-year-old competitive swimmers with this condition, and at least 80% of swimmers have suffered from tendinitis of the supraspinatus at some time during their careers. With the advent of T-ball there has been a substantial decrease in clinical presentation of this condition in young pitchers.

Chronic rotator cuff problems are most prevalent in athletes over 40 years of age. It is not uncommon for individuals involved in manual labor to be avid recreational or weekend athletes. Injuries occurring at work may diminish recreational performance and vice versa. About half of the patients remember a specific episode that caused injury. The other half recall minor problems with the shoulder in the past such as bursitis, A/C joint arthritis, impingement, calcium deposits, and tendinitis treated successfully by steroid injections. If athletic trauma initiates acute change in a chronic situation, complaints could be either trivial, such as a dull pain in the side of the arm and night pain developing after a racquetball injury, or more significant, such as feeling something tear while sliding into second base. Presentation varies: The patient may complain of a dull ache in the shoulder, night pain, pain in reaching overhead, pain after activities such as tennis, weakness and early fatigue, or inability to raise the arm. These complaints mirror the spectrum of the disease.

Pathogenesis

There are many conditions that lead to supraspinatus tendinitis, all problems of use: misuse, disuse, abuse, and overuse. Injury to the supraspinatus can occur with contusion, as in tackling someone with the shoulder or falling on one's shoulder in rugby, football, or hockey. In young

athletes, overuse is the predominant cause, because there are commonly no bony changes associated in athletes under 16. Many young junior high school and high school swimmers rotate their arms through a million cycles per year. Incline bench pressing and wide-grip bench pressing in weight training place the shoulder in a critical position that leads to impingement against the acromion. Asking a young athlete to throw repetitively or to go through repetitive motions while preparing for such athletic activity will easily produce rotator cuff tendinitis due to fatigue and muscle imbalance.

If the humeral head is not well contained in the shoulder socket by the internal and external rotators, or if the humeral head is not pulled back properly during throwing activity, the supraspinatus and biceps must compensate, which leads to fraying or breakdown of the supraspinatus at the greater tuberosity insertion. This usually produces a partial-thickness internal rotator cuff tear (Figure 7.1). As the subluxation continues, that is, as the capsule gets looser over time, the humeral head tends to progressively migrate toward the acromion, leading to further erosion on the outside of the cuff (Figure 7.2). This will compress the bursa between acromion and cuff, leading to fibrosis initially and then breakdown ultimately.

Clinical complaints are due primarily to friction of the supraspinatus tendon against the overlying coracoacromial arch, which consists of the two projections of the scapula, the coracoid, and the acromion, as well as to the span of tissue in between,

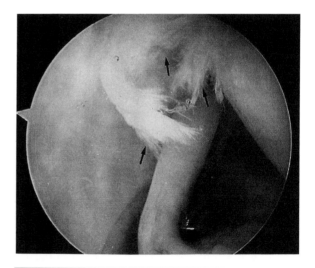

Figure 7.1 Toggle tear, a partial-thickness intra-articular tear due to disruption of normal force-couple and superior structural supporting mechanism, seen through arthroscope.

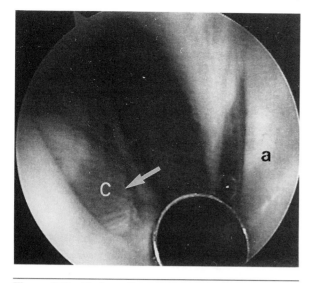

Figure 7.2 Early cuff wear through inferior bursal wall at greater tuberosity, seen through subacromial bursoscopy (a = acromion, c = cuff erosion).

the coracoacromial ligament. Overuse may cause wear or impingement against these structures. The thin lubricating serosal sac, which covers the acromion on one side and the supraspinatus on the other, may initially become edematous, may become fibrotic, may break down into thickened bands, or may invaginate into the acromion and thicken its undersurface (Figure 7.3, a-c), worsening impingement and leading to an "onion-skin" erosion of the supraspinatus near the greater tuberosity. Invagination of the serosal sac may also lead to calcific and ossific extension or thickening of the acromion and to spur formation (Figure 7.4, a and b).

Spurs and subacromial tissue thickening or remodeling into the Type III acromial form may develop to stop concurrent subluxation or to act as a tissue spacer to center the humeral head while the arm is down at the side. These compensation mechanisms nevertheless lead to progressive wear into the supraspinatus with overhead activity (Figure 7.5). Subluxation, increased wobble of the glenohumeral joint due to wearing and stretching of the superior capsule and superior suspension mechanism, stretching of the underlying capsule, fibrosis, or synovitis of the posterior capsule (which leads to central stiffness and peripheral overuse of the scapulothoracic joint) all lead to further impingement.

The actual pathology that occurs in the impingement area is a combination of inflammation, fibrosis, and erosion. The bursa may be primarily inflamed. More commonly the rotator cuff may be jammed up into the acromial surface, either due to a fall or due to subluxation of the glenohumeral joint. A bony spur may develop in these locations: under the acromion at the origin of the coracoacromial ligament, from the coracoid at the insertion of the coracoacromial ligament, as a traction phenomenon at the anterior acromial origin of the deltoid tendon, or on either side of an arthritic A/C joint, causing supraspinatus penetration. Spurs also develop at the rotator cuff insertion into the greater tuberosity due to microtrauma, partial-thickness rotator cuff tears, and subsequent calcific tendinitis or calcific necrosis.

The serosal walls of the bursa, which attach to the coracoacromial ligament, have fine cross-striations in youth, but these usually degenerate in the early teenage years. Serosal walls may get inflamed, showing mono- and polymorphonucleocyte invasion in early athletic overuse, and then thicken as cross-striations between the bursal walls, coalescence of the walls, or erosion occurs. With repetitive use, the central subacromial bursa tends to wear out with peripheral thickening of the wall and eventual separation of the subacromial space from the subdeltoid space. Coalescence of the wall may pull the rotator cuff up toward the acromion, increasing impingement (Figure 7.6, a and b).

Wear of the bursa on the side of the greater tuberosity may be associated with invagination of the opposite bursal wall into the acromion. The anterior rim hypertrophy and fibrous change that occur with erosion into the acromion may lead to a process similar to enchondral ossification (Figure 7.7, a-c), thickening the acromion and causing further wear into the rotator cuff. This may in fact be an adaptive process to contain the humeral head, but it is counterproductive when the arm is raised and there is further impingement near the greater tuberosity.

The opposite process also occurs when there is calcification near the greater tuberosity due to calcific tendinitis or calcific necrosis associated with partial-thickness cuff tears. Both the coracoacromial ligament and the rotator cuff can be found with focal areas of collagen necrosis as impingement proceeds (Figure 7.8). There is collagen breakdown early on, and calcium deposition in the reparative process. This may cause local inflammation leading to fibrotic replacement, or calcific degeneration may continue where the coracoacromial ligament ossifies (Ciullo & Guise, 1981a).

Encroachment of body spurs into the supraspinatus outlet wears into the rotator cuff, roughening its surface so that it no longer glides smoothly

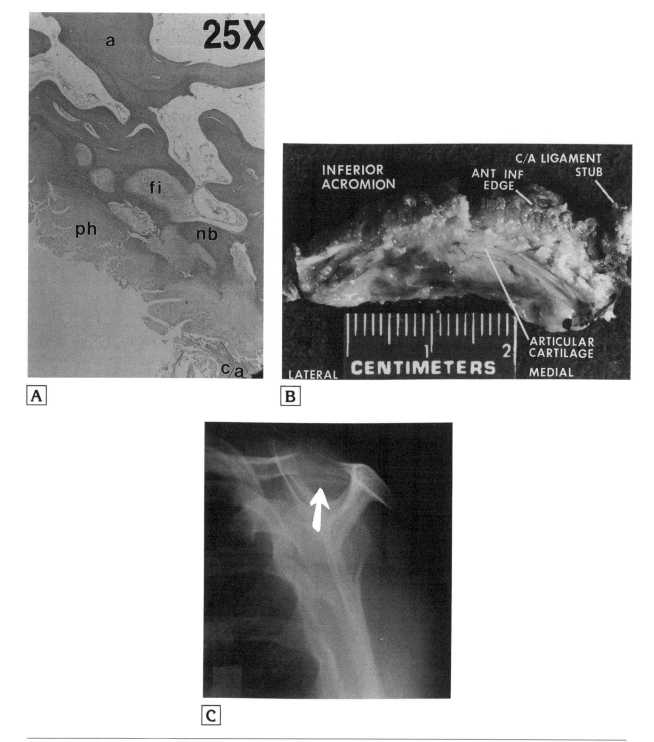

Figure 7.3 Infra-acromial thickening into supraspinatus outlet.

[A] Histology: Invagination and soft-tissue fibrotic build-up under acromion (a = acromion, fi = fibrous invasion, ph = periosteal hypertrophy, nb = new bone, c/a = coracoacromial ligament origin).

[B] Surgical specimen: Fibrous build-up under acromion gives appearance of a joint surface.

[C] X-ray: Fibrous subacromial build-up undergoes enchondral ossification leading to more rigid protrusion into the supraspinatus outlet.

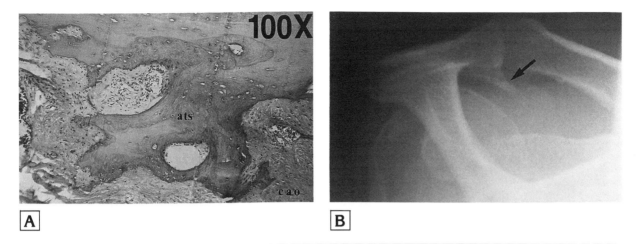

Figure 7.4 Coracoacromial ligament traction spur.

[A] Histologic early traction spur (ats = acromial traction spur, cao = coracoacromial ligament origin).

[B] X-ray demonstrating spur.

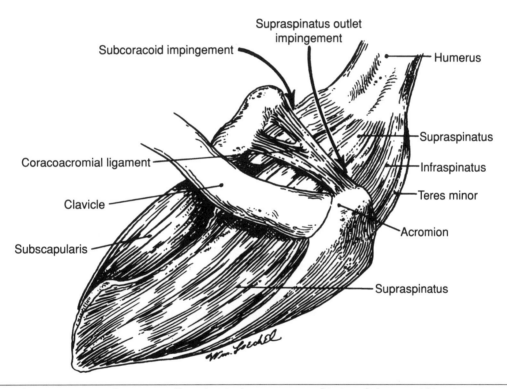

Figure 7.5 Impingement and rotator cuff tendinitis due to wear or friction. Subcoracoid impingement of subscapularis presents clinically much less often.

under the acromion. Such spurs commonly occur under the inferoanterior acromion, inferoposterior clavicle, or the A/C joint itself (Figure 7.9, a-c).

Histologic changes within the tendon itself mimic the changes that are found in the coracoacromial ligament. The bursal hypertrophy is a short-staged phenomenon. Erosion of the bursa may leave a few bands (Figure 7.10) until central cross-striations wear away and the bursal wall hypertrophies.

Continued impingement against the acromion, A/C joint, clavicle, and coracoacromial ligament leads to a hyperemic blush on the rotator cuff (Figure 7.11, a-c). The parallel, wavy, collagen-bundle structure is lost; there is an edematous change between these fibers, collagen necrosis, and even

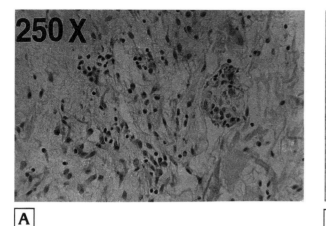
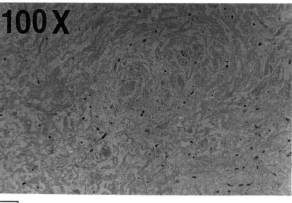

Figure 7.6 Bursal wall changes.

[A] Early bursal inflammation and hypertrophy.

[B] Later bursal fibrosis.

focal calcification. Cellularity is diminished, and there is very little evidence of repair. A/C arthritis or coracoacromial ligament bony traction spur formation intensifies impingement.

Superficial erosion may be partial thickness in a primary impingement problem with wear slightly more proximal than the greater tuberosity insertion. Laxity of the superior glenohumeral joint, with the biceps and the cuff pulling in a tandem arrangement, can lead to an internal partial-thickness tear through the tendon.

Muscles must be balanced to effectively contain the shoulder. If internal and external rotation strength is lost, the humeral head is not depressed properly, and this may propagate superior migration, allowing further wear of superior capsular structures. As the supraspinatus and biceps tendon wear, the humeral head rides higher. With the erosion progressing into the short depressors—the subscapularis, infraspinatus, and teres minor—they may lose their depressor function. In fact, because of angular change, they may start working as elevators, further accentuating the process and leading to *end-stage impingement*, wearing all the way through the supraspinatus, and allowing the humeral head to articulate with the acromion. This relationship will be explored in chapter 11. As the humeral head migrates superiorly it loses its instant center of rotation, the deltoid becomes a less effective elevator and more of a compressor, and wear continues. Friction of the humeral head against the acromion transmits further energy to the A/C joint and causes progressive breakdown and more inferior spurring, which leads to further erosion into the rotator cuff.

The cuff may finally wear through. Codman (1934) pointed out that rotator cuff tears can start from a *rim rent*. He pointed out that there can be partial-thickness tears of the rotator cuff on the inside of the tendon, partial-thickness tears on the outside of the tendon, intratendinous tears, and full-thickness tears (Figure 7.12).

An oblique hole pattern can account for night pain in that bursal fibrosis, along with superior compression afforded by hydrostatic pressure of the deltoid pumping during the day, is relaxed at night. This allows the hole to open somewhat and joint fluid to leak out, causing a chemical irritation inside the deltoid to its root, or insertion into the humerus (Figure 7.13).

Natural History

If rotator cuff strain is left untreated, a vicious cycle is set up: Either calcific changes occur at tendinous or ligamentous insertions, which are abrasive and allow rotator cuff wear, or muscle atrophy leads to stiffness, particularly in the back of the shoulder, which can progress to further weakness, further superior humeral head migration, and further subluxation and stretching of the joint capsule. Although impingement in athletes can occur on its own, more commonly it is a result of subluxation allowing the humeral head to slide forward and hit the acromion; weakness of surrounding muscles and progressive superior migration lead to additional stretching of the capsule, which in turn allows progressive impingement. Abnormal wear against the acromion transfers to the A/C joint and can cause breakdown there as well. Of course,

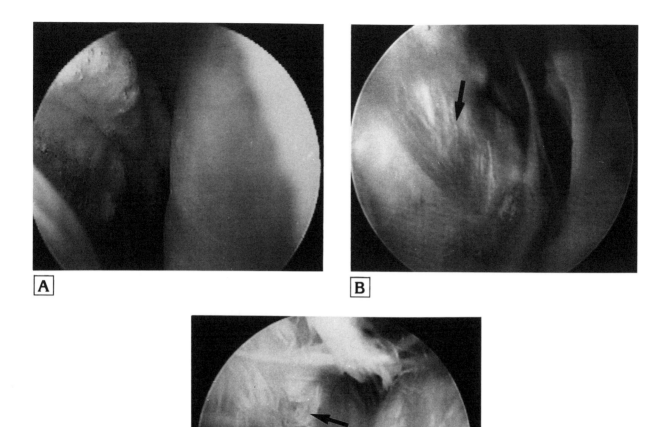

Figure 7.7 Acromial changes associated with impingement.

[A] Fibrous build-up acting as a "speed bump" may undergo enchondral ossification, leading to wear of the rotator cuff with overhead activity.

[B] Meniscoid wear at the anterior acromial edge. Extension of coracoacromial ligament may thicken and ossify as well.

[C] "Crabmeat" appearance of inferior acromion due to friction against bursa and cuff.

previous trauma to the A/C joint could lead to arthritis and cause wear into the rotator cuff, thus starting the cycle in reverse. Regardless, the end stage seems to be subluxation of the glenohumeral joint, erosion of the rotator cuff, and breakdown of the A/C joint. This triad degeneration can be initiated by repetitive overhead use, common in swimming and pitching, and commonly by improper body mechanics or by attempting activity that the shoulder is not prepared for.

Diagnosis

In early clinical presentation, the athlete complains of a vague pain deep within the shoulder after athletic activity, often described as a "toothache" type of pain. This pain is most pronounced in the overhead position, for example, at the point of releasing the baseball in throwing or when the hand touches the water in swimming. If the athlete attempts to bear the pain, it may eventually affect

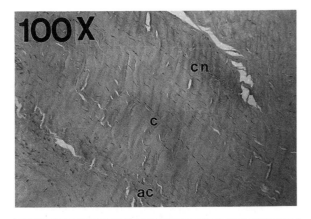

Figure 7.8 Histology of coracoacromial ligament in impingement shows mixoid degeneration and focal calcification, which may eventually contribute to spur formation or increased friction against the rotator cuff (cn = collagen necrosis, c = calcification, ac = attritional changes).

his or her ability to participate in the sport. Be careful when the athlete states that it feels as if the arm is "going dead" in addition to pain, weakness, snapping, or stiffness; this indicates subluxation.

History. In diagnosing chronic rotator cuff strain injury it is mandatory to listen to the patient's history. The spectrum of complaints corresponds fairly well to the amount of tissue damage. The condition may be annoying, that is, pain the day after sport activity with no loss of function; it may be aggravating in that there is progressive night pain that may have the edge taken off by aspirin; or it may have led to progressive inability to use the arm for functional activity. The patient may state that the pain had been annoying for some time, may have responded to cortisone injections or rest, yet continued to worsen over time. The patient may relate an episode when something subsequently "popped within the shoulder" while swinging a bat, sliding into base, or swinging a racquet. It is usually the change in symptoms that brings the athlete with chronic symptoms to the office. There may have been pain before, but he or she is no longer able to lift the arm. The dull pain after activity may have progressed to night pain or constant pain when attempting to lift the arm or with overhead activity, implicating propagation of the original tear. Not all full-thickness tears can be attributed to propagation of a smaller tear. Clinically acute trauma can cause tearing, popping, and immediate inability to lift the arm. Erosion into the long-head biceps tendon may lead to sudden rupture, which may be the athlete's presenting complaint.

Physical Examination. On physical examination there may be point tenderness in the interval between the acromion and coracoid process, or near the greater tuberosity, and the pain may worsen with forward flexion and internal rotation. In pure rotator cuff tendinitis, raising the arm in palm-down abduction may be painful between 80° and 120°, which allows the greater tuberosity to impinge against the acromion. Turning the hand over in palm-up abduction usually eliminates the pain. If palm-up abduction is more painful, subluxation of the glenohumeral joint is most likely the etiology of the impingement and should be treated primarily rather than the impingement.

Midrange abduction is the key to assessment. Pain in the 60° to 100° range palm-down that is relieved palm-up indicates primary rotator cuff tendinitis. Inability to abduct more than 40°, hiking the shoulder to produce this scapulothoracic abduction, implicates a full-thickness rotator cuff tear, subdeltoid fibrosis, or soft tissue catching within the glenohumeral joint. Capsulitis occurs in the healing process of even a partial-thickness tear. There is usually a loss of some motion in the termination of abduction, of forward flexion in the 30° to 40° range, or of 4 to 12 vertebrae of internal rotation. There may even be an inability to break the plane of the body when testing internal rotation behind the back.

Even though the supraspinatus is the most commonly strained muscle in the human body, it heals most of the time. Even an incomplete peripheral healing response may leave scar tissue and cause a blockage of some motion or contracture about the capsule, which most commonly leads to posterior shoulder pain. There may be tenderness over the A/C joint that is made worse with horizontal flexion, but hyperabduction is often difficult to assess with motion blocked in the upper range. Supraspinatus testing in functional abduction thumb-down against resistance demonstrates no weakness early on, but as pathology progresses resistance is easily overcome.

Fine crepitation may be felt when rotating the shoulder, which correlates with bursal sclerosis, inflammation, intra-articular labral interposition, or bands of adhesions within the subacromial bursa. Generalized grinding at 90° of abduction with internal rotation may be due to wear of the acromion against the roughened cuff and may occur in a pure impingement phenomenon. Testing in functional abduction in line with the scapula, thumb toward the floor, pushing up against resistance (Jobe's test, see Figure 3.11 in chapter 3), may cause pain to the root of the deltoid, the most common area of referred pain. In fact, the patient

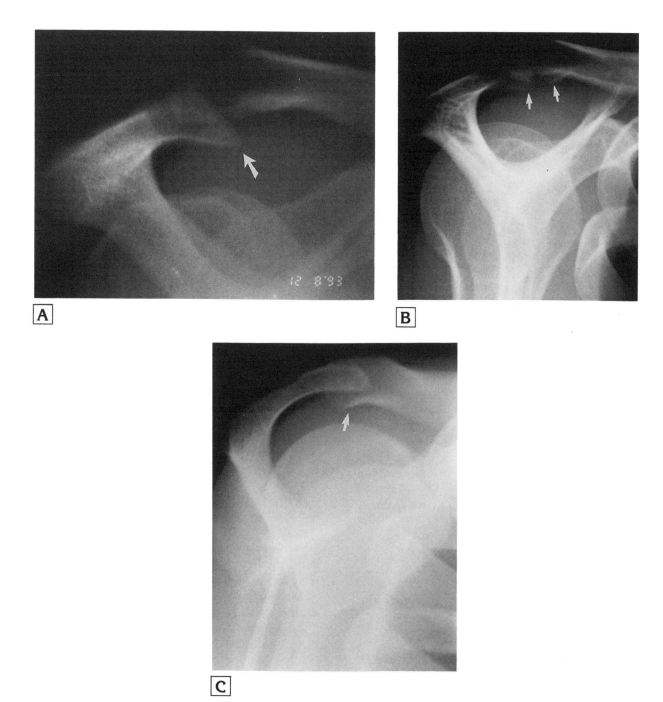

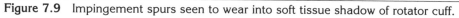

Figure 7.9 Impingement spurs seen to wear into soft tissue shadow of rotator cuff.

[A] Acromion.

[B] Both acromion and clavicle.

[C] Clavicle.

may complain of a toothache-like pain near the deltoid insertion as the presenting symptom.

The examiner must assess for instability, because there is a high correlation with rotator cuff disease. Instability may initially lead to secondary impingement. However, once there is progressive thinning of the rotator cuff or a full-thickness hole develops, the humeral head is no longer centered or may lose its negative pressure fit within the joint, leading to further instability. Instability therefore can be a cause of tendon disease or may result from or be worsened by tendon disease.

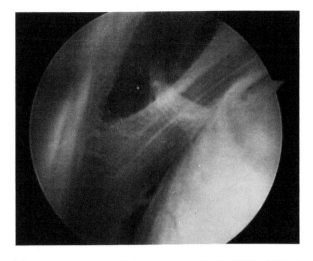

Figure 7.10 Subacromial bursoscopy of bursal bands that may be the result of trauma or the remnants of tissue under the acromion, which can cause snapping and are amenable to endoscopic resection.

Check for anterior-to-posterior subluxation with the arm at the side (Hawkins's test) as a sulcus sign (Warren's test), because glenohumeral subluxation is often the primary cause of secondary cuff impingement. Muscle imbalance also develops, increasing both instability and impingement. A containment maneuver may be useful (see page 93). Pain with resisted palm down 90° abduction indicates impingement. Pain with the palm up shows instability.

Radiographic Assessment in Early Tendinitis. A four-view X-ray study is useful to check for underlying A/C joint arthritis (which may cause or contribute to impingement or wear into the rotator cuff), to check for subluxation signs, and to look for inferior acromial architectural changes common with impingement. Mound atrophy and supraspinatus insertional sclerosis, originally described by Codman (1934), are signs of traction at the greater tuberosity and of inflammation leading to subacromial trabecular absorption of bone. Small spurs on the coracoid process or greater tuberosity, or calcification of the coracoacromial ligament may be seen in midsubstance or at the acromial insertion. Erosion into the acromion or small spur formation, particularly on the AP film angled down 15°, may indicate a deltoid traction spur or a density under the acromion associated with traction hypertrophy at the origin of the coracoacromial ligament. Calcific tendinitis in the supraspinatus is due to the impingement phenomenon and to localized necrosis that may further cuff degeneration (Figure 7.14, a and b).

Advanced disease may develop in which the humeral head is seated well in the socket on AP X-ray but may ride through a hole in the cuff in an attempt to push off from a chair, showing a loss in the humeral acromial distance and a break in Maloney's line. Narrowing or sclerosis at the A/C joint, spurring under either side of the A/C joint (particularly with impingement), and tension of the coracoacromial ligament causing significant traction spurring near the ligament's origin or insertion may result. Progressive pressure on the coracoacromial arch can lead to focal necrosis and tearing of the rotator cuff.

The arthrogram tells definitively whether there is partial-thickness intra-articular or full-thickness rotator cuff tear. Depending on the radiologist's skill, diagnosis of a large full-thickness tear is accurate 95% to 98% of the time. It is key to determine whether or not a full-thickness tear is distracted. Partial-thickness intra-articular tears, however, are less defined, and the superficial erosion is usually missed unless a bursogram is done. Changes within the biceps tendon and irregularities on the cuff can be seen on an arthrogram, giving evidence of chronicity.

A CT-arthrogram is very useful in early stages of the disease when internal partial-thickness tears and concurrent subluxation can be documented with increased joint volume and labral pathology. If there is a full-thickness tear in the cuff, the CT aspect of labral assessment is not good, because the dye leaks out of the joint. An arthrogram is effective in assessing the size of a rotator cuff tear and whether the tear is significantly displaced from the greater tuberosity. Adhesive capsulitis is not unusual in the healing of a cuff tear and may compromise arthrotomographic assessment.

A bone scan can help to document early inflammatory arthritis changes within the A/C joint or glenohumeral joint degeneration associated with cuff pathology. It can show synovitis or tendinitis but is not a very specific test. An MRI, on the other hand, if done on one of the newer generation machines, can help to identify edematous change within tendon, fibrotic replacement of tendon, subacromial spurs, arthritic changes that cause indentation of the rotator cuff, arthritic change within the A/C joint and glenohumeral joint, and even avascular necrosis of the humeral head. However, radiologists commonly overread MRIs.

Injury Classification. Classification of rotator cuff impingement has been best described by Neer (1983), who subdivided rotator cuff tendinitis or impingement into three stages. Stage 1 is reversible

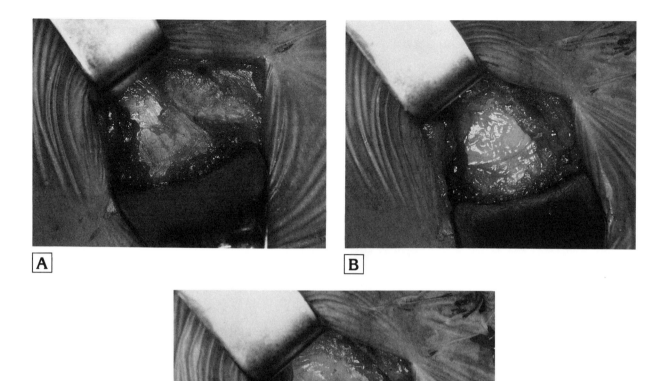

Figure 7.11 Gross findings of early impingement.

[A] Hypertrophy of coracoacromial ligament can be resected, demonstrating

[B] fibrotic bursa, which when resected shows

[C] hyperemic blush of rotator cuff in early impingement.

edema and hemorrhage of the rotator cuff but should also include inflammation of the serosal and peripheral bursa that commonly occurs in patients under 25 years of age. This can be considered a subacute stage, because many athletes will ignore it. Stage 2, fibrosis and tendinitis occurring in patients from 25 to 40 years of age, is the usual status at initial clinical presentation. The bursa is no longer inflamed, and fibrotic changes may have already occurred within the bursa and the rotator cuff near the greater tuberosity. Stage 3 tendinitis commonly occurs after age 40 and implies structural change, including bony changes and tendon ruptures, chronicity, and increased need for surgical intervention.

There is a great deal of overlap in this classification scheme, and damage is most highly correlated with the amount of overuse occurring at any age. The fact that the athlete may initially try to work it off may mean that he or she may not present until a later stage.

Further subdivision is necessary, however, because structural cause must be identified in order to suggest the proper conservative or surgical method of treatment. Stage 3, or chronic tendinitis of the rotator cuff, is a progressive phenomenon. At this stage the factors that lead to progressive rotator cuff trauma may be clumped into three groups: group A—factors above the cuff, group

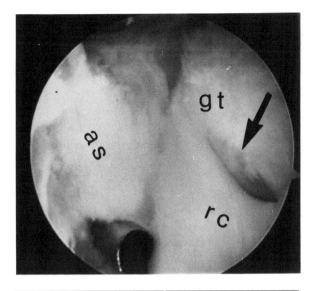

Figure 7.12 Subacromial bursoscopy of a rim rent. A small, full-thickness tear may allow joint fluid extravasation, causing night pain but no decrease in strength because the supraspinatus is still relatively attached on both sides of the tear (rc = rotator cuff, gt = greater tuberosity, as = acromial spur).

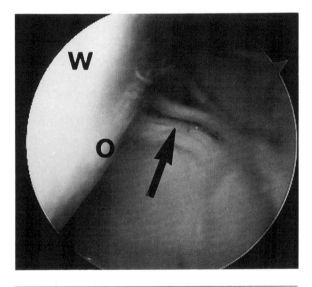

Figure 7.13 Oblique full-thickness tear, seen by glenohumeral arthroscopy, may work as a trapdoor, allowing joint fluid to leak out at night when the deltoid is relaxed (arrow = oblique multilayer rotator cuff insertional tear seen inside joint, w = superior humeral articular cartilage wear, o = early osteophyte formation).

B—factors below the cuff, and group C—factors central to the cuff (Table 7.1). In actuality, these groups are interrelated, and it is often difficult to separate cause or effect within these groups because they overlap.

Above the Cuff. In group A, factors above the cuff, the coracoacromial arch and subacromial bursa are affected. The acromion may protrude on the cuff and bursa, causing erosion from development of traction spurs (within the anterior deltoid, within the lateral deltoid, or at the origin at the coracoacromial ligament) or central erosion caused by shape change due to superior migration of the humeral head combined with hypertrophy of anterior acromial bone. This hypertrophy may in fact be a braking mechanism that develops in an attempt to minimize anterior subluxation at the glenohumeral joint. The acromion helps to contain the humeral head in its socket, although this function may be lost from the effects of a nonfused apophysis, an apophyseal line loosened posttrauma, or continued superior pressure from a loose glenohumeral joint. A ridge forms at the posterior aspect of the nonfused apophysis, which can also cause impingement. Fractures of the acromion or coracoid as well as degenerative arthritis and inferior spurring at the A/C joint can cause encroachment into the supraspinatus outlet. With continuous inferior pressure due to loss of humeral head depression the acromion may thin and lose its containment ability, thus allowing further superior migration of the head and erosion of the cuff.

The serosal walls of the bursa may invaginate the acromion, grow into trabecular interstices, develop a fibrocartilage layer that thickens the acromion, and allow further erosion into the cuff, as discussed on page 129. The bursa may wear away except for a few fibrous bands that snap as the athlete elevates his or her arm. In response, the athlete may subconsciously throw more to the side and change normal shoulder mechanics. This in itself can lead to further impingement by rotation of the scapula, further wear at the A/C joint, and so on. Although the bursa initially hypertrophies, at a chronic stage it becomes more fibrotic, especially peripherally, which significantly interferes with its sliding function. Again, normal biomechanical shoulder motion is disrupted. Thickening or fibrosis of the bursa and edema of the injured rotator cuff put pressure on the coracoacromial ligament, which may initiate traction spur formation under the acromion and at the coracoid. These bony changes are even more traumatic to the cuff and further accelerate disease. Fibrosis of the bursa is common in diabetics even if they are athletic.

If the athlete begins activities such as pitching or swimming at a young age, the coracoid may be pulled on and actually curve, leading to impingement against the cuff (Figure 7.15). If there is weakness or damage to the humeral head depressors,

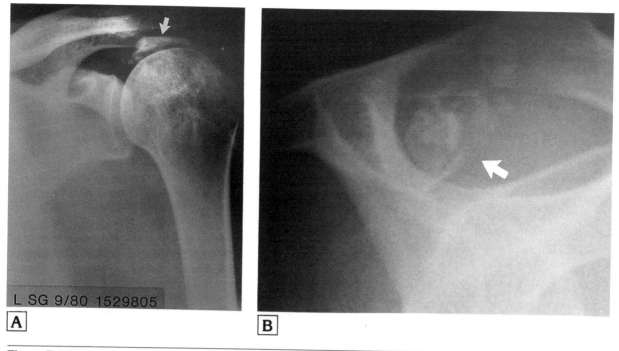

Figure 7.14

[A] Calcific tendinitis within supraspinatus tendon due to progressive focal necrosis.

[B] Here radiographic changes assumed to be due to calcific tendinitis are found associated with an acromial osteochondroma. Not all calcification about the shoulder is calcific tendinitis.

especially with a hooked coracoid, subcoracoid impingement is not uncommon.

Subcoracoid impingement occurs when the subscapularis is injured or partially thinned, specifically when there is synovitis or contracture at the posterior capsule, which pulls the glenohumeral joint posterosuperiorly. With a lax superoglenohumeral ligament or an anterior joint capsule with an enlarged interval defect (common in glenohumeral subluxation), this allows preferential superoanterior shifting of the humeral head, jamming it into the coracoid (Figure 7.16). Pain radiating down the medial aspect of the upper arm is characteristic of impingement against the coracoid and conjoined tendon. The cycle continues as impingement causes further erosion of the superior subscapularis fibers.

Below the Cuff. In group B, factors below the cuff, either damage to the superior suspension mechanism (associated with pitching or athletic trauma enlarging the rotator interval), stretching the coracohumeral ligament and damaging the biceps stabilizing mechanism, or glenohumeral laxity (which can eventually stretch out the superior capsule) leads to wear of the rotator cuff. Here, the initial partial tears are internal or are the rim rents that Codman first described (1934). The biceps and

associated coracohumeral stabilizing ligaments are unable to stabilize the top of the joint when there is either posterior contracture of the capsule, anterior laxity of the superoglenohumeral mechanism, or failure of the supraspinatus or infraspinatus to depress the humeral head.

This increased motion at the top of the joint leads to microinstability, superior wobble, and supraspinatus insertional attrition near the greater tuberosity that tends to propagate with time. Breakdown in this area is also accelerated by glenohumeral arthritis in two ways. First, thinning of the glenohumeral articular surface, which can occur with loaded activity such as weight training, gymnastics, and handball, can change the instant center of the humeral head so that additional pull is necessary by the supraspinatus, leading to wear. Second, bony hypertrophy along the articular edge, which increases surface contact, can wear the rotator cuff from the inside as the cuff is sandwiched between the spur and the acromion.

Objects within the joint, such as a stub of a biceps tendon, a loose body, or a fragment of a torn labrum, can shift the humeral head out of the socket just slightly, causing functional subluxation and an abnormal pull at the supraspinatus insertion, which shifts the humeral head toward the

Table 7.1 Factors Related to Rotator Cuff Disease

Group A (above cuff) Coracoacromial arch and subacromial bursal factors

Acromial encroachment
  Deltoid traction spurs
  Coracoacromial ligament origin spurs
  Apophyseal stress fractures
Coracoid fractures or curve
A/C arthritis
Acromial thinning and decreased containment
Subacromial bursal thickening
Scapular rotation
Posterior glenohumeral capsular fibrosis
Loose coracohumeral ligament

Group B (below cuff) Intra-articular glenohumeral factors

Superior mechanism sprain
  Superior glenohumeral ligament
  Superior capsular
Enlargement of rotator interval
Glenohumeral laxity
Cuff thinning, rim rents, partial thickness tears
Functional subluxation
  Loose bodies
  Torn labrum
  Cuff partial tears
  Biceps stub
Glenohumeral degenerative joint disorder (DJD) with change of instant center

Group C (central cuff) Intrinsic cuff lesions

Supraspinatus static thickness
  Thickening (edema)
  Thinning (erosion)
Supraspinatus plasticity decrease
  Scar
  Calcium deposits
Supraspinatus disability
  Suprascapular nerve dysfunction
Loss of biceps humeral head depression
Coracohumeral sprain and loss of superior mechanism

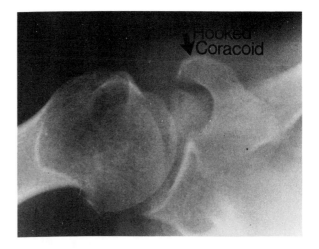

Figure 7.15 Hooked coracoid or remodeling of bone due to impingement forces in 12-year-old swimmer may lead to subcoracoid symptoms later in life.

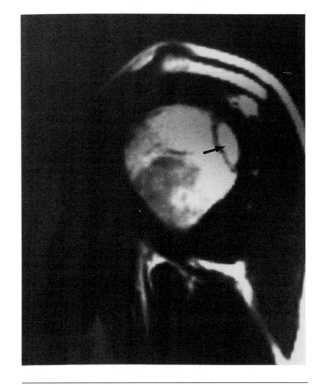

Figure 7.16 Subcoracoid impingement. Wobble at the top of the joint leads to erosion into superior subscapularis fibers and impaction against the coracoid and to associated vascular changes of the humeral head, noted here on MRI.

coracoacromial arch and leads to erosive wear. With joint laxity the acromion may change shape, increasing slope in order to stabilize the humeral head. Unfortunately the change in slope of the acromion with the arm at the side may not be the best functional adaption for activities in forward flexion, in which the cuff will be brought into contact with this adapted acromial shape (Ciullo, 1989a).

Central Cuff Disease. Group C includes changes of the rotator cuff itself. Early edema within the cuff will increase friction between the acromion and humeral head. Partial tearing, either superficial or deep, may cause a catching sensation that will change the normal smooth mechanics in activities such as throwing or lifting, and altered mechanics may perpetuate the impingement process. Ingrowth of scar in the healing process may inhibit motion, which leads to selective atrophy of the muscle fibers that are no longer exercised through their full range, thus further altering mechanics and leading to further impingement. Interstitial tearing within the cuff, even without external or internal partial erosion, can lead to fusiform dilation that interferes with smooth motion. When the sliding motion of the supraspinatus under the acromion is lost, secondary muscles may be overused, leading to breakdown of other structures, the best example being periscapular muscle spasm. Calcific changes due to necrosis of the cuff near the greater tuberosity, traction spurring of the greater tuberosity, and avulsion fractures near the greater tuberosity insertion all interfere with normal mechanics and lead to impingement and subsequent wear of the cuff. A tear may heal with a fibrotic component that may be thickened and prone to further erosion. The long biceps tendon can be considered part of the rotator cuff. Its rupture can lead to loss of humeral head depression, allowing further superior migration of the humeral head and further wear of the remainder of the cuff.

Differential Diagnosis

Stiffness, arthritis, and referred pain, primarily of neurologic origin, can lead to similar symptoms and confuse diagnosis. Because effective treatment is founded on accurate diagnosis, it is important to differentiate wear of the rotator cuff from other causes of symptoms in order to suggest effective management.

Neurologic Problems. Because any nerve that passes a joint branches off to that joint, it is not uncommon to have pain referred to the shoulder from other sources. It is important to rule out a cervical radiculopathy, cubital tunnel syndrome at the elbow, or carpal tunnel syndrome at the wrist. Irritation at one of the other sources can amplify symptoms at the shoulder, a condition called *shoulder/hand syndrome*, or *double crush phenomenon*

(Osterman, 1988), which is considered to be impedance of axonal flow from two separate compression areas of the same nerve. Irritation of a nerve in two areas amplifies symptoms considerably; treatment of one area may radically diminish pain in the other area, and subsequent treatment in the second area may not be necessary.

MRI, lateral X-rays of the neck, and especially EMG may be useful in defining a C5-6 radiculopathy; the EMG can assess other nerve compression syndromes in the extremity as well. The muscles innervated by the C5-6 nerves may become unbalanced and lose their depressor function if denervated, and impingement may be the result. The age group susceptible to such radiculopathy, especially with athletic trauma, is also susceptible to rotator cuff disease, and these conditions can coexist. An EMG, myelogram, or MRI can help identify radiculopathy originating in the neck. Nevertheless, if there is also a positive arthrogram, both conditions should be worked up concurrently. There is no reason to hold up a shoulder arthroscopy or shoulder surgery to await complete resolution of neck symptoms.

Inability to lift the arm may be due to a "frozen shoulder," disruption of normal muscle force couples, a SLAP lesion, or rotator cuff pathology. Suprascapular nerve entrapment as a component of brachial neuritis or secondary to rotator cuff tear, retraction of cuff material, and fibrosis in an aborted healing process can lead to pain in themselves or to weakness of the humeral head depressors; EMG can help define the situation.

A/C Joint Arthritis. A/C joint arthritis may cause pain in the shoulder as either an isolated phenomenon or from erosion into the cuff; a 15°-angled-up AP film can help define involvement. History of previous trauma to the A/C joint is important.

Bone scan can be, but is not often, helpful in differential diagnosis. Arthrography can be helpful, however. Selective injection to the A/C joint of Marcaine or Xylocaine can help define whether symptoms arise primarily from A/C joint pathology. The problem here is that the disk is worn out with arthritis, and injection into the joint may flow freely into the subacromial space; pain from a cuff tear may be masked. Primary A/C joint arthritis can respond to a conservative program of horizontal flexion and hyperabduction stretching, strengthening, and anti-inflammatory medication. If it does not, and the patient comes to surgery, it is mandatory to explore the cuff concurrently and repair a hole if found. There may be a role for arthroscopic dome decompression of the arthritic change under the A/C joint to minimize A/C joint symptoms and decelerate cuff changes.

Calcific Tendinitis. Calcific tendinitis, although within the spectrum of rotator cuff disease, can be evident on X-ray. With limited motion, when pain is more clinically evident than expected with a cuff tear, further work-up of the cuff tear, such as arthrography, is not necessary and should be held off. Anti-inflammatories such as sustained-release Indomethacin, local modalities, mobility and strengthening exercises, and even needling or arthroscopic debridement of the calcific deposit may be considered first prior to further diagnostic work-up of cuff disease.

Instability. The most important factor to assess in differential diagnosis is the stability of the glenohumeral joint. The patient with a positive impingement test as well as a positive apprehension sign that is minimized by anterior pressure on the shoulder (the containment maneuver; Ciullo, 1989a) has subluxation as the etiology of impingement, and treatment should be geared toward subluxation rather than impingement (Ciullo, 1989b). Arthroscopy is important here to assess the progression of degeneration in the subacromial space; when conservative treatment fails, concurrent subacromial decompression and glenohumeral stabilization may be necessary.

Triad Degeneration. Injury leads to disuse and associated decrease in strength. With weaknesses comes muscle imbalance and progressive wear of the rotator cuff so that it does not slide as well under the acromion.

When A/C joint breakdown has also occurred it must also be addressed. Loss of motion, particularly reverse extension or horizontal extension to the 90° abduction point, seriously compromises the ability of the muscles about the shoulder to depress the humeral head, due to loss of muscular integration or balance. Motion and strengthening must be sought first, prior to consideration of surgical intervention; retraining muscles to work efficiently may avoid the need for surgery. Until motion is full the patient is a less ideal surgical candidate, because the muscles cannot be maximally strengthened without a full range of motion; superimposed postoperative adhesions may complicate the picture even more.

Arthritis in either the glenohumeral or the A/C joint can minimize motion and produce findings similar to impingement, such as grinding throughout the range of motion in horizontal flexion. Apprehension and hyperabduction testing for the glenohumeral and A/C joints, respectively, should be done.

Advanced Cuff Disease. Although a full-thickness rotator cuff tear is part of the spectrum of injury, it is treated much differently than early inflammatory tendinitis. Surgical intervention is more likely to be considered for the full-thickness tear. Ultrasound, arthrography, or arthroscopy can help in differential diagnosis. Isolated biceps tendinitis is extremely rare but can have similar symptoms, and testing palm-up forward flexion against resistance may help define this entity when found painful.

Reflex Sympathetic Dystrophy. It is important to rule out reflex sympathetic dystrophy syndrome (RSDS). Diminishing use of the arm can minimize muscular pumping action to return blood to the heart. Pooling of blood in the extremity can lead to mottling of the skin and edema in the digits, as well as temperature change and sensitivity to weather, which are the hallmarks of reflex sympathetic dystrophy syndrome. If diagnosis of RSDS is suspected, a triphase bone scan that finds a defined blush on the early phase is 98% effective for confirmation. RSDS is treated by vasodilatory drugs in a pain clinic or with the help of experts and by antianxiety medication in conjunction with psychiatric service.

Management

In managing impingement it is important to first rule out subluxation. Ideally, subluxation is treated first, and the secondary impingement should diminish as the shoulder becomes more stable. If there is significant wearing into the cuff or concurrent A/C joint arthritis, such factors may need to be dealt with as well if surgery is indicated. Horizontal flexion, hyperabduction, and reverse extension stretching for the A/C joint can help regain the motion necessary to strengthen the internal and external rotators that depress the humeral head and minimize impingement. Posterior bursal and subscapular adhesions that pull the humeral head up and back, causing subacromial compression, must be eliminated (Table 7.2).

Early Cuff Disease. Most often the athlete will present with early impingement symptoms. In these cases conservative management is most appropriate and usually effective. As disease progresses, however, arthroscopic intervention may be considered.

Conservative Management. In primary impingement, which is markedly more uncommon than

Table 7.2 Conservative Rehabilitation Program for Acute Rotator Cuff Strain or Impingement

---

Stage 1   Weeks 0-2   Immobilization

Anti-inflammatory medication and icing.

Sling until deep pain gone.

Start dependent pendulum exercises to prevent stiffness.

Stage 2   Weeks 2-4   Mobilization

Remove sling and advance to wall climbing.

Passive supine stretching with forward elevation and external rotation.

Cane exercises in front of body or towel exercises behind body to maintain motion. (Use of myostimulation on deltoid may be initiated to prepare for upper range activity.)

Stage 3   Weeks 3-9   Strengthening

Emphasize posture and start isometric training.

Internal and external rotation strengthening to depress humeral head. Start at 0° abduction; advance to 90°.

Stage 4   Weeks 4-12   Return to activity

Full painless motion.

At least 90% of external rotation strength and 100% of internal rotation strength.

Emphasize maintenance program of flexibility and strengthening to promote endurance and help prevent reinjury.

Return to training or recreational sports.

---

impingement related to instability, it is important to mobilize the shoulder and strengthen the rotator cuff muscles, particularly the supraspinatus, throughout the full range. The deltoid must also be strengthened, the anterior and posterior slips to help balance the shoulder and the medial slip to help lift. Mobilization of the A/C joint, particularly with horizontal flexion to help stretch out the posterior capsular structures, may help balance the shoulder and prevent impingement. Anti-inflammatory medication, mainly aspirin or nonsteroidal anti-inflammatory drugs, is useful. In a sports clinic setting, certain medications have been found effective for specific conditions. These include Naprosyn for capsulitis and tendinitis symptoms, Indomethacin if A/C joint arthritis or calcific tendinitis is a concurrent entity, or a general anti-inflammatory drug, such as Diclofenal Sodium or Ketoprogen, if arthritis coexists in both the A/C and glenohumeral joints.

Swimmers and throwers, if they are diagnosed early in the course of disease, respond well to rest, nonsteroidal anti-inflammatory medication, and therapeutic strengthening. Modalities such as ice before and after activity, decreasing activity to about half the practice level at which symptoms occurred, and stretching and then strengthening while progressively increasing activity as symptoms diminish are usually effective. Eccentric muscle strengthening is often best tolerated in early impingement rehabilitation.

If physical therapy in the first 8 weeks helps to regain motion and strength, proceed with further therapy for an additional 8 weeks: Progress toward a home program with a return to full activity when the strength deficit is less than 20% of the opposite shoulder or less than 20% of what is normal for the patient's height and weight. If there is no initial response to physical therapy at 6 weeks or if the patient is too uncomfortable, proceed with a CT-arthrogram alone for the younger athlete, and include a bone scan for the older athlete because A/C joint arthritis may be of some concern. CT-arthrography helps define a full-thickness tear of the rotator cuff or signs of labral damage that indicate subluxation. Capsular redundancy in subluxation or decreased joint space in adhesive capsulitis can be defined.

Injection. It is important to avoid steroid injections in treatment of bursitis or cuff disease. By decreasing inflammation, injection may minimize not only pain, but also the healing response. Steroids abort the healing process, unravel collagen, and may contribute in effect to subsequent propagation of the tear in areas of fiber fatigue. Pain is a protective mechanism and if taken away may not protect the athlete against the offending activity that can make the impingement worse. Kennedy and Willis (1976) injected steroid into healthy tendon and noticed that it unraveled collagen and made the tissue more edematous; reorganization of the collagen took 6 or more weeks. If the pain response is diminished, the athlete has a tendency to return to activity prematurely and perhaps cause more damage. If a decision is made to use cortisone injection, it is important that the athlete understands that it leaves the muscle fibers at risk. Steroid injections should be used judiciously.

The physician returns the athlete to practice. The athlete's coach or club pro allows the athlete to return to competition when appropriate. Shoulder biomechanics and proper technique of the sport must be assessed to help avoid future irritation of the rotator cuff. An exercise program recommended by the physician and therapist must be maintained.

Surgical Intervention. When there is no response to conservative management—that is, continued pain in spite of increased motion and strength in therapy—then surgery may be an option. Try to avoid surgery unless preceded by mobilization; operating on a stiff joint may lead to an even stiffer joint. Surgery consists of evaluation under anesthesia, manipulation to regain remaining lost motion, arthroscopic assessment, and perhaps either inferior arthroscopic acromioplasty or endoscopic debridement of arthritis or spurs at the A/C joint. Judgment should be made about what part of the acromion is offending the cuff and whether the coracoacromial ligament is involved.

Removing the weight and placing the arm through a range of motion at the time of arthroscopic analysis to check where impingement occurs can aid in assessment by defining corresponding worn areas of the acromion and cuff. The weight is returned to give clearance for surgery, and the affected area of bone or soft tissue (bursal adherence to the undersurface of acromion or thickened bursa) is debrided. The weight is again removed, and if there is further impingement, then bone in the area of irritation is also debrided. This usually includes just the anterior rim of the acromion; however, if there is A/C joint arthritis, a dome decompression at the undersurface of the joint or joint resection can be useful to remove impinging osteophytes and regain A/C joint motion. When the coracoacromial ligament is involved, cauterization is generally necessary to diminish bleeding, unless one of the newer fluid management systems is utilized.

Partial-thickness tears of the rotator cuff can be dealt with arthroscopically. The internal articular side tears are debrided to prevent irritation of the biceps tendon and catching within the joint. Loose, frayed material is not debrided to stimulate healing but to better assess whether there is a full-thickness tear. Debridement of intra-articular amplifying factors, such as labral tearing, frayed superior gleno-humeral ligament tissue, and so on, can help minimize symptoms in rehabilitation.

If there is any question of whether a full-thickness tear exists in the supraspinatus due to obliquity of fiber failure, an injection of weak (10%) methylene blue dilution into the glenohumeral joint during endoscopic assessment of the subacromial space can show thinness of the remaining cuff or a complete cuff tear. A needle through the A/C joint into the intra-articular component of the tear can help identify the extra-articular component during subacromial bursoscopy. A very small full-thickness rotator cuff tear or partial erosion on the bursal side may respond dramatically to a subacromial decompression.

The actual areas of impingement can be defined by removing the weight at time of arthroscopy. The undersurface of the acromion that directly contacts the edematous or worn part of the rotator cuff usually has a "crabmeat" appearance. Debriding this acromial segment alone is all that is necessary to minimize symptoms. This is safely accomplished by keeping the arthroscopic debrider flat on the scapular spine posteriorly and working from the back of the A/C joint forward toward the front (Figure 7.17, a-c).

Subacromial bursal bands and thickening or fibrosis of the bursa that minimizes the smooth lubricated motion of the cuff, if found, should be debrided. Primary bursal fibrosis is not uncommon in conditions such as diabetes. Smoothing of a flap near the eroded area of the cuff, debridement of acromial and clavicular spurs, and debridement of irregular bursal tissue can give smoother motion, which minimizes wear-related pain in athletic activity, particularly in the recreational athlete. When discomfort is minimized, stretching, strengthening, and rehabilitation are more likely to be successful (Table 7.3).

The majority of patients will have partial-thickness intra-articular or occasional extra-articular tear of the rotator cuff under previous impinging acromial or clavicular spurs. Even with a very small hole, most patients respond to endoscopic debridement as previously outlined. They require therapy, stretching, and strengthening, but usually no additional surgical intervention. If additional surgery is required, after passive (and, with luck, active) motion is regained in therapy, then open repair, decompression with or without a Mumford procedure, or concurrent stabilization of the glenohumeral joint may be indicated as a second surgical stage. The mobilized tissue is easier to repair. Elimination of stiffness ensures a better postsurgical result.

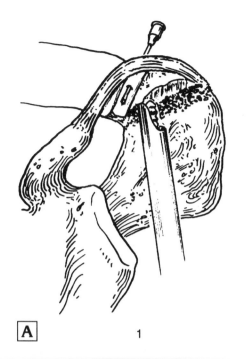
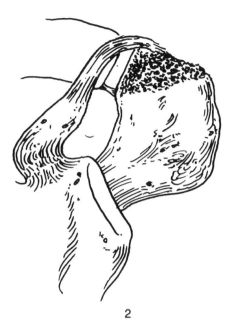

[A]   1   2

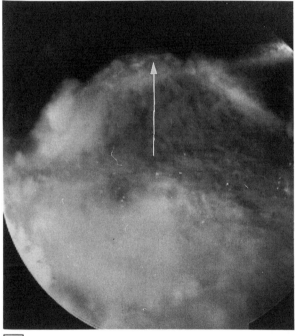

[B]

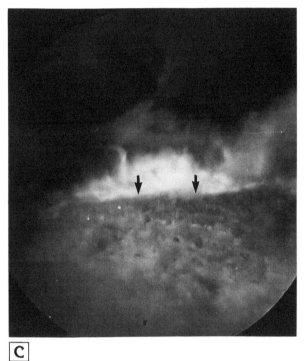

[C]

Figure 7.17 Endoscopic acromioplasty.

[A] Technique. Note needle through A/C joint for orientation.

[B] Size of spur being resected.

[C] Completed acromioplasty.

If surgery is done, rehabilitation is mandatory, first to regain motion and then strength. Mobilization is important to help prevent recurrence of adhesions and fibrosis; work toward internal and external rotation with the arm at the side and then use functional abduction exercises. Keeping the muscles balanced, that is, progressing toward a home maintenance exercise

Table 7.3 Postoperative Impingement Therapy Plan

With arthroscopic acromioplasty

Preoperative training and pendulum exercises, elastic tubing exercises in internal and external rotation, interior and external rotation cane exercises, posterior towel exercises, and Codman exercises.

Postoperative sling immobilization overnight.

Active range of motion out of sling at day 1. Start passive range of motion in therapy within first 4 days, progressing to active, five times a week for 2 weeks if significant pain or with lack of motivation.

Active strengthening at 2-4 weeks 3 times per week minimum.

Overhead strengthening at 4-8 weeks when motion is full and when internal and external rotation strength at side are equal.

If still painful at 12-16 weeks, consider open cuff imbrication and use postoperative open cuff repair plan.

Following arthroscopic decompression, with or without distal clavicle resection, or with miniarthrotomy cuff repair

---

Same preoperative plan as following arthroscopic acromioplasty.

Sling overnight but avoid active motion above 60° for the 1st week until skin incisions are less painful.

At day 10, start assisted range of motion, external rotation cane exercises, and internal rotation towel exercises behind back.

Strengthening exercises at 3-5 weeks below 60° until pain has been advanced to 90° or above.

Strengthening at 4-6 weeks, emphasize endurance exercise. Progress to proprioceptive neuromuscular facilitation (neuromuscular reorganization), then open kinetic chain exercise, finally plyometrics.

Return to sport with activity level regulated by return of external rotation strength and endurance in overhead range.

Following open cuff or cuff imbrication repair

Same preoperative exercise training as following arthroscopic acromioplasty.

In sling for 4 weeks to allow deltoid healing in stable cuff repair or imbrication. Six weeks immobilization necessary for repair done under tension to allow cuff to heal.

Pendulum exercises out of sling the day following surgery.

Passive external rotation at 2 weeks and passive supine elevation at 4-6 weeks when out of sling.

External and internal rotation strengthening with arm at 0° abduction at 6-8 weeks.

Cross-pattern and abduction strengthening at 8-10 weeks.

Proprioceptive neuromuscular facilitation (neuromuscular reorganization and coordination), advancing to open kinetic chain exercise and plyometrics.

Return to sport if cuff repair is stable and strength and endurance have been recovered. Otherwise consider change to sport with less strenuous overhead activity.

---

program, is mandatory to help avoid recurrence of impingement.

A mesoacromion or a nonfused acromial apophysis that demonstrates significant motion after debridement of the soft tissue of the undersurface of the acromion may indicate a more serious problem, which may necessitate compression screw and tension band fixation if debridement alone is not satisfactory. Such problems necessitate open repair, in which the excess bone from the resected A/C joint can be used as bone graft for fixation of the meso-acromion. In this case treatment is the same, whether symptoms are acute or chronic. If arthroscopic subacromial decompression is not sufficient to diminish symptoms, open reduction and internal fixation of the loose anterior acromial fragment can be considered.

Advanced Tendinitis. Management of chronic rotator cuff change depends on the extent of symptoms. Most patients who have been treated for "bursitis" or "bicipital tendinitis" have in fact had rotator cuff disease. Treatment is geared first toward restoration of motion. Fibrosis or a partially "frozen" shoulder must be overcome in an effort to rehabilitate the shoulder. Once motion is regained, then muscular strength can be worked on. It must be emphasized to the patient that the minor snapping caused by residual bands of scar tissue within the shoulder is of no considerable consequence unless it hurts.

Late Conservative Management. Of prime importance is strengthening of the humeral head depressors. Even if the supraspinatus static depressor is thin, preferential strengthening of the subscapularis and infraspinatus can hold the humeral head down and minimize symptoms. The use of a 5-lb (2.25-kg) weight on the wrist or elbow in rehabilitation can pull the humeral head down slightly, diminish symptoms, and minimize supraspinatus grinding. Strengthening of the deltoid, biceps, triceps, and periscapular stabilizers can significantly minimize supraspinatus symptoms. Working on flexibility can help minimize subsequent propagation of a tear.

When conservative management is not effective in alleviating the pain associated with partial- or full-thickness cuff tears, or if there has been no improvement in active elevation of the arm after a complete tear (i.e., surrounding musculature does not compensate for the tear), surgery is indicated. Endoscopic bursal surgery is useful in resection of pathologic changes that lead to wearing of the rotator cuff. Resection of bony spurs from the acromion, A/C joint, and clavicle or of a calcified or thickened coracoacromial ligament can be accomplished.

Arthroscopic Mobilization. Any athlete who intends to remain active and has pain or loss of motion related to rotator cuff disease is a surgical candidate. In treatment of chronic impingement, a two-staged surgical approach should be considered. In the first stage, arthroscopy is done along with an evaluation under anesthesia to regain motion. Manipulation breaks scar tissue and will speed recovery more than if management is accomplished with physical therapy alone. Concurrent glenohumeral arthroscopy allows treatment of amplifying factors such as labral sprains or SLAP lesions. Arthroscopic debridement within the joint, SLAP lesion repair when necessary, and assessment of the rotator cuff is then followed by bursoscopy of the subacromial space with acromioplasty and resection of bursal and subdeltoid adhesions. Adhesion resection can increase mobility of the rotator cuff significantly. A second stage, open cuff repair, is often avoided due to the relief of pain from mobilization and debridement alone.

Open Exposure. With a large tear or significant wearing into the cuff under the A/C joint, a utility incision is most useful for open repair. This is an incision in line with the end of the clavicle across the acromion; the deep incision is in line with the skin incision but curves at the end of the acromion down into the deltoid, paralleling fiber arrangement (Figure 7.18b). This wide exposure allows resection of the A/C joint and cuff repair or imbrication. With coexistent glenohumeral pathology a saber incision is used so that both conditions can be dealt with concurrently (Figure 7.18c).

Cuff Imbrication. Significant erosion into the cuff thins the cuff and makes balancing and containing the humeral head more difficult. Bone and tissue protrusion into the supraspinatus outlet can cause a worn area in the rotator cuff. This ulcerative area usually becomes less symptomatic after arthroscopic subacromial decompression, dome decompression of the A/C joint, or endoscopic or open distal clavicle resection. Scarring in the healing process, however, may minimize motion and lead to the need for further physical therapy, manipulation under anesthesia, or arthroscopic debridement of the new scar. The worn area may not heal even if full motion is restored, in which case the patient may complain of a constant dull ache directly under the previously impinging A/C joint area that gets worse with weather change, leading to the need for open repair of the ulcer. Surgical imbrication of the worn cuff may be necessary to restore a smooth surface to ride under the acromion so that scapulothoracic overuse can be minimized (Figure 7.19, a-c).

Cuff Repair. Repair of the hole in the cuff is very effective in decreasing the pain that radiates to the root of the deltoid. In a younger individual the cuff may have been pulled off by acute trauma, and repair without decompression may be all that

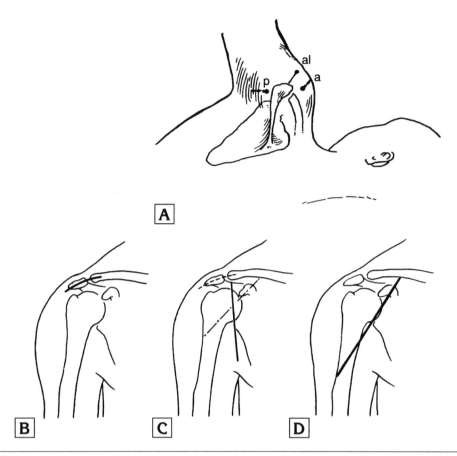

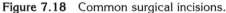

Figure 7.18 Common surgical incisions.

[A] Arthroscopic portals can be extended for open repair. Posterior portal (p) extends into posterior saber incision for posterior capsular plication. Anterior portal (a) extends for anterior saber capsular approach. Anterolateral portal (al) extends toward acromion for miniarthrotomy in line with deltoid fibers.

[B] Utility incision through both skin and deltotrapezial periosteum.

[C] Saber incision allows both deltopectoral and utility approach.

[D] Deltopectoral incision for shoulder replacement and fracture work.

is necessary. If soft tissue or bony changes have developed, they must be dealt with concurrently. This would mean appropriate acromioplasty (either anterior, medial, or lateral depending on the size of the spur), stabilization of a mesoacromial apophyseal nonunion (which uncommonly co-exists with glenohumeral instability or superior impact injury), distal clavicectomy for A/C joint arthritis, tightening of the coracohumeral suspensory system, or capsular stabilization of the gleno-humeral joint when appropriate. Lack of attention to the associated or modifying factors can lead to failure of the repair of the rotator cuff.

A very small rotator cuff tear can be ignored if amplifying factors are removed in either an open or endoscopic procedure. Arthroscopically assisted surgery has the potential of minimizing irritation of the deltoid muscle, which is important in rehabilitation. A very small hole can be usually ignored but is easily repaired through a mini-arthrotomy incision, which is an extension of the anterolateral portal toward the A/C joint. A moderately sized hole of 1 to 3 cm, especially if it exists as a sleeve or has been identified by arthrogram as nondisplaced or minimally displaced, can be repaired through a mini-arthrotomy (Figure 7.20a).

Interscalene or regional block can yield enough pain relief to allow miniarthrotomy to be done as an outpatient procedure. Rather than the traditional method of making a trough, which needs significant advancement of tissue, merely abrading the greater tuberosity area, sinking a subcortical anchor, and bringing the rotator cuff to this freshened area can yield enough tissue to close a small or moderate-size tear (Figure 7.20, b and c). The patient is immobilized for 4 weeks, pendulum

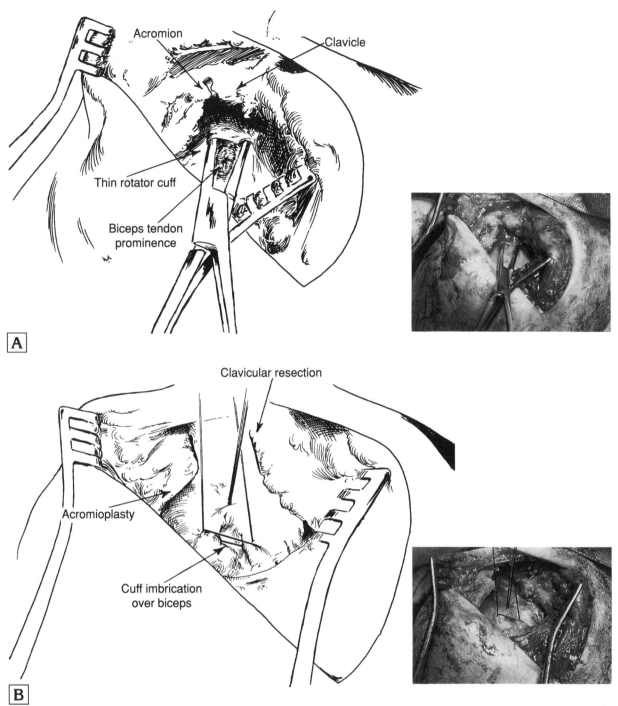

Figure 7.19 Imbrication of rotator cuff in area over the long biceps tendon worn into by previous A/C joint spurs in functional elevation.

[A] Thin area of cuff through which biceps tendon is easily palpated.

[B] The walls of the ulcer are brought back together to thicken tissue and to yield stability to the top of the joint.

(continued)

exercises can be started the following day, and relief of pain from the chemical irritation of joint fluid leaking out of the hole is almost instantaneous. A bolus of I.V. antibiotics is usually given in the outpatient center prior to discharge. Outpatient endoscopic rotator cuff repair without mini-arthrotomy is an experimental technique (Figure 7.21, a-c).

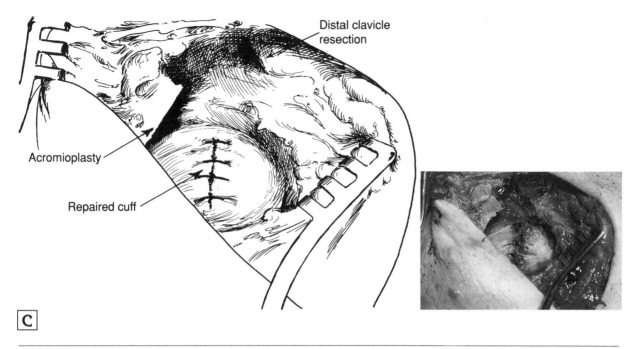

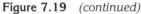

Figure 7.19 *(continued)*

[C] Imbricated rotator cuff reestablishes depressor function, and a soft tissue spacer protects the biceps tendon and may tighten the superior joint capsule to eliminate constant dull ache.

A larger hole, however, necessitates greater exposure, usually by stripping the deltoid from the acromion and distal clavicle, and is therefore more painful (Figure 7.22). Hospitalization is necessary for patient-controlled anesthetic pain relief and I.V. antibiotics. The length of time for postoperative immobilization and initiation of pendulum exercises is usually the same as for an outpatient procedure. It may be extended by 2 weeks if there is some tension on the repair. The use of an abduction splint is no longer advocated, because a muscle healing in an abducted position most likely will rip as the arm is brought down to the side when the brace is removed.

Many "irreparable" rotator cuff tears can be repaired by subdeltoid adhesion resection and mobilization of tissue (Figure 7.23, a and b). Endoscopic Mumford distal clavicectomy or dome decompression of inferior acromial spurs can be done. Removal of inferior acromial spurs can be done concurrently. If arthroscopic distal clavicle resection and inferior acromioplasty has been done, often a short, 3-cm anterolateral incision, extending the anterolateral portal distally from the edge of the acromion toward the A/C joint marking needle, is all that is needed for a short tear.

With repair, the transposed muscle may be pulled apart with early use or may no longer pull in the same direction, so that motion will be jeopardized. A large tear that cannot be easily closed should most likely be left alone to obtain the best functional result. As the individual ages, motion is more important than attempting to regain power. Golf and doubles tennis may be substituted for overhand throwing and weight training.

Irreparable Cuff Debridement. Although subdeltoid adhesion resection may change the situation, occasionally a massive tear may not be repairable. Debridement of irregular cuff edges, the inferior acromion, the undersurface of the acromioclavicular joint, bursal edges, and so on or SLAP lesion repair can decrease friction and minimize symptoms. These can be done arthroscopically or as open procedures. Arthroscopic debridement has the advantages of concurrent debridement of the glenohumeral joint and not having to take down the deltoid, but open debridement has the advantage of allowing at least partial repair of the rotator cuff, salvaging whatever strength can be recovered along the normal pull of the muscle. Transposing a tendon may alter the effective vector of its pull, and even though some strength may be regained, a decreased amount of motion is usually associated. Trying to close a large defect may minimize function.

A surprising number of elderly recreational athletes with large, full-thickness rotator cuff tears are so pleased with arthroscopic debridement that

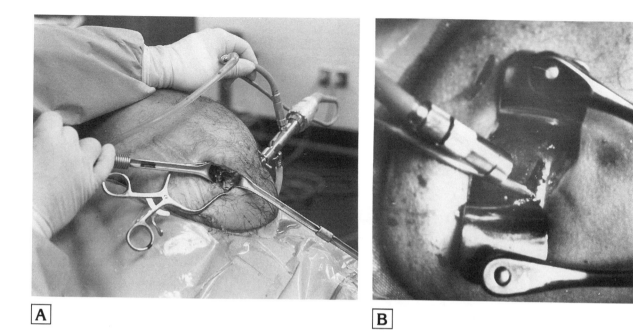

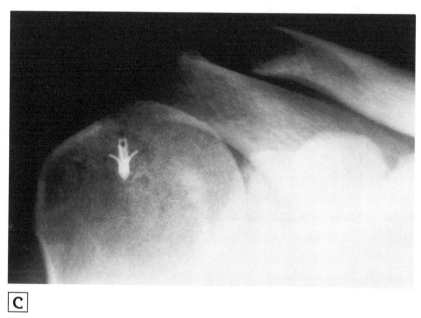

Figure 7.20 Miniarthrotomy extension of anterolateral portal allows repair of moderate rotator cuff lesions.

[A] The arthroscopic tools are useful to help light, irrigate, and debride during the open procedure. The same lateral decubital arthroscopic position can be used for open repair.

[B] Debridement of greater tuberosity using an Acromionizer (Dyonics, Smith & Nephew Endoscopy, Andover, MA).

[C] Advancement of rotator cuff to area of freshened greater tuberosity secured by Superanchor (Mitek, Norwood, MA).

they do not wish to go on to further attempted open surgery and go back to playing golf, tennis, swimming, bowling, and so on with minimal discomfort. Arthroscopic debridement may be a temporizing maneuver until the tear propagates further. However, with adequate flexibility and strengthening from exercising the remaining tissue, very few of these athletes come back with clinical propagation of a tear or clinical complaints. They tend to be slightly weaker than patients who have had cuff repair, but they have more motion, which is ultimately more important.

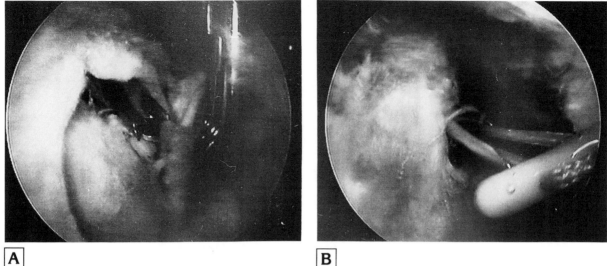

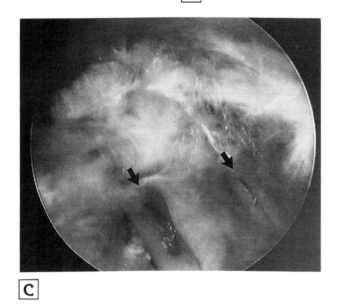

Figure 7.21 Experimental endoscopic rotator cuff repair, using technique developed by Jerome Jennings, MD, Winston-Salem, NC.

[A] Guide utilized for percutaneous drill holes through greater tuberosity.

[B] Advancement of implant through edge of rotator cuff (T-Fix, Acufex, Smith & Nephew Endoscopy, Andover, MA).

[C] Sutures are tied; implant fixes the advanced cuff to the freshened greater tuberosity.

Salvage Arthroplasty. Subacromial decompression, either open or arthroscopic, is most effective when there has been no superior up-riding of the humeral head. Once the humeral head has buttonholed through the rotator cuff defect, which implies failure of the humeral head depressors, it is very difficult to decelerate the degenerative cycle. This leads to end-stage impingement disease in which the humeral head articulates with the acromion, coracoid, or undersurface of the clavicle. The athlete may possibly have to give up active partici-pation in athletics before this occurs, so the goal in treatment should be to avoid this stage. Salvage, pain relief, and return to daily activities, rather than return to athletic activity, become the goals.

Total joint arthroplasty is not effective in taking care of these problems, because the supraspinatus static depressor is no longer effective, the subscapularis active depressor is commonly stretched or frayed, and the teres minor and infraspinatus depressors are usually contracted. The best that can be done is to use a large hemiprosthesis of the

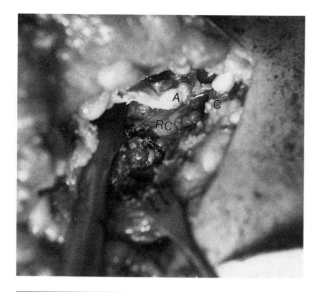

Figure 7.22 Open rotator cuff repair for large lesions needs greater exposure; a half-inch curved osteotome turned upside down acts as a retractor and can be used to lyse subdeltoid adhesions in order to advance the tendon edges (A = acromion, C = clavicle, RC = rotator cuff).

humeral head to help regain an instant center and to help the deltoid and remaining muscles to function near their optimal length. Even with end-stage impingement, subacromial decompression can be effective in pain relief, although it is much less predictable (Figure 7.24, a and b). Much depends on retraining the deltoid to elevate in the lower range, but this cannot always be accomplished.

Complications

If impingement is allowed to proceed, muscle activity is compromised: The ability to depress the humeral head is minimized, subluxation may get worse, or postural changes may slump the scapula forward, leading to further impingement. Again, the superior migration of the humeral head wears further into the supraspinatus and eventually leads to a full-thickness rotator cuff tear. Complications also arise in treatment.

Early Cuff Tendinitis. If the rotator cuff is strengthened in therapy primarily by exercising the supraspinatus and deltoid muscles, the imbalance of the internal and external rotators (common in subluxation) may get worse, and the patient will complain of more pain in therapy than before therapy, a condition also found with a SLAP lesion or functional subluxation. When this occurs check for subluxation, and instruct the therapist to work only on over-the-top inwardly rotated pendulum and Codman exercises, with the left shoulder clockwise and the right shoulder counterclockwise. Rotation in the opposite direction mimics the abducted, externally rotated apprehension maneuver and will make the patient feel more uncomfortable when subluxation is the underlying problem. In this situation, therapy is completely reversed, with internal rotation strengthening done first, progressing toward external rotation balancing, and then external rotation in functional

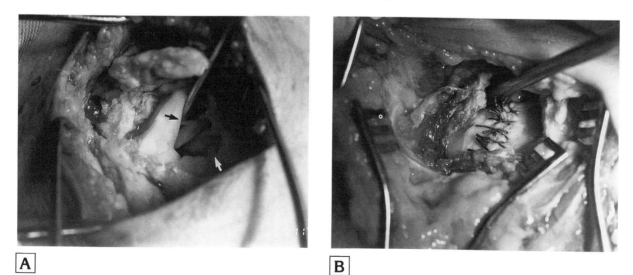

A   **B**

Figure 7.23

[A] Edges of massive "irreparable" rotator cuff tear are mobilized by endoscopic resection of subacromial adhesions, which

[B] allows tissue to be anchored at the decorticated greater tuberosity to yield a watertight repair.

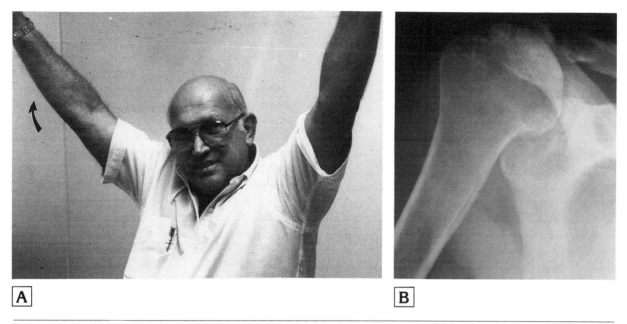

Figure 7.24 End-stage impingement in this high school athletic director and wrestling coach led to stiffness and adhesive capsulitis; he was only able to shrug the shoulder.

[A] The postoperative result was increased range of motion without pain with slight decrease in strength compared to opposite shoulder.

[B] X-ray appearance after arthroscopic debridement and endoscopic distal clavicectomy.

elevation. Exercise the supraspinatus and medial deltoid elevator muscles only after the depressor muscles of the cuff (infraspinatus, subscapularis, and anterior and posterior deltoid) are stronger.

Arthroscopic surgical decompression may make the underlying subluxation worse by allowing further superior migration of the humeral head. Ideally, relief of secondary impingement symptoms will allow the patient to return to strengthening exercises to depress the humeral head and treat the primary glenohumeral instability problem. If therapy fails in this case, however, subsequent tightening of the shoulder capsule may be of some benefit. The anterior acromial hook may be overlooked if it is within the deltoid muscle and will not be uncovered at time of arthroscopic subacromial decompression when following around the front of the tendinous insertion and removing the rim of thickened tissue. Even in an open acromioplasty it is very important not to take out too much acromion, because the anterior acromial hook may have developed as a stabilizer to prevent anterior-to-posterior subluxation of the shoulder. Removal of the hook may unmask the underlying instability or make it worse, leading to the need for open stabilization.

Chronic Cuff Pathology. With full-thickness rotator cuff tearing, the initial presentation may be handled effectively by conservative management. Propagation of the tear, however, may lead to subsequent reinjury. The supraspinatus is the most commonly strained tendon in the body. Early edematous changes are most likely reversible, and clinical symptoms may be minimized even in full-thickness tears if secondary factors can be stabilized, that is, if the humeral head depressors are strengthened and accessory muscles retrained. Massive full-thickness rotator cuff tears usually will not heal; however, the body has an amazing potential to recover. The author has seen two cases of greater than 3-cm tears that were considered irreparable, one in a 17-year-old high school wrestler and one in a 49-year-old recreational racquetball player who underwent arthroscopic and open debridement, respectively. Motion was lost postoperatively, and at subsequent endoscopic resection of subdeltoid adhesions, the cuff tears had fibrosed in and no hole was identified. After adhesion release, motion recovered; the extra scar, an apparently excess part of the healing process, was an effective patch of the rotator cuff.

Tear Propagation. Complications occur from treatment and from lack of treatment. A tear in the rotator cuff may propagate while the patient is in therapy, and the patient must be warned ahead of time that this is a risk. Of course, therapy is ordered in the hope of avoiding such propagation by stretching, strengthening, and exercises for humeral head depression, but this is not always effective in the long run. Too aggressive or unsupervised physical therapy or improper use of isokinetic testing equipment for therapy may lead to surgical failure (Figure 7.25).

Misdiagnosis. Too generous an acromioplasty, either arthroscopic or open, can lead to further superior migration of the humeral head and accelerate the degeneration process both within the glenohumeral space and of the rotator cuff (Figure 7.26). Failure to properly diagnose, that is, operating on a clinical rotator cuff tear when adhesive capsulitis, instability, cervical radiculopathy, or tumor is the actual cause, can also lead to failure of management. It must be remembered that not all shoulder pain is impingement (Figure 7.27, a-c).

Although most soft tissue problems about the shoulder are not well defined on X-ray, the plain X-ray is an important part of the orthopedic examination (Figure 7.28).

Neurologic Dysfunction. Fibrosis in retracted rotator cuff tissue may mean that function of the suprascapular nerve is lost and may not recover. Even if the hole is closed, loss of supraspinatus and infraspinatus innervation may mean no return of motor function. One must also deal with the

patient's goals and explain that regular function may not recover.

Loss of Motion. Presenting with pain and loss of motion, the athlete may expect both to recover after repair. With a massive tear, fiber orientation gets altered in an attempt to close the hole. Repair may limit joint fluid from leaking out and minimize pain. However, the change in orientation of fibers necessary to accomplish this means that muscles are now pulling in different directions from the way they were meant to; therefore, motion is compromised. The repaired tendon in a full-thickness tear is by no means a normal tendon. Even with stable fixation to a roughened bone trough area (which is made to encourage healing), acromioplasty, subacromial decompression, and adequate immobilization, the advanced tissue may not hold, and failure of the operative repair is a possibility.

Failed Tendon Repair. The main complication of rotator cuff repair is cuff failure. This is due to many factors: the tissue paper–like cuff often found at time of repair, reorientation of remaining cuff fibers in closing the gap, significant strain on tissue when it is advanced down to a bone trough, postoperative adhesions, infection, deltoid retraction or detachment, denervation of the rotator cuff muscles or deltoid, limited results compared to

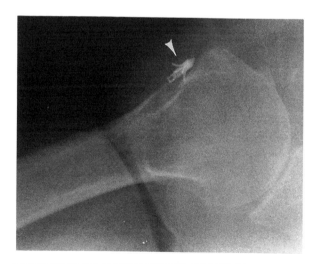

Figure 7.25 At 4 months following miniarthrotomy and repair of the rotator cuff, the therapist insisted on the last 10° of abduction. Pain returned, the patient was no longer able to lift her arm or to swim, the anchor rivet pulled out, and the rotator cuff tore again, which necessitated re-repair, resulting in full function without return to therapy.

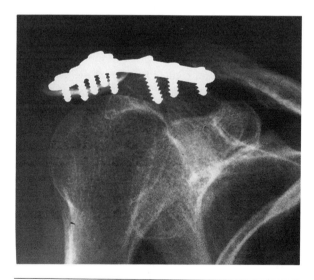

Figure 7.26 Impingement pain in a 25-year-old tennis player led to total acromionectomy. Pain continued, leading to reflex sympathetic dystrophy and fibrosis between the exposed deltoid fascia and rotator cuff. The patient did not work for 13 years. Reconstruction of the acromion utilizing iliac crest graft and plate fixation led to resolution of pain and symptoms as well as return of function.

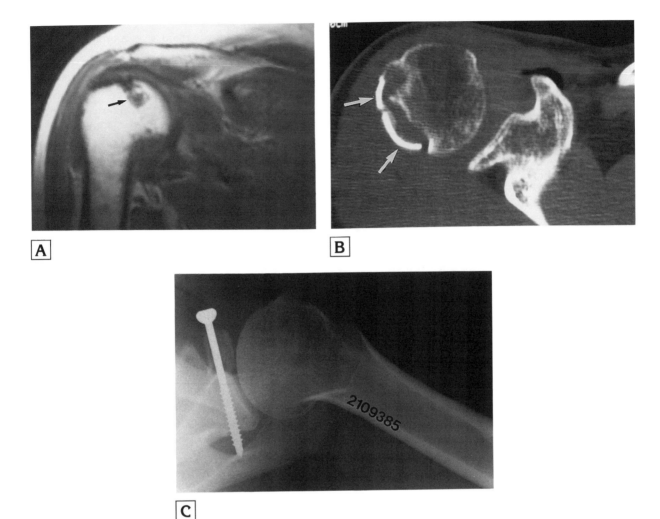

Figure 7.27 Clinically misdiagnosed "impingement" found to be due to other causes.

[A] Atypical humeral head intraosseous ganglion cyst with resting pain found on MRI.

[B] Nondisplaced cortical fracture of the greater tuberosity appears normal on plain X-ray, but causes point tenderness over greater tuberosity on MRI.

[C] Following coracoid transfer for glenohumeral stabilization, the patient is referred for "anterior and posterior impingement pain," which completely resolves with removal of the screw.

the patient's expectation, sterile drainage and dehiscence in spite of adequate decompression, concurrent cervical radiculopathy, or syringomyelia.

Prognosis

Most young athletes who have not developed thickening or fibrosis of the subacromial bursa, bony spurs under the acromion, or significant erosion of the rotator cuff do well in therapy consisting of diminishing their activity level, rest, nonsteroidal anti-inflammatory medication, mobilization, and strengthening within 6 to 8 weeks. It is important to emphasize to these young athletes that they need to continue these stretching and

strengthening exercises at home or before and after sport activity so that the pain does not return. It is important to correct the improper mechanics that caused the problem, such as insufficient body roll in swimming or throwing too hard without proper strengthening of the internal and external rotators in pitching, again so that symptoms do not redevelop.

If conservative management is not effective, arthroscopic intervention can be done for subacromial decompression, and therapy modified accordingly. That is, if anterior subluxation signs are found, internal rotation strengthening is done first, working toward external rotation strengthening and then elevation strengthening. Even with

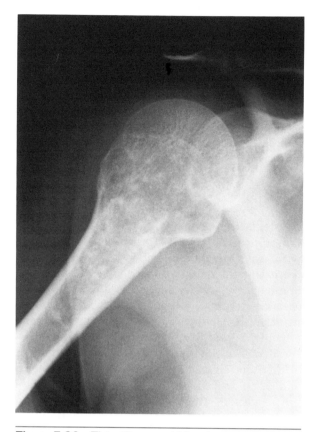

Figure 7.28 This 45-year-old bowler complained of shoulder pain for 2 years and did not respond to cortisone injection or 18 months of physical therapy. She was referred for endoscopic subacromial decompression, when an X-ray was taken for the first time, demonstrating chondrosarcoma. Not all shoulder pain is "impingement pain."

primary impingement, debridement of the acromion must not be so aggressive as to allow initiation of laxity of the joint where the postoperative response is more variable. Returning to sport activity may take from 2 days to 9 months even after arthroscopic subacromial decompression.

Open procedures that encompass A/C joint surgery and rotator cuff repair will take longer to recover from if the deltoid is taken down in exposure. Deltoid function is important in rehabilitation, and the muscle must heal before attempting strengthening exercises. Obviously, less wear from the A/C joint into the tendon means less injury and an overall better result. One cannot make new tissue where it does not exist. If there has been significant wear of the cuff, it is often useful to retrieve the eroded edges and bring them together, in effect thickening the cuff so that it is better balanced and rides more smoothly under the acromion and the muscles work more normally due to centralization of the humeral head.

When treating associated impingement, one is tempted to take down the fibrous area of the non-fused symptomatic acromial apophysis to develop bleeding edges of bone for the healing response. This does not work out well if percutaneous pins and screws are all that is used for acromial fixation, because there is significant motion across the front of the acromion in the activities of daily living. Leaving the bone in place and merely placing compression lag screw or Herbert screw fixation across the nonfused apophysis can be effective (Figure 10.31, a-c) as can a central rotational bone plug. Open reduction and internal fixation have a better chance of leaving a stable acromial edge that will no longer wear into the underlying supraspinatus.

Associated degenerative arthritis of the acromioclavicular joint must be dealt with effectively and concurrently; otherwise, the mobilization and strengthening necessary to overcome impingement cannot proceed or at least is much less predictable. Continued mobilization and strength to minimize recurrence of symptoms is important, especially to elite athletes.

In the advanced disease state, subacromial decompression or rotator cuff debridement or repair almost universally decrease pain. Subsequent mobility and return to athletic activity are directly related to the integrity of the tissue and of the repair and to the amount of motion possible post-surgically. The larger the tear and the poorer the tissue at the time of repair, the less successful the return to athletic activity. Better quality repair and lack of thinning of the cuff or of superior migration of the humeral head have a higher correlation with successful return to athletic activity.

Cost Containment

To contain costs, various studies, including arthrography, ultrasound, bone scan, and MRI, may not be immediately necessary. Four-view X-ray studies are useful in screening. If an ultrasound shows no ectogenic changes of the cuff, an MRI is perhaps not necessary. Because there is a high correlation of subluxation with impingement, however, the author prefers the CT-arthrographic study if further investigation is considered. The sooner the athlete is treated, the less likely the need for surgical intervention and costly diagnostic tests.

Patient Education

The physician must inform the patient that, even if symptoms are relieved, it is important to continue strengthening and stretching to help prevent them from recurring. The athlete who has undergone surgical intervention for symptoms must also be warned that he or she needs to maintain strength and mobility on a lifetime basis to help avoid recurrence of symptoms. The main cause of patients returning to the clinic after successful management of an impingement problem is noncompliance with a home exercise program. Most such athletic failures respond to a very short refresher course of therapy, and patients are more conscientious about their maintenance programs afterwards. If the patient has not improved dramatically in response to physical therapy, it is important to analyze why this is the case and to modify therapy accordingly. If the patient is merely given a hot pack on the shoulder and instructed to do unsupervised exercises with 5-lb weights, the patient needs to go to another therapy facility where hands-on treatment is available. Sending a patient back for therapy for 6 months straight that was not effective right from the beginning is a counterproductive, discouraging waste of time and money and even may make the injury worse. On discharge from therapy it may be advisable to have the patient either join a health club or get home exercise equipment, which can range from 2- and 5-lb cuff weights, elastic bands, or a heating pad, all the way to a home gym multistation machine.

Prevention

It appears that many progressive rotator cuff injuries are preventable and that stretching the joint capsule and humeral head depressors can diminish or prevent the initiation of impingement symptoms. Proper body mechanics in athletic endeavors is also mandatory. Icing the shoulder before and after activity, stretching, weight training, and weighted pendulum or Codman exercises can also diminish symptoms if done routinely. Horizontal flexion and hyperabduction stretching, internal and external rotation strengthening, and functional abduction strengthening are all useful to help avoid impingement symptoms.

Biceps Strain

Strain injury to the biceps tendon spans a continuum that includes avulsion, tendinitis, subluxation, adhesive tenosynovitis, and so on. Carter Rowe, in teaching his residents and fellows, has stated that "the biceps is often implicated but rarely found guilty" (personal communication, 1982). Inflammation of the biceps tendon is usually

secondary to some other problem; in treating the primary condition, bicipital inflammation will usually clear on its own.

Epidemiology and Etiology

Biceps symptoms are commonly found in association with rotator cuff thinning or impingement and tendinitis, glenohumeral subluxation, and inflammatory conditions such as adhesive capsulitis. Therefore, patients who participate in throwing or pitching sports or swimming, especially at an elite level, are prone to bicipital tendinitis. Weight-training activity has the highest incidence of tendon rupture in the athletic population, especially with heavy weight and inadequate spotting assistance. Underhand activity, in which the biceps tendon may ride within a constricted groove, can be associated with symptoms in sports such as underhand softball pitching, curling, horseshoes, and bowling. Rotational activities of the upper arm associated with extension at the elbow and shoulder at the same time can lead to bicipital symptoms and occur in activities such as karate and judo arm extension, table tennis, and competitive video arcade activity. One other symptom-producing activity is the use of hand weights while fast walking, step training, or aerobic dancing. This practice must be condemned, because the upper and lower extremities should be in balance. Overweighing the upper extremities can jeopardize normal, balanced crossed-extensor activity and energy amplification, potentially increasing risk of injury.

Pathogenesis

There is a very wide variety of "normal" anatomy of the bicipital groove that may lead to a deficient medial wall of the lesser tuberosity (Fisk, 1965; Hitchcock & Bechtol, 1948). The coracohumeral ligament either swings over from the coracoid process, exists partially as a slip of the pectoralis minor, or may be the second muscle belly of the pectoralis minor. It inserts just above the transverse humeral ligament, actually coalescing to form the transverse humeral ligament in many individuals. The transverse humeral ligament works as a retinacular structure to hold the long biceps tendon in the bicipital groove. Fibers covering the biceps tendon therefore attach both to the lesser tuberosity and to the greater tuberosity, and wear through either tuberosity can eventually cause inflammation of the biceps tendon. The long tendon of the biceps is an integral part of the superior suspensory mechanism. It originates in most cases from the posterosuperior labrum, but in less than 2% of cases it originates entirely from the supraglenoid tubercle or directly from the rotator cuff. Less commonly, it can originate from both (Figure 7.29).

In approximately 5% of arthroscopic specimens there are multiple slips of the long biceps tendon, the major one attaching to the superior labrum and the minor slips attaching directly to the rotator cuff (Figure 7.30). Only 0.1% of individuals have two or more firm, large bicipital tendon origins within the joint (Figure 7.31). In 0.5%, no intra-articular tendon exists; the biceps merges with the rotator cuff or has no intra-articular presence whatsoever (Figure 7.32).

The tendon is usually tubular both within the joint and within the extra-articular walls of the bicipital groove, which span this tendon as the arm functionally abducts. Injury to the superior suspensory mechanism may cause it to flatten, especially if it subluxates out of the groove (a Type I or Type II injury, discussed later; Figure 7.33). Trauma may be affected by underlying congenital variation or may produce abnormal bicipital variations (Figure 7.34).

As the arm abducts, the intra-articular extent of the biceps tendon will shorten. This is technically not muscle excursion but merely the fact that the

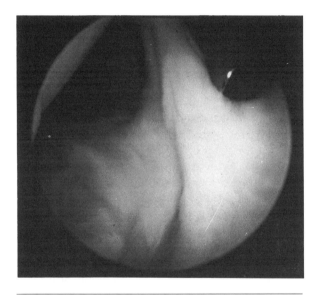

Figure 7.29 Bicipital origin half from superior glenoid tubercle, half directly from rotator cuff.

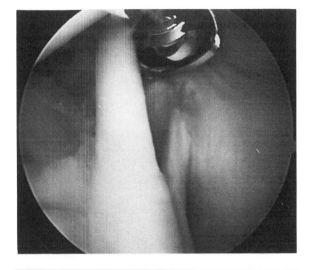

Figure 7.31 Two intra-articular biceps tendon origins, one through cuff and one through bicipital tunnel.

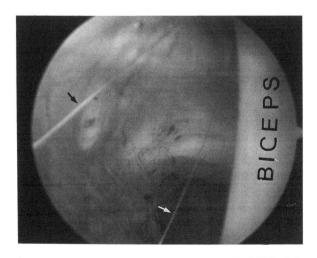

Figure 7.30 Major bicipital tendon attaching to superior labrum, minor tendon slips directly to cuff.

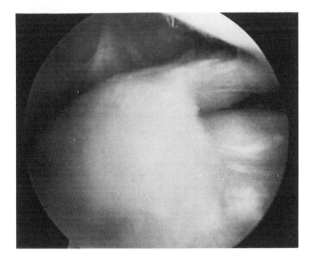

Figure 7.32 No biceps attachment to superior labrum, which exists here as a SLAP lesion directly attached to the anterior joint capsule through the superior glenohumeral ligament.

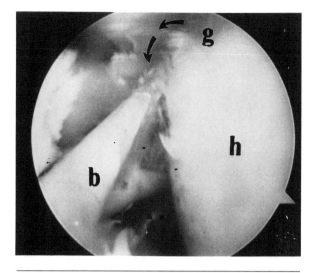

Figure 7.33 Combination Type I and Type II injury with biceps tendon eroded, flattened, and anteriorly subluxated out of groove, dissecting under subscapularis tendon (b = biceps, g = greater tuberosity, h = humeral head).

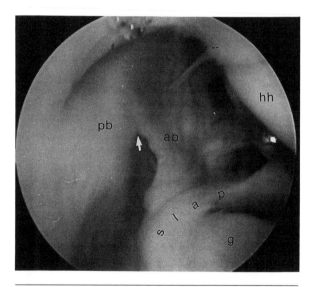

Figure 7.34 Intra-articular biceps split. Anterior biceps segment attached to detached superior labrum, posterior segment detached from labrum but attached to superior tubercle and rotator cuff. Note split up the biceps tendon. Trauma may be superimposed on congenital variation here (ab = anterior biceps, SLAP = avulsed anterior superior labrum, pb = posterior biceps, hh = humeral head, g = glenoid).

tendon will ride within the intertubercular groove of the humerus, much like a monorail, depressing the humeral head through the range of motion. In the act of throwing, with the humeral head riding forward, due to the proprioceptive function of the anterosuperior capsular structures, the biceps may fire to help centralize the head, stabilize it, and effect superior containment. In most cases, this will cause traction on the superior labrum. With enough force, the superior labrum can detach from the glenoid. If force is placed on the anterior capsule while the biceps is firing to help centralize and depress the head, a Bankart lesion type of anterior capsular avulsion may propagate around the top of the rim, causing a SLAP lesion. This is common if the arm is forced into abduction and external rotation. If the arm is in reverse extension or slightly forward when the biceps is firing, a reverse Bankart lesion may extend into a SLAP lesion. Therefore, in a throwing activity or a fall, a SLAP lesion by itself may initially occur, but when the biceps is firing it may extend into the capsule or labrum anteriorly or posteriorly. With repetitive tugging of the biceps in one direction and the rotator cuff in another, there will be progressive loosening of the anterior capsule and superior glenohumeral ligament. Subluxation will be associated with the biceps symptoms, which in turn lead to increased instability under the acromion and resultant impingement symptoms.

If injury occurs to the coracohumeral ligament, increased play in the superior capsule may occur, the biceps tendon may slide totally out of the groove or partially subluxate, arthritis may develop at the corners of the coracohumeral insertion and cause spurring, and the tendon substance itself may progressively change and fray or rupture. Erosion into the lesser tuberosity area, loosening the superior glenohumeral ligament and subscapularis, will allow the biceps tendon to slide out of the bicipital tunnel; soft tissue may need to be reattached to this top corner to stabilize the biceps tendon and keep it in the tunnel. As commonly occurs in throwing activity, the biceps pulls in one direction on the superior labrum to attempt to hold the humeral head in place while the supraspinatus pulls in another direction; a traction injury may occur in the rotator cuff or biceps due to this force-couple arrangement (see p. 128). This may pull the labrum off, causing a SLAP lesion that may extend into the biceps tendon substance itself (Figure 7.35).

Superior laxity of the shoulder mechanism leads to an unstable pivot point at the superior capsule and may extend into a Bankart lesion either anteriorly (when the biceps pulls while attempting to stop abducted external rotation) or posteriorly (when the biceps fires in internal rotation trying to stop forward momentum). Attempting to counterbalance a superior subluxation may lead to more extensive tearing peripherally or into the

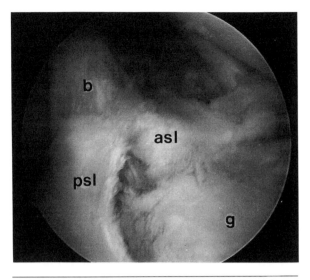

Figure 7.35 Grade IV SLAP lesion erosion into biceps tendon (b = biceps, g = glenoid, psl = avulsed posterior superior labrum, asl = avulsed anterior superior labrum).

biceps. The superior glenohumeral ligament, which is an interior counterpart of the coracohumeral ligament, may stretch out and no longer help anchor the biceps insertion or function in proprioception. When this occurs, the humeral head is not well maintained in the socket and wobbles superiorly, leading to compression of the rotator cuff against the acromion and transmission of energy into the A/C joint. Cuff impingement, cuff thinning, and subsequent A/C joint symptoms develop. As the cuff progressively erodes, the biceps becomes relatively uncovered or unprotected; the biceps can actually be felt to roll under the fingertip of the examiner with internal and external rotation. When the cuff thins or tears the biceps has been known to lose its normal, roundish shape and to flatten, a phenomenon related to its increased function as a head depressor in this circumstance.

Fraying at the arthritic corners of the bicipital groove can lead to erosion of the biceps tendon, and a sudden pull can avulse the tendon, causing either avulsion at the superior tubercle or a SLAP lesion. Primary avulsion near the top of the labrum requires significant sudden stress to pull tissue off; this commonly occurs in a flexed-elbow position with the arm down at the side, when the superior structures are unable to help share the load. Because excursion is not significant in most cases, avulsion at the musculotendinous junction can occur. Adhesive changes about the joint in an effort to heal a rotator cuff tear are associated with synovial disease and capsulitis and cause stenosis near the greater tuberosity and friction within the bicipital

tunnel. Stretch of the coracohumeral mechanism can lead to subluxation of the bicipital tendon and accelerated disease.

Natural History

Bicipital tendinitis in most cases is secondary to subluxation, adhesions, or rotator cuff impingement and inflammation. Symptoms may worsen if the primary problem gets worse but will decrease in intensity if the primary problem is treated accordingly. Erosion into the rotator cuff can lead to initial inflammation around the biceps tunnel and eventually to bicipital avulsion. Subluxation can cause wearing at the bicipital tunnel opening. As the tendon wears or is irritated by an inflamed tenosynovium, it no longer rides smoothly within the bicipital groove. The tendon may widen to replace the static function of the thinned or torn rotator cuff, may avulse off the supraglenoid tubercle or superior labrum, may fray and finally tear within the bicipital tunnel, or may even tear at the musculotendinous junction extra-articularly. Intra-articular pain of biceps origin may occur when the rotator cuff is torn and the biceps flattens to attempt to cover a wider distance to depress the humeral head.

Diagnosis

Because the etiology of bicipital lesions involves many factors, a myriad of clinical presentations can occur. It is critical to pay attention to the athlete's stated history and tie it to the clinical examination to come up with the proper diagnosis.

History. The patient may describe an impingement or subluxation phenomenon that gradually increases at the front of the shoulder. He or she may describe an acute injury or minor complaints for some time preceding a specific injury that caused something to pop and led to a physical deformity or bleeding. The patient may describe early fatigue with the arm giving out or with a feeling of something moving in and out of the joint, specifically with subluxation of the tendon. He or she may describe a popping within the joint with some ecchymosis that gradually resolved over a few weeks or may complain of pain developing about the shoulder with a snapping sensation following an acute fall on an outstretched arm.

Physical Examination. In an acute case physical examination will reveal tenderness along the bicipital groove, which is located approximately 30°

lateral to the supinated forearm. It is very important to test both arms, because the bicipital tendon may be tender normally in many individuals. As the arm internally rotates, the pain should change in position along with the interval between the greater tuberosity and lesser tuberosity. Having the patient "make a muscle" or pull his or her hands behind the head may show an abnormal bulge of the biceps, implicating musculotendinous or intratendinous rupture that leads to recoiling within the upper arm.

Moving the elbow into extension as the arm supinates against resistance (the *Speed test*) can define tenderness along the biceps. Testing a flexed elbow against resistance in supination (*Yergason's test*) may demonstrate pain near the bicipital tunnel. A positive impingement test with point tenderness over the coracoacromial ligament or coracoid process shows an interrelationship between biceps strain and concurrent impingement or rotator cuff pathology. Atrophy of the supraspinatus and infraspinatus muscles may occur if erosive injury to the tendon itself was caused by rotator cuff thinning.

Imaging. The four-view office X-ray series is mandatory in assessing disease of the biceps tendon. Osteopenia from disuse associated with adhesive capsulitis, A/C joint arthritis associated with energy transmission through the acromion and with subluxation, and subacromial spurs associated with impingement are X-ray changes that demonstrate the originating factors that lead to secondary bicipital tendinitis. The Fisk view, usually done in conjunction with an arthrogram, is an X-ray done tangentially down the bicipital groove with the patient in a prone position, holding the X-ray cassette in his or her supinated forearm (Fisk, 1965). With dye surrounding the tendon this view can demonstrate whether the biceps tendon is present and is subluxated or dislocated out of the groove (Figure 7.36, a and b).

Ultrasound may demonstrate subluxation of the tendon out of the groove. A SLAP lesion can be identified on the plain, 15°-downward-angled X-ray, if there is an associated avulsion fracture at the top of the joint. A SLAP lesion can be identified on a CT-arthrogram if the radiologist is aware of this lesion and specifically looks for it. Because this study is usually done with the arm at the side, allowing the capsule to be pulled down superiorly and interfering with the flow of dye into the bicipital-labral base, overhead motion is necessary to distribute the contrast dye in an effort to identify a SLAP lesion. The MRI has not been used primarily for biceps tendon lesions, mostly because it is not cost effective and has not been proven to show accurate detail of this lesion. As surface coils are perfected and analysis done throughout a range of motion, the MRI, probably with use of contrast, may become the most useful means to evaluate bicipital trauma. The current diagnostic standard is arthroscopy, through which intra-articular pathology can be identified by examining the biceps through a range of motion, examining the size of the bicipital tunnel opening, and defining the relationship of its injury to concurrent precipitating problems of subluxation or impingement.

Injury Classification. In addition to trying to find the precipitating cause of injury, the injury itself can be graded into one of six categories depending on the zone of injury (Figure 7.37), which

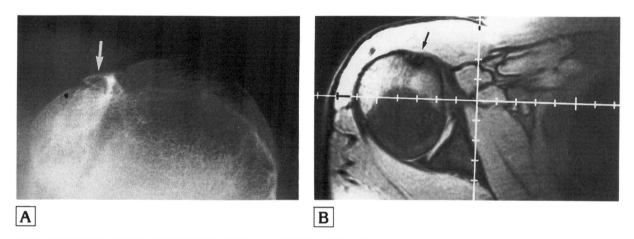

Figure 7.36 Fisk view.

[A] Arthrogram and

[B] MRI showing biceps tendon within tunnel.

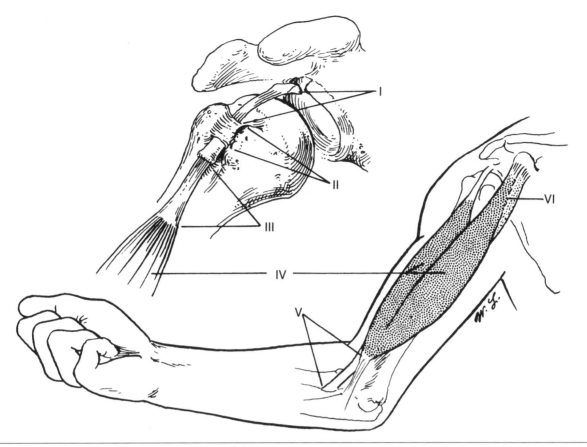

Figure 7.37 Zone classification of injuries of the biceps.

is important in determining the proper course of management.

Zone 1. Zone 1 injury is intra-articular and can include avulsion from the supraglenoid tubercle since this is an occasional area of attachment. More commonly, it involves loss of injury to the bicipital anchor, that is, a stretched superoglenohumeral ligament or stretched coracohumeral ligament that leads to an enlarged tunnel seen arthroscopically (Figure 7.38). When this is associated with a SLAP lesion the superior labrum may not be attached well; this may be due to the biceps firing at the time of initial injury, which pulls the labrum off, in the attempt to stop a fall or to stop forward momentum of the humeral head. A stretched biceps tunnel opening is commonly associated with intra-articular fraying of the rotator cuff just posterior to the bicipital tunnel, a traction injury incurred as the force-couple of the biceps and the supraspinatus pull in opposite directions, being out of phase due to injury.

If subluxation proceeds, repetitive trauma in this area can lead to splitting of the labrum up into the bicipital tendon. Fraying of the tendon itself can occur proximally near the labral insertion or at

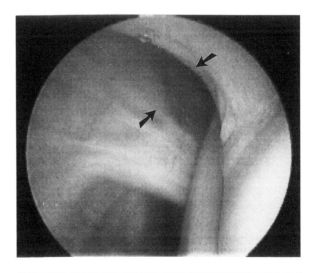

Figure 7.38 Enlarged bicipital tunnel due to incompetent superior mechanism, seen arthroscopically, leads to an unstable biceps tendon and symptoms of bicipital tendinitis.

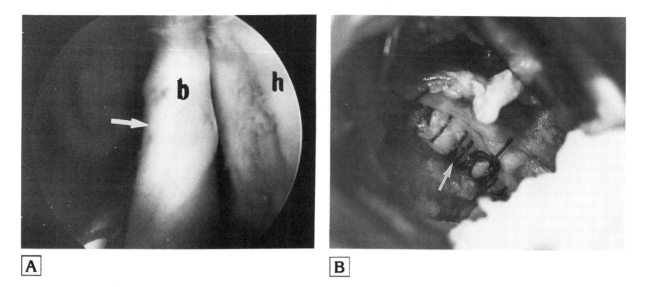

Figure 7.39 Zone I mid–biceps tendon wear, seen arthroscopically.

[A] Tendon erosion (b) due to continued impingement following full-thickness tear of rotator cuff; note superior chondral erosion of humeral head (h).

[B] Whip-stitch repair of biceps tendon restoring tubular shape during open cuff repair.

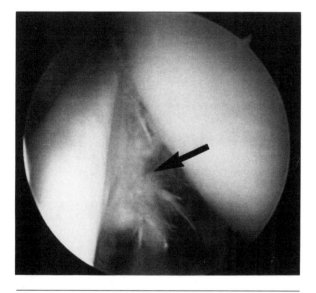

Figure 7.40 Biceps tendon fraying near tunnel opening, often associated with osteophytes within the tunnel, seen arthroscopically.

midlength if due to impingement (Figure 7.39, a and b), particularly if there is a hole in the rotator cuff that leaves the biceps unprotected. Fraying may be associated with trauma against osteophytes near the bicipital groove (Figure 7.40), bordering on a Zone II injury.

Zone II. The second zone is movable; that is, it includes injuries to the bicipital sulcus area, because the walls of the sulcus, coalescing to become

the transverse humeral ligament, should be buttressed both deeply and superficially by an intact coracohumeral ligament. This embracement, like a monorail track, allows the biceps tendon to be contained as the arm is abducted and the intra-articular portion shortens to depress and center the humeral head. Thinning of the rotator cuff and supporting structures near the bicipital tunnel opening will be documented arthroscopically as an enlarged bicipital tunnel opening. Stabilizing spurs that have developed near the bicipital tendon exit from the groove will cause progressive wear and ultimate rupture; a short-tendon stub (Zone I injury) may remain within the joint and can act as a functional subluxator (Figure 7.41).

If erosion of the coracohumeral ligament or a shallow medial wall of the groove is injured further by forcing the adducted or partially abducted arm into external rotation with continuing resistance of the biceps, as may occur in arm wrestling, the biceps may tunnel through the transverse humeral ligament to lay on top of the subscapularis and become subluxated or subluxatable; or, it more likely may tunnel under the subscapularis to lie loose within the joint, leading to very atypical presentation patterns in examination. Zone II will be the most painful area when adhesive capsulitis involves the biceps. Pain in the bicipital groove is amplified by attempting to supinate and extend the forearm against resistance. Synovial inflammatory conditions, including gout, rheumatoid disease, tuberculosis, and pseudogout, mimic the tunnel stenosis of adhesive capsulitis.

Zone III. Zone III injuries are injuries to the tendon beyond the bicipital groove up to the musculotendinous junction and unfortunately occur frequently. They may be due to anchoring down the tendon in the bicipital groove, which occurs with inflammatory disease combined with a sudden pull on the arm. They may be due to overuse of the biceps to retain and center the humeral head when a massive rotator cuff tear exists, which leads to injury at the musculotendinous junction. Zone III is a common site for sudden avulsion in young and middle-aged athletes, which unfortunately makes the ability to repair the tendon by sewing directly to muscle almost impossible (Figure 7.42).

Zone IV. Zone IV injuries occur within the muscle belly itself as a result of direct trauma, such as a

karate kick or sudden force of the forearm as in body building. Direct muscle-to-muscle repair has a dismal prognosis, and need not be attempted.

Zone V. Zone V injuries at the distal musculotendinous junction, the tendon substance itself, and the tendon's insertion to the elbow warrant early surgical repair (Figure 7.43). Late salvage is not that effective. Zone VI injuries, or injuries to the short head of the biceps within the conjoined tendon, will be subsequently discussed in this chapter.

Differential Diagnosis

In differential diagnosis it is important to first identify the primary cause of bicipital inflammation; subluxation, rotator cuff impingement or full-thickness tear, and adhesive capsulitis must first be ruled out. Inflammatory disease involving the bicipital groove, including gout, pseudogout, and adhesive capsulitis, can cause similar symptoms. Subluxation, which can stretch the bicipital tendon or involve the bicipital anchoring point (commonly found with a SLAP lesion), must be ruled out. With the increased wobble of the shoulder in subluxation, impingement can develop against the undersurface of either the acromion or coracoid, so assessment of both areas must be done. Subcoracoid impingement involves the superior subscapularis insertion into the lesser tuberosity. Progressive wear in this area can weaken the coracohumeral ligament anchor and lead to subluxation of the tendon out of the groove. Erosion of the superior fibers of the subscapularis will diminish its depressor function and lead to superior pull of the subscapularis, which will work in tandem with

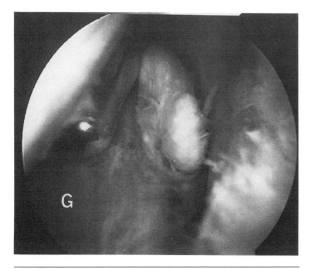

Figure 7.41 Stub of biceps tendon following rupture, here seen arthroscopically, may lead to functional subluxation and painful click due to interposition within joint (g = glenoid).

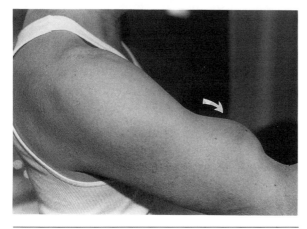

Figure 7.42 Clinical presentation of common musculotendinous rupture of long biceps tendon.

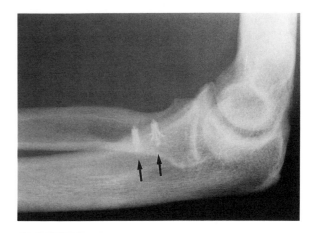

Figure 7.43 Distal biceps tendon repair to radial tuberosity area or to tendon stub by elevating cortical trapdoor or by distributing force through use of subcortical anchor.

the depressor function of the biceps tendon. This superior pull will gradually increase erosion through the medial wall of the bicipital groove and start another cycle of subluxation and bicipital tendon involvement. Neurologic involvement, including cervical radiculopathy, thoracic outlet syndrome, or brachial plexopathy, all of which can be associated with subluxation around this area, and scarring or stretching of nerves in the injury process must also be ruled out.

Management

Management of acute subluxation of the biceps tendon out of the groove means immediate surgery for stabilization, although late repair usually is found effective by the same surgical technique (Figure 7.44, a-c). The biceps tendon is placed back in the groove, the transverse humeral ligament is shortened, and the upper edge of the subscapularis is reattached to the freshened bone in this area to stabilize the tendon.

An anchor or subcortical fixation is useful, although suture through bone is just as effective. Of course, the underlying cause of bicipital subluxation has to be assessed. If a factor such as rotator cuff tearing or subcoracoid impingement led to avulsion of the intact biceps tendon out of the groove, it could be corrected by repair of the coracohumeral suspension system and subscapular erosion superiorly. More commonly the symptom of pain radiating down the biceps is associated with superior labral avulsion or SLAP lesion. In this case, the present procedure of choice is reanchoring the SLAP lesion anteriorly and posteriorly after curettage of the superior cortex of bone and arthroscopic advancement of the superior glenohumeral ligament (see Figure 6.38 in chapter 6).

When a SLAP lesion or bicipital subluxation is found in conjunction with other capsular laxity, an open capsular tightening should be done concurrently. When rotator cuff tear or wear leading to increased force on the biceps tendon seems to be associated with the pain, then cuff repair or imbrication may be the treatment of choice. Concurrent manipulation and evaluation under anesthesia at the beginning of such a treatment can break scars significantly within the bicipital tunnel and help the gliding of the tendon. Unfortunately, these injuries frequently are not recognized, primarily because soft tissue detail is not well demonstrated on plain X-ray films.

If the biceps tendon is avulsed, either at the musculotendinous junction or off the top of the labrum, open repair techniques do not work well; for cosmesis it is best to anchor the biceps tendon into the bicipital groove, if there is enough tendon substance to do this. With loss of humeral head depression, rupture of the proximal tendon at the musculotendinous junction or within the muscle belly itself is in effect an irreparable lesion, decreasing strength ultimately by about 18%, which is usually acceptable in recreational athletes. Other factors that will maintain the humeral head in place, such as stability or repairing the rotator cuff, should be the focus of treatment instead. These factors will not make the motion or stability of the shoulder normal, however. Decelerating glenohumeral arthritis or wear of the cuff by acromioplasty or distal clavicular resection is the primary goal.

Complications

The major complication in the treatment of bicipital tendon injury is the inability to diagnose the underlying problem, which can lead to secondary bicipital inflammation. Evaluation and manipulation under anesthesia, including palm-up abduction and forward flexion, and an arthroscopic analysis in conjunction with a physical examination will help to identify the underlying problems. One complication of reattaching a biceps tendon stub into a keyhole in the bicipital groove for cosmesis is that its function of depressing the humeral head remains lost; trading a scar on the front of the arm for a bump may not lead to any functional improvement and may allow continued wear of the humeral head. Occasionally in surgery to repair the underlying laxity of the capsule, to reattach the tendon of the subscapularis for stability, or to tighten the tendon near the coracohumeral ligament, an inflammatory condition can occur within the bicipital sheath and symptoms will be aggravated.

Prognosis

With avulsion of the biceps tendon, the humeral head depressor function of the long biceps tendon is lost. A pull on the biceps producing a SLAP lesion leads to an injury that will not heal on its own because of the poor blood supply to the labrum; such lesions warrant an attempt at arthroscopic repair, or debridement if stable. Leaving a lesion of this type alone will limit the patient's ability to reach overhead, to exercise with weights, or even to use vibrating tools, impact devices, and torque wrenches at work.

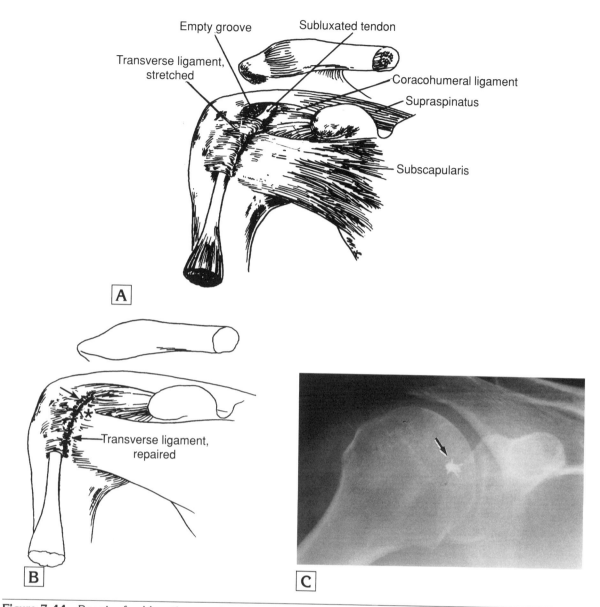

Figure 7.44 Repair of subluxating proximal long biceps tendon.

[A] Pathology.

[B] The transverse humeral ligament is tightened and, along with the superior edge of subscapularis tendon, anchored to the freshened superior edge of the lesser tuberosity to recreate a medial buttress.

[C] Radiographic position of suture anchor.

If the tendon needs to be reanchored within the bicipital groove, it should be done quickly; otherwise progressive erosion across the superior edge could lead to progressive tearing of the biceps, particularly if osteophytes develop. Surgical management would be the cautious approach before returning the patient to sport. If a repair is done, soft tissue needs to heal; if repair is done for a concurrent Bankart lesion, the athlete may be out of activity for 6 months to a year. Strength must be regained prior to the return to sports. Proper throwing mechanics must be established through proper coaching and motion analysis, and if it has taken some time to identify the problem, muscle weakness will have to be overcome. This may end a competitive athlete's career, but most likely he or she may return to recreational sports with time.

If the superior anchor of the biceps tendon is not repaired at the time of capsular stabilization, long-term problems may result: Superior laxity may progress, erosion into the biceps may develop, and outright avulsion of the tendon at the superior labrum may eventually occur. Progressive subluxation into the joint may cause wearing near the subscapularis and make repair more difficult. Failure to recognize the underlying subluxation or rotator cuff pathology may lead to less effective management of the underlying problem in the long run and thus to progressive dysfunction.

Cost Containment

Costs can be contained by avoiding expensive tests such as an MRI or bone scan. Ultrasound can be used as an effective screening technique if the radiologist has considerable experience, but do not rely on the results of such a test if the radiologist is still within the learning curve, generally less than 50 cases.

Patient Education

If the patient has pain as he or she reaches in front of the body in horizontal flexion and internal rotation and does not respond to internal and external rotation exercises, then he or she must be made aware that surgery is a method of treatment. Arthroscopically introduced absorbable rivets or implants will help anchor the superior mechanism for most of these injuries, leading to recovery in 8 weeks following acute injury. If there is subluxation out of the bicipital groove, open surgery and repair of associated problems, such as partial avulsion of the subscapularis or glenohumeral instability, should be undertaken before erosion and tearing of the bicipital tendon lead to a more unsatisfactory result. For an older athlete in the late 60s or 70s, for whom strength above horizontal flexion may not be that important, conservative management of the associated rotator cuff tear may be effective if the athlete is willing to limit postoperative overhead activity.

Prevention

There is no effective means of prevention of bicipital tendon lesions other than keeping the shoulder strong and flexible. If primary subluxation and rotator cuff pathology can be avoided, so can secondary involvement of the biceps tendon. The postsurgical patient must be fully rehabilitated before attempting to return to sport.

Other Strains

Muscles about the shoulder other than those previously discussed can be injured, but such injuries are relatively rare. Identifying them is important, however, because early treatment is the only effective way of trying to return to full capacity; late treatment with more than limited results is almost impossible in most cases. If muscles are not properly stretched, they may avulse or tear on sudden trauma, such as a parachute cord contusion at the front of the biceps or rupture of the pectoralis muscle when jerking a weight. One major problem with superficial muscles about the shoulder is that bleeding can cause a tense hematoma so that a palpable structural gap may initially go unrecognized. Strength testing, aspiration of clot, and selective injection may be useful to avoid problems in diagnosis.

The following muscle injuries are discussed in decreasing order of frequency; all are rare. A high index of suspicion is mandatory, and history and clinical examination are the first lines of defense. These types of injuries are not preventable, so patient education should emphasize early repair or reconstruction before muscle atrophy and fibrosis jeopardize results.

Pectoralis Major

Pectoralis major injuries are rare. They occur in arm wrestling, weight training, and hockey. In the author's limited experience, injuries to the pectoralis major in arm wrestling tend to occur in individuals who lose their match. Body builders tend to sustain their avulsion when the bar is off balance. Either there is a sudden pull on one side, which leads to avulsion from the bone, or the bar contacts a tense muscle, which leads to musculotendinous junction injury; inevitably, the spotter is blamed for the injury. Body builders may decline surgery, stating that they do not want a surgical scar, until the hematoma resolves and the deformity is more defined, at which point surgery is not as successful. It is not uncommon to see athletes with only partial tearing, and tenderness with no outright avulsion at the insertion into the lateral lip of the bicipital groove.

One jogger who was referred after being hit by a car was noted to have complete avulsion of the clavicular and costosternal pectoralis origins, which was repaired at time of thoracotomy by the thoracic surgeon. Tenderness at the distal insertion was not accompanied by a palpable defect and was treated conservatively.

Pectoralis major injuries generally occur in young athletes between the ages of 18 and 35. The athlete usually complains of an audible pop and a sudden traumatic avulsion near the humerus. He or she may not initially feel a defect, and ecchymosis may develop within the first 20 minutes or up to 72 hours. There is usually a palpable defect or visual abnormality interfering with the normal axillary web, but this may be gone as soon as hematoma develops; the hematoma may hide the defect. Affected patients have complained of inability to do wide-grip bench pressing or internal rotation of the arm in dumbbell work.

X-rays are not helpful; however, ultrasound can help define the hematoma, and fine point ultrasound as used in obstetrics can actually reveal whether the rupture is partial or total. MRI has been found useful to distinguish tears at the bony insertion, which are repairable, from tears at the musculotendinous junction or within the muscle itself, for which surgical repair is not that effective.

Partial ruptures are best managed with rest and sling immobilization for 2 weeks. This should be followed by passive and then active motion and then by gradual internal rotation strengthening. Although late surgery can be done, early surgical repair gives the best results. Not all tendon injuries can be repaired, or repair might not hold up, because the tendon is short and musculotendinous tears will not hold a suture well. Multiple sutures and an elevated flap to bury soft tissue, subcortical anchors rather than multiple drill holes, or a combination of these techniques can lead to a successful surgical result (Figure 7.45). Fine point ultrasound can help define the actual injury pattern and with luck avoid unsuccessful surgical attempts.

Triceps

Triceps injuries generally occur in body builders, who in general are a very difficult group to treat. Some tend not to follow postoperative instructions. Triceps injuries seem to have a high correlation with the use of anabolic steroids. At the time of surgery, avulsion of the tip of the olecranon or associated soft tissue leaves retraction from 0 to 7.5 cm proximally.

One individual who had won the Mr. Universe contest 4 months earlier brought in a beautiful MRI that disclosed a 7.5-cm retraction proximally and good definition of muscle tissue (the same information could be obtained with a routine X-ray; Figure 7.46). This was repaired through a 2-cm incision by pulling the bony stub down to its previous insertion, anchoring it with absorbable suture, and closing subcuticularly. He took the extension cast off at 2 weeks at the recommendation of a friend, who had gone through a biceps repair some years before, and returned to exercise. This patient

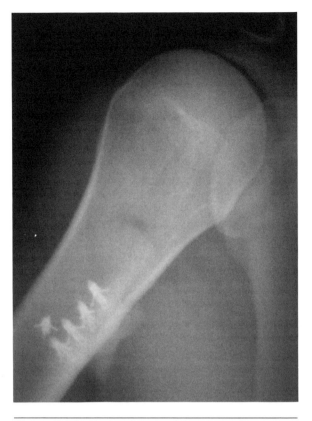

Figure 7.45 Reattachment of the pectoralis major through a cortical trapdoor with anchoring rivets enhances the chance of healing of an avulsed short tendon in a professional hockey player.

placed within the top 10 in the Mr. Universe competition the following year.

An individual who previously held the America Cup body building title was treated for an acute distal triceps avulsion, kept the cast on for 4 weeks with a removable night cast after that, and returned to training at approximately 6 weeks (Figure 7.47).

One individual who avulsed his triceps insertion at the elbow attempted to rehabilitate the arm, which had no strength in extension, for 1-1/2 years before seeing a physician. He was promptly referred to an orthopedist by his family doctor. This avulsion was repaired with an incision larger than those required in the cases above, and he regained essentially normal strength but lost considerable muscle definition after this prolonged detachment (Figure 7.48). Within a year he partially avulsed the opposite triceps at the elbow, and this was treated in a cylinder cast for 8 weeks. He was diagnosed as being in kidney failure 3 years later, although all lab studies had been essentially normal at the time of his surgical revision. He underwent kidney transplant, and 4 months later he returned to body building and the use of anabolic

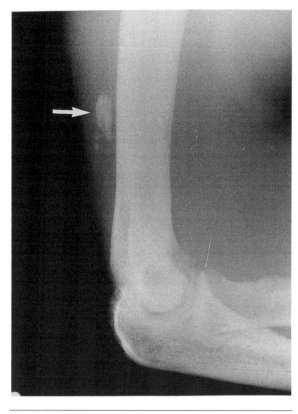

Figure 7.46 Distal triceps tendon insertion retracted proximally 7.5 cm, with fleck of bone, seen in X-ray.

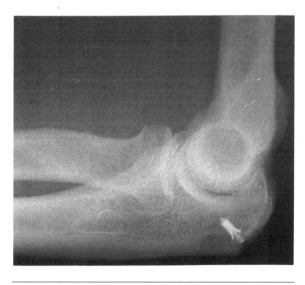

Figure 7.47 Reattachment of distal triceps to olecranon tip in professional body builder.

steroids, the suspected cause of both problems. Central necrosis of the tendon seen surgically at the time of repair in these cases also correlates with the use of anabolic steroids.

Partial rupture of the triceps insertion at the distal arm into the olecranon is best managed with

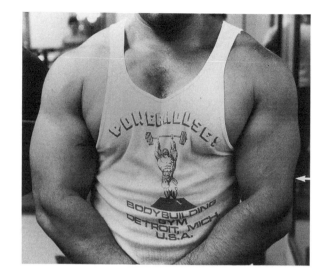

Figure 7.48 Late repair of distal triceps 1-1/2 years following injury allowed return of function and ability to weight train, yet bulk is permanently diminished.

cylinder cast fixation for 4 to 6 weeks. Total disruption is best managed with repair as soon as possible, with cylinder cast fixation for at least 6 weeks. After the initial immobilization, the patient is taken out of the cast and works on flexion on his or her own for an additional 4 weeks. At this time, physical therapy may be initiated if range of motion has not returned to normal. Most of these athletes will not undergo physical therapy and will quickly attempt to return to weight training.

Proximal avulsion of the triceps is even more rare (Figure 7.49). With one- or two-head involvement, overall function may not be much impaired. Musculotendinous injury or involvement of all three heads may not be a repairable injury.

X-ray and MRI are the best ways to assess triceps avulsion. If a bony block is obvious and soft tissue planes are well defined on X-ray, the MRI may not be necessary. The main complication is overlooking the lesion, because a hematoma may form. This oversight can be avoided by getting an X-ray and by having the patient attempt to push the examiner away with the elbow in a flexed position; inability to do so indicates a significant injury.

Subscapularis

Subscapularis avulsion is most commonly seen in body building, baseball, and arm wrestling. Trying to lift too heavy a dumbbell can force the arm into abduction and external rotation with a sudden avulsion of the subscapularis. If the athlete cannot actively bring the arm away from the body while it is behind the back, this is an ominous sign of

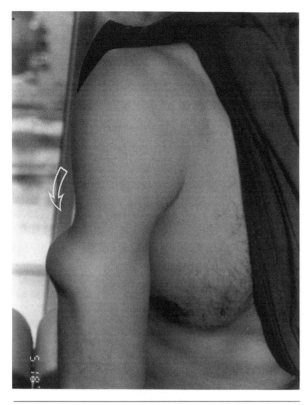

Figure 7.49 Clinical presentation of proximal triceps avulsion.

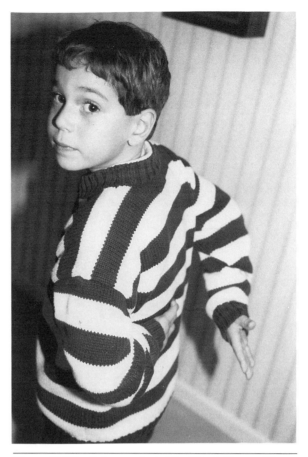

Figure 7.50 Subscapularis lift-off test. Normal function of an attached subscapularis is necessary to elevate the arm away from the body behind the back.

subscapularis disruption. Ability to lift the arm off the back indicates that the subscapularis is still intact (Figure 7.50). Repair of the subscapularis (Figure 7.51, a-c) generally allows return to activity, even weight training, in 3 to 4 months.

The author has treated two baseball players who sustained avulsion of the subscapularis tendon 1 to 2 years after surgical reconstruction of other shoulder problems. The first occurred following a Magnuson-Stack operation; the second, after a Bankart operation. The first occurred without obvious glenohumeral dislocation merely by having the athlete's arm pulled away from his body, and the second occurred with a new glenohumeral dislocation (Figure 7.52, a and b). Both were treated with a revision Bankart, the first with removal of staple and replacement of the subscapularis in its normal position.

One soccer player avulsed the subscapularis from under a staple 4 years following a Magnuson-Stack operation. He developed significant instability and unfortunately slipped in the hospital shower 2 days after revision surgery, avulsing the subscapularis and dislocating his shoulder again. He subsequently had a revision Bankart procedure and reattachment of the subscapularis and has had no problems for at least 10 years postoperatively.

One 15-year-old avulsed his lesser tuberosity while arm wrestling (Figure 7.53). He could not pitch overhand for 3 months afterward but declined surgical osteotomy and reimplantation, electing to give up pitching instead. Subcoracoid impingement symptoms remained.

Treatment of subscapularis rupture is acute surgical repair. Clinical examination may reveal significant hemorrhage in the front of the shoulder and always reveals considerable loss of power in internal rotation. History of previous surgery to the subscapularis, such as in anterior stabilization of the shoulder, may help in diagnosis.

Beware of considerable deficit in strength in internal rotation and a clinically subluxating shoulder. At time of the Bankart reconstruction (which is a layer-by-layer approach to help define pathologic conditions and to repair the conditions found) it is not uncommon to find the upper third to two thirds of the subscapularis avulsed. It is often avulsed under the fascia so that the subscapularis seems very thin. In this case the muscle itself

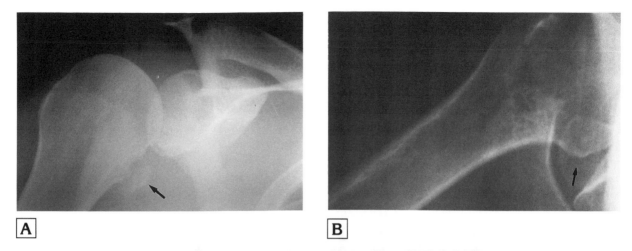

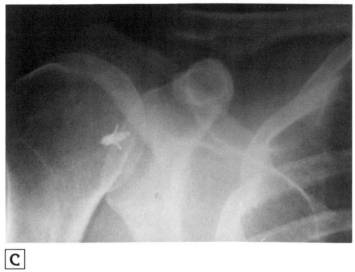

Figure 7.51 Avulsion of the subscapularis tendon can lead to anterior glenohumeral instability.

   [A] Lesser tuberosity avulsion with subscapularis strain.

   [B] Anterior instability is best assessed on axillary view.

   [C] Reattachment of subscapularis to lesser tuberosity with anchor following an acute injury in a body builder (Superanchor, Mitek, Norwood, MA).

must be advanced, reattached to the fascia, and repaired to regain strength and stability. Full function may return from 6 to 9 months following such surgical repair.

Conjoined Tendon

In the past 12 years, the author has treated only five significant injuries to the *conjoined tendon*. One was an iatrogenic release of the tendon apparently caused by harvesting the coracoid tip for an isolated bone block modification of a Bristow reconstruction, which generally moves the conjoined tendon and the bone block together. One injury was a partial strain without a palpable defect that was obtained by direct compression in a kick

boxer. Two were sustained in falls associated with concurrent glenohumeral dislocations, probably in the anterosuperior quadrant area, because coracoid fractures occurred. Musculocutaneous nerve dysfunction with paresthesia in the forearm was noted in both these individuals initially. The 57-year-old elected to leave this as it was and recovered 80% normal motion; although musculocutaneous sensation in the forearm has returned to normal, bicipital weakness persists. The 15-year-old, initially seen 5 months postinjury with fractures to both the coracoid and the anteroinferior third of the glenoid (rotated 180° on a hinge of labrum; Figure 7.54, a and b), responded to open reduction, internal fixation of the glenoid with absorbable pins, and a concurrent capsular stabili-

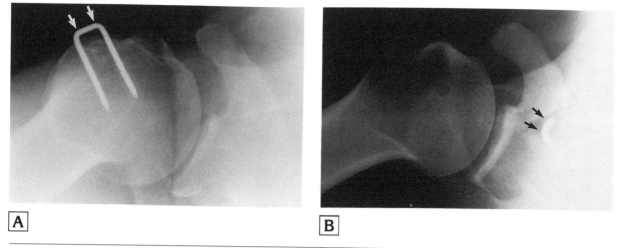

Figure 7.52

[A] Glenohumeral instability in abducted external rotation may be limited by Magnuson-Stack lateral transfer of subscapularis tendon fixed by metal staple.

[B] Motion returned as staple avulsed and migrated within soft tissue.

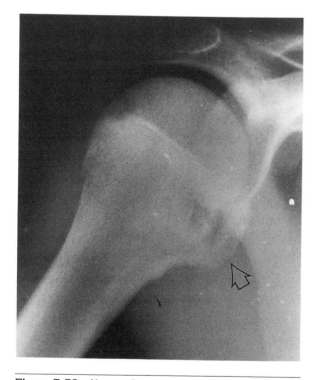

Figure 7.53 X-ray of an arm wrestling injury that led to avulsion of subscapularis tendon and associated lesser tuberosity and to malunion, interfering with the internal rotation and pitching ability of a 15-year-old male.

zation procedure, and was back to essentially full activity at 5 months.

A high jumper jamming his extended arm upward while landing had avulsed his conjoined tendon and sustained a SLAP lesion, effectively avulsing both heads of the biceps. This was repaired by arthroscopically reattaching the SLAP lesion with absorbable rivets (Figure 7.55, a and b) and concurrently making a skin incision to attach the conjoined tendon to the coracoid process with the use of a metal subcortical anchor (Figure 7.55c).

Considerable loss of internal rotation with a history of subluxation or dislocation of the glenohumeral joint and fracture of the coracoid either at the tip or the base may give evidence of conjoined tendon injury.

Serratus Anterior

Only one sports-related injury to the *serratus anterior* has been reported in the literature (Hayes & Zehr, 1981). This occurred in a 25-year-old all-terrain-vehicle rider, who sustained a displaced fracture of the inferior angle of the scapula when his vehicle rolled over. He was treated conservatively in a sling and was noted to have subscapular bursitis, easy fatigue, and winging of the scapula. At 9 months postinjury he underwent exploration, at which time both the rhomboids and the serratus anterior were found detached. The bone fragment was removed from the inferior scapula, and direct reattachment of these muscles to bone allowed him to return to full activity as a carpenter, reportedly without restriction.

Hematoma is commonly associated with underlying full disruption. This may cause one to suspect musculotendinous disruption, and further workup might include fine point ultrasound, CT, or

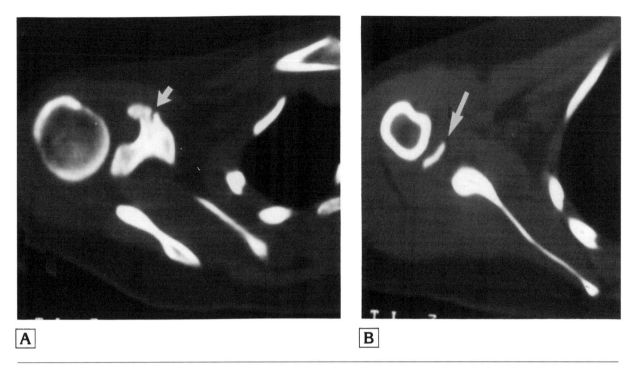

Figure 7.54 A 15-year-old with anterior dislocation into coracoid tip sustained partial avulsion of the conjoined tendon.

[A] Repair of tendon and fractured coracoid base by suture, seen in CT scan.

[B] Retrieval of one third of glenoid articular surface (arrow). Repair by absorbable pin fixation led to return of full function within 5 months (Orthosorb Absorbable Pin, Johnson & Johnson Orthopaedics, New Brunswick, NJ).

MRI. Early recognition and treatment will give best results. Delayed treatment is feasible but runs the risk of permanent atrophy, fibrosis, and compromised results.

Deltoid

Contusion injury to the *deltoid* muscle, which commonly occurs in football, leads to a temporary axillary nerve palsy, humeral subperiosteal hematoma, and occasionally a residual bony deformity, or "helmet exostosis," in spite of adequate padding. Contusion is best managed with early motion, icing, and progressive strengthening until the return to full activity.

The author has seen only one more-significant deltoid strain. The athlete was a runner who decided to race across the street in front of a bus while slightly intoxicated. He lost the race, and after 74 units of blood and repair of the subclavian artery, orthopedics was consulted in the operating room. A pelvic external fixator was applied, which immediately stopped the bleeding, an open Monteggia fracture was debrided and repaired at the elbow, and on removal of the drapes the extremely swollen lower extremities and right shoulder justified split-wick catheterization assessment

for compartment syndrome. The legs went through routine fasciotomy. The deltoid had a compartment pressure of over 110 mmHg, greater than 50 mmHg above diastolic, and a fasciotomy of the deltoid allowed evacuation of hematoma and investigation of muscle rupture. Sixteen weeks later the patient walked into the orthopedic office to schedule removal of the pelvic fixator and within 6 months of injury returned to jogging. No dysfunction of the deltoid was found. Iatrogenic deltoid avulsion can occur following rotator cuff repair or subacromial open decompression. This is difficult to attach and is best avoided. If attempt is made to reattach, subdeltoid adhesions must be released, and postoperative immobilization enforced.

Summary

Strain injury about the shoulder is perhaps the most common injury that occurs in the athlete. The supraspinatus is the tendon most often involved, with injury labeled as impingement. As is clearly seen in analysis of injury to the supraspinatus,

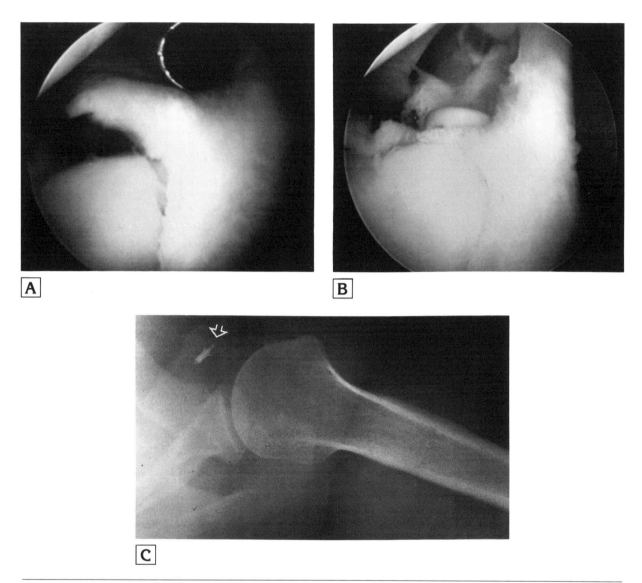

Figure 7.55 Avulsion of both heads of the biceps.

[A] Biceps long head detached at base as SLAP lesion.

[B] Repair of long biceps base by arthroscopic absorbable rivet fixation of SLAP lesion.

[C] Reattachment of the conjoined tendon and biceps tendon to the coracoid process assisted by a subcortical anchor (arrow).

strain injury about the shoulder is often a combination injury; instability and impingement commonly coexist. Treatment of one may not be effective without concurrent treatment of the other. Isolated muscle injuries about the shoulder are somewhat uncommon, because a complex balancing mechanism is necessary for effective athletic performance.

The key to effective management of shoulder strain injury is listening to the athlete's complaint. Examination must be tied to a thorough knowledge of anatomy and to an understanding of the activity in which the injury occurred. With these parameters in mind, effective treatment can be established.

Assessment and treatment of strain and sprain injury have been discussed in this and the preceding chapters. These long and detailed chapters have dealt with the most common use and overuse shoulder problems. Nevertheless, other injuries occur as well and will be discussed in the following chapters. Although these injuries are less common, the treating team must hold a high clinical suspicion of other causes in an effort to best assess the athlete's injury.

8

Fibrosis, Inflammation, and System Breakdown

There is a complex interrelationship among the structures of the shoulder. The *bursa*, fine striations of tissue directly under the acromion that project outward under the deltoid early in youth, will occasionally thicken but normally wear out under the acromion. The bursa under the acromion becomes an essentially separate compartment, isolated from the subdeltoid bursa by thickening of the peripheral walls at the edge of the acromion. Occasionally, the subacromial and subdeltoid areas are completely congested with scar. This bursal thickening is associated with disuse, diabetes, and cortisone injections. Fibrosis of the supraspinatus outlet will prevent the normal sliding of the supraspinatus under the acromion and A/C joint. Motion becomes abnormal. The patient starts to hike the shoulder by using the scapulothoracic mechanism instead, leading to periscapular muscle spasm or neck pain. The sternoclavicular joint may also be overused. Treatment must be geared toward the primary problem, that

is, subacromial fibrosis, in order to relieve the secondary overuse symptoms.

There is a broad category of what might be considered active or burnt-out inflammatory conditions about the shoulder that have been called periarthritis in the past but more correctly are labeled as conditions of the synovium, capsule, or bursae. These conditions include adhesive capsulitis, capsulitis, inflammatory capsulitis, supraspinatus syndrome, bicipital tendinitis, adhesive bursitis, calcific bursitis, bicipital tenovaginitis, calcific tendinitis, primary frozen shoulder, secondary frozen shoulder, stiff shoulder, and so on.

Histories of inflammatory or fibrotic conditions vary considerably. The athlete may complain of severe posterior shoulder pain immediately following a game, the day after a game, or interfering with performance during a game. He or she may have pain halfway into the game or after specific methods of throwing or other athletic motions. The exact mechanism is important, because the muscular imbalance leading to posterior or generalized joint inflammation should be identified. Inadequate flexibility and unbalanced musculature will lead to injury.

Because most of the conditions in this chapter concern soft tissue, very little can be demonstrated from plain X-rays. Of course, osteopenia from disuse can occur in any of these problems. Laboratory studies may be of some use in diagnosing inflammatory or fibrotic conditions and are limited to the rheumatoid panels: sed rate, rheumatoid factor, HLA B27, LE prep, and so on. These may define an underlying disease state that is not caused by the athletic endeavor but can hamper athletic performance. The patient presenting with bilateral spontaneous capsulitis should have lab work to rule out diabetes.

The relatively simpler clinical problems of synovitis, capsulitis, and bursitis will be dealt with first. The more advanced clinical presentations of levator scapulae syndrome, fibrositis, and variations of reflex sympathetic dystrophy syndrome will be dealt with later in this chapter.

In understanding advanced system breakdown, it is important to remember that all joints are linked together and work in concert to allow athletic performance (Nicholas, Grossman, & Hershman, 1977; Jackson & Ciullo, 1986) through a system of energy amplification (Ciullo & Zarins, 1983) and coordination of eccentric and concentric muscles. This coordination is accomplished through crossed-extensor and lagged reciprocal crossed-extensor reflexes. Through these reflexes, motion and sport activity become possible (Ciullo & Jackson, 1985). Muscular activity has energy needs that can be met only by an integrated circulatory mechanism that can deliver nutrients and eliminate waste products. When systems are caught out of phase, some structures may be overtaxed in an effort to compensate. Overuse and pain syndromes develop.

It is not uncommon that an athlete presenting with elbow pain in fact has restricted shoulder motion that has caused overuse at the elbow to compensate in activities like throwing. Due to the properties of linkage, an injury to the knee that restricts the motion needed for energy amplification in throwing can lead to overuse and breakdown of the shoulder. Restoring proper mechanics is the basis of rehabilitation and is necessary to help prevent pain syndromes and avoid reinjury.

Although athletes often ascribe to the "no pain, no gain" attitude, it is not uncommon to find pain well out of proportion to clinical findings in sports medicine. This is extremely common in injuries

about the shoulder, in which psychological factors may amplify symptoms considerably. Pain patterns influence active mobility and lead to system breakdown and overuse of secondary structures or of secondary muscle groups. Muscular pain syndromes thus involved have been labeled as conversion reaction, differential sympathetic dysfunction, enthesopathy, fibromyalgia, fibromyositis, fibrositis, levator scapulae syndrome, muscle knots, myofascitis, myofibrositis, nonrestorative sleep disorder, osteopenic disorder, pain amplification syndrome, polymyalgia rheumatica, polymyositis, pressure point syndrome, psychosomatic illness, reflex sympathetic dysfunction, reflex sympathetic dystrophy, shoulder-hand syndrome, Sjogren's syndrome, tension myalgia, and trigger point phenomenon, among other names. All these syndromes can probably be classified into seven main divisions that range from mostly mechanical in origin to physiopsychological involvement.

Synovitis

Pitchers and throwers are particularly prone to posterior inflammatory conditions about the shoulder. These conditions are most often due to overload of the short external rotators; the external rotators are weaker than the internal rotators and fatigue more quickly. Overload of the external rotators leads to anterior pulling without proper posterior balancing; synovial inflammation develops superiorly along the superior glenohumeral ligament, posterior joint capsule, and superoposterior glenoid labral rim (Figure 8.1). A traction phenomenon develops a partial rotator cuff tear just behind

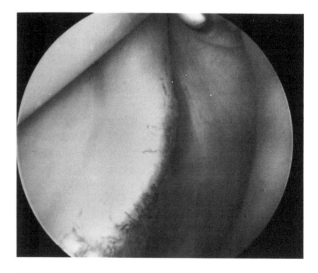

Figure 8.1 Arthroscopy through posterior portal shows synovitis and early glenoid rim osteophytic spur.

the entrance to the bicipital tunnel intra-articularly (Figure 8.2a), while a fibrous inflammatory response develops in the subacromial space extra-articularly (Figure 8.2b). This is the initiation of superior capsular laxity and is commonly associated with a SLAP lesion caused by unbalanced biceps pull. Concurrent synovitis along the posterior rim of the glenoid is also caused by traction phenomenon and external rotator fatigue. This synovitis, different from generalized synovitis, which occurs with early degenerative arthritis, may be aggravated by early rheumatoid disease and may not be caused by athletic activity. Synovitis may be due to chondral overload, as seen in racquetball and handball.

History

In the case of generalized inflammation there may be a history of a rheumatoid or nonrheumatoid variant disease, diabetes, or, very rarely in the athlete, septic arthritis. Loaded activity, such as handball or stopping oneself from falling while being tackled, can lead to shedding of articular cartilage and generalized synovitis. The athlete may volunteer history of a specific traumatic event.

Pathogenesis

Pitting erosion at the entheses, particularly near the humeral articular rim, can be seen radiographically with synovitis. A generalized synovitis is markedly different than the posterior synovitis

that develops from throwing overuse. *Generalized synovitis* tends to originate from irritation by chondral debris related to articular cartilage degeneration. *Posterior synovitis* is more a traction phenomenon caused by imbalance of internal and external rotators or superior mechanism disruption that leads to traction on the posterior capsule as the biceps pulls in one direction while the rotator cuff pulls in the opposite direction. Fraying of the rotator cuff may develop, which can irritate the bicipital tendon in its role of stabilizer and humeral head depressor. Inflammation about the bicipital tunnel, or tenosynovitis, can lead to degeneration of the bicipital tendon or to a generalized fibrotic pattern throughout the capsule, of which the bicipital tunnel is a part.

Synovitis, or generalized inflammation of the glenohumeral joint, can be confused with septic arthritis, initial synovial chondromatosis, pigmented villonodular synovitis, tumor, massive rotator cuff tear, and fracture of the greater or lesser tuberosities. X-ray to rule out fracture and bone scan to delineate synovial pattern versus septic arthritis or localized tendinitis pattern are often helpful in differential diagnosis.

Management

Initial immobilization is not advocated in any of the inflammatory or fibrotic conditions about the shoulder. It is important to keep mobility, either active or passive, to help prevent the loss of motion

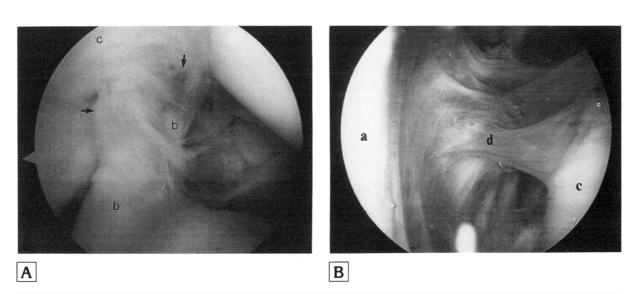

A **B**

Figure 8.2

   [A] Posterior arthroscopic view of a partial-thickness intra-articular traction cuff tear near bicipital tunnel.

   [B] Tear shown in [A] may lead to extra-articular subacromial fibrous ingrowth in an attempted healing process (a = acromion, b = biceps, c = cuff, d = adhesion to external cuff from bursal remnant).

associated with muscle atrophy and prolonged recovery. Generalized synovitis is treated with nonsteroidal anti-inflammatory drugs, gentle motion, and progressive strengthening. If there is no considerable response, then arthroscopic assessment and synovectomy are warranted. In the posterior synovial pattern, external rotation strengthening must first be sought and then balancing of internal and external rotation strength to depress the humeral head and prevent secondary impingement symptoms. When this is not successful, it is followed by arthroscopic assessment and minimal debridement of synovitis over the stretched superior glenohumeral ligament. A partially torn rotator cuff, any synovial inflammation of the anterosuperior or posterosuperior quadrants, and adhesions to the bicipital tendon should be resected. Early motion should be emphasized immediately afterward, progressing toward strengthening. Eight to 12 weeks of physical therapy is mandatory, and up to 6 months is not unusual prior to consideration for arthroscopic assessment or debridement.

Early on, active inflammation of the shoulder due to synovitis can be a self-limiting problem, but if left untreated or neglected, can lead to capsulitis and loss of motion or to a change in body mechanics such that secondary structures are overused and athletic performance impeded. The pitcher may start throwing more side-armed, and periscapular spasm of the levator scapulae and trapezius may become evident. The main problem in synovitis may be iatrogenic. Immobilization enforced by the physician can lead to an adhesive capsulitis.

With synovitis, the prognosis is good if early mobilization and nonsteroidal anti-inflammatory medication can be utilized. Again, it must be stressed to the primary care physician that immobilization can make the condition worse. Mild stretching progressing toward strengthening is the preferred course of treatment.

Capsulitis

Capsulitis may be perceived by the athlete as restriction of joint motion and may be due to capsular fibrosis. It is most common in athletes with diabetes and in recreational athletes, particularly in middle-aged female swimmers, tennis players, and cross-country skiers. Any restricted motion, either active or passive, is considered capsulitis. Capsulitis may be spontaneous, it may be due to repetitive microtrauma, or it may be a secondary result of a major traumatic event.

Diagnostic History

Capsulitis may follow a traumatic event such as subluxation due to capsular laxity or functional interposition. It may even follow self-enforced rest due to perceived problems in the shoulder, such as radiculopathy or referred pain from pectoralis strain or cardiopulmonary problems. It may also follow surgery.

Diagnostic Imaging

A break in Maloney's line (that is, the arch drawn from the undersurface of the humerus to the bottom of the glenoid) can occur when the humerus rides a few millimeters high in association with adhesive capsulitis or cuff tear. As the capsulitis resolves, the humeral head can regain its normal position on the anterior X-ray; this is seen even after manipulation or arthroscopic subdeltoid adhesion resection. In the initial inflammatory phase of capsulitis, a bone scan will be positive but will be negative as inflammation subsides. This differs from synovitis, in which there will be a generalized inflammatory pattern, or from the localized pattern near the greater tuberosity associated with tendinitis. An arthrogram demonstrating less than 10- to 12-mm filling capacity, loss of the axillary fold, and lack of filling of the subscapular bursa are pathognomonic for adhesive capsulitis (Figure 8.3).

Injury Classification

Capsulitis can be classified as either idiopathic or traumatic. The idiopathic type is usually unilateral,

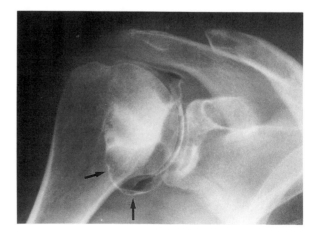

Figure 8.3 Arthrogram demonstrating decreased volume and loss of inferior pouch in adhesive capsulitis.

although 20% of those affected will subsequently develop stiffness of the opposite shoulder. If the patient is diabetic, there is greater than 70% incidence of subsequent contralateral involvement. Once the symptoms resolve they very rarely recur (Rizk, Christopher, Pinals, Higgins, & Frix, 1983). When bilateral stiffness exists, the physician must rule out systemic diabetes. There are three phases of nontraumatic, or idiopathic, capsulitis.

A *painful phase* initiates spontaneously and symptoms develop gradually. Like a rotator cuff tear, the pain is worse at night, and like an A/C joint problem, the pain is worse when sleeping on the affected shoulder. This phase may last from 2 to 9 months (Reeves, 1975).

The second stage is the *freezing phase*, which lasts from 2 to 10 months. The patient complains of inability to perform activities of daily living, including reaching into the back pocket, fastening a bra, or combing hair. There has been a considerable loss of motion, both glenohumeral and scapulothoracic, such that abduction is commonly limited to 40°. Horizontal flexion appears clinically to be primarily scapulothoracic motion (Figure 8.4, a and b). This is due primarily to bursal thickening, leading to fibrosis and adhesions between the scapular spine, rotator cuff, and deltoid. Secondarily, and actually less commonly, the glenohumeral capsule may be fibrotic.

The patient may have considerable difficulty reaching behind his or her back, with internal rotation limited to breaking the plane of the body or lower lumbar spine. Internal rotation is usually the first motion to go and the last to come back; however, some patients present with normal internal rotation but difficulty in abduction and pain with palm-up forward flexion. These patients usually have involvement of the bicipital tunnel as

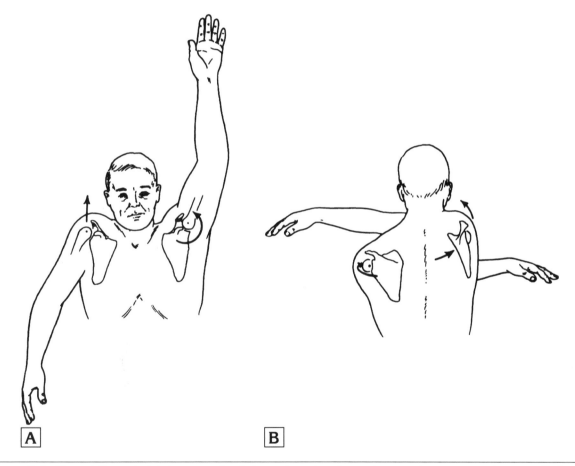

Figure 8.4 Scapulothoracic joint overuse leads to neck and periscapular muscle overuse and spasm. Rather than normal motion centered through the glenohumeral joint,

[A] scapulothoracic retraction is emphasized in abduction and

[B] scapulothoracic protraction is emphasized in horizontal flexion.

Scapulothoracic overuse is accompanied by pathology such as rotator cuff tearing, subacromial impingement, subdeltoid adhesions and adhesive capsulitis, labral interposition, SLAP lesions, or even A/C joint arthritis.

part of the capsulitis syndrome. The patient may complain that he or she can no longer serve overhead and is finding it more difficult to swing at the side in racquet sports.

The final idiopathic stage of capsulitis is that of *thawing*. With increased motion comes decreased pain. This stage ranges from a few weeks to over a year. In some cases, motion has not completely returned to normal, but over time, the patient perceives that he or she has much more motion than he or she actually is capable of exhibiting; the patient has learned to accommodate the loss of motion. After the stiffening stage the patient may have noted a slight difference that he or she feels is a great improvement.

Posttraumatic capsulitis differs from the idiopathic type in that the patient can usually identify an inciting event, such as a particular athletic overuse situation, the onset of bursitis, symptoms of A/C joint degeneration, a rotator cuff tear, contusion, or history of a fracture. Symptoms may also be traced to initiation of C-spine pathology or radiculopathy, recent surgery including breast or cardiac procedures, lymph node biopsy, localized chest or back muscle flaps, and so on. Immobilization, such as that following perceived shoulder pain associated with heart disease, can induce stiffness as well.

Differential Diagnosis

Capsulitis must be differentiated from synovitis as well as from shoulder dislocation, hemarthrosis, subacromial impingement, fibrositis, thoracic outlet syndrome, hyperparathyroidism, avascular necrosis, pancoast tumor, myocardial infarction, reflex esophagitis, diaphragmatic herniation, gallbladder disease, gastric ulcer, fibromyositis, osteopenia, suprascapular nerve palsy, shoulder-hand syndrome, reflex sympathetic dystrophy, or psychosomatic disorders. Careful examination, X-ray evaluation from at least two different planes (i.e., AP and axillary), sed rate, rheumatoid workup, blood panel, selective injections, and assessment in a pain clinic may be of some use.

Management

Capsulitis that does not respond to conservative management—using anti-inflammatory medication and passive motion advancing to active motion and then strengthening—will respond to endoscopic management. Manipulation under anesthesia, when necessary to regain motion, will break adhesions in the subacromial and subdeltoid spaces three times as often as rupturing the inferior intra-articular joint capsule (Figure 8.5).

Resection of peripheral scarring under the acromion (essentially bursal wall thickening that bridges the deltoid to the rotator cuff; Figure 8.6, a and b), and acromioplasty and A/C joint resection when indicated, are highly successful following manipulation under anesthesia. Arthroscopic debridement of the ends of adhesions helps to ensure that the shoulder does not scar again. The associated arthroscopy can help define the possibility of intra-articular pathology (a SLAP lesion, multidirectional instability, pigmented villonodular synovitis, etc.), which may have led to secondary fibrosis in the subacromial space. In late stages, the intra-articular joint capsule may need arthroscopic release.

After this manipulation and resection of tissue primarily in the subacromial space, the patient does well with return to the conservative management program (Table 8.1).

Although there is occasionally a considerable difference between passive and active motion in the capsulitis syndromes, early mild mobilization in physical therapy can possibly avoid the full-blown cycle of freezing then thawing stages. Failure to diagnose the actual cause of the scapular snapping or of the secondary scapulothoracic overuse may lead to prolongation of symptoms or even to inappropriate surgery.

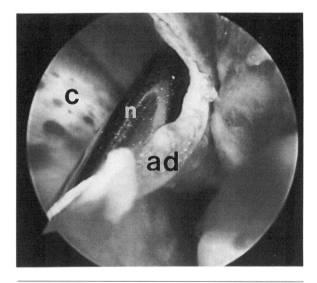

Figure 8.5 Subacromial bleeding due to breakage of subacromial adhesions, seen here through subacromial endoscopy, is three times as common as inferior intra-articular capsular rupture in management of capsulitis (c = cuff, n = A/C marking needle, ad = subacromial adhesion broken by preoperative manipulation).

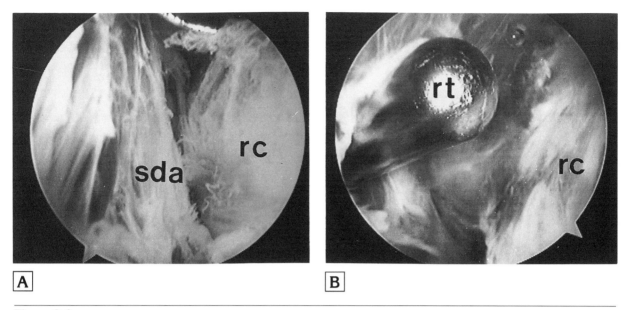

Figure 8.6

[A] Thickening of bursa can bridge the rotator cuff to both the subdeltoid fascia and subacromial surface, limiting motion (seen arthroscopically) and capturing the shoulder.

[B] After resection of adhesions, the gliding plane for motion of the supraspinatus muscle under the acromion is restored (seen through subacromial endoscopy), posterior shoulder pain is eliminated, and neck muscle spasm is usually gone (sda = subdeltoid adhesion, rc = rotator cuff/supraspinatus, rt = resecting tool).

As in synovitis, there is no role for total immobilization. The older theories that capsulitis may be a self-limiting problem that will resolve over 12 to 18 months are incorrect. Motion may be markedly limited in the long run, but the athlete's expectations may have changed: He or she may change sports or may decide that throwing more side-armed is acceptable. The athlete might also give up athletics or decrease the level of competition.

Capsulitis may be real or perceived. Regardless, lack of motion leads to muscle imbalance. This in turn leads to earlier fatigue, and the cycle of disuse is perpetuated. A significant restriction for more than 3 years is not uncommon if the condition is left untreated.

Subacromial Bursitis

For all practical purposes, what has been called *subacromial bursitis* is, in actuality, partial or complete tearing of the rotator cuff. The subacromial bursa loses its fine cross-striations between the two bursal walls by the time the average individual is 20 years old, or even 12 years old in competitive swimmers. Wear of muscle under the acromion and the inflammatory response cause pain.

Pathogenesis

In the attempted healing of a worn supraspinatus, peripheral remnants of the bursa are the origin of a vascular scar growing in to patch the eroded area. This scar is necessary for the healing process; however, as the scar matures it loses its blood and nerve supply and thickens. Over time, scar tissue developing from the back wall of the remaining bursa may build up and bridge the deltoid and rotator cuff, attaching the cuff to the back of the acromion or scapular spine (Figure 8.7, a and b). This scarring thickens the bursal wall and pulls the humeral head posterosuperiorly, restricting motion and capturing the shoulder. It also pulls the humeral head upward, increasing impingement, causing contracture, and leading to postural change and enforced overuse of the scapulothoracic joint to accommodate loss of the normal supraspinatus-subacromial sliding mechanism.

Diagnostic Imaging

Radiographic assessment of rotator cuff wear is limited to calcific changes in the rotator cuff tendons on plain X-ray, spotty inflammation demonstrating tendinitis on the bone scan, and changes generally associated with rotator cuff disease on arthrogram or MRI.

Table 8.1 Rehabilitation Program Following Manipulation and Arthroscopic Debridement for Stiff Shoulder

Preoperative

Physical therapy for range of motion progressing toward strengthening in an attempt to avoid surgery or to teach postoperative program. Continue until plateau using TENS, but avoid ultrasound.

Consider manipulation under neurogenic block for 1 to 5 sessions; follow with physical therapy if mobilized.

If patient is diabetic, emphasize weight loss and tight glucose control preoperatively.

Day 0-4

Arthroscopic debridement of peripheral adhesions through the supraspinatus outlet, protruding bony spurs or A/C arthritis, and intra-articular synovitis; inject with Marcaine.

Wake up in recovery with wrist immobilized above head postoperatively until patient realizes position. Ice bag on shoulder.

Arm lowered and placed in ice cuff and sling. Ice q. 6-8 hours times 3 days.

Out of sling first postoperative day.

Start physical therapy on day 1-4, 5 times a week for 2 weeks, then 3 times a week for 6 weeks, for full, immediate, passive, supine forward flexion and external rotation with arm at the side. Advance to active motion.

Weeks 2-6   Strengthening

As active motion progresses, continue passive motion, start internal and external rotation strengthening with elbow at side, and increase strengthening in abduction as tolerated.

Consider deltoid myostimulation if motion above 90° has been restricted longer than 6 months.

Weeks 6-16   Endurance and maintenance

Continue strengthening, balancing internal and external rotation, and passive-to-active flexibility exercises.

Continue strengthening of both shoulders to prevent recurrence in affected shoulder and to prevent similar symptoms in opposite shoulder.

Return to recreational activity such as golf when strength deficit less than 20% at the side and 30% overhead. Emphasize maintenance program to prevent atrophy, recurrence of stiffness on ipsilateral side, or stiffness on opposite side.

Management

Rotator cuff wear is best treated as described in chapter 7 for rotator cuff tendinitis. Since inflammatory tendinitis in the subacromial area is commonly associated with subluxation, the underlying laxity problem must be treated first. Just as in subscapular bursitis (discussed next), the primary condition must be sought and dealt with effectively.

When this is done, the secondary bursitis commonly disappears. If fibrosis in the subacromial area, a change in biomechanics, or the presence of calcific or fibrous densities under the scapula persists after treatment of the primary problem, then they may need to be dealt with secondarily. They may also be treated concurrently with the primary condition.

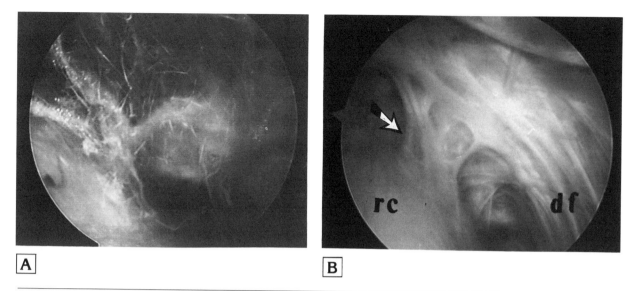

Figure 8.7

[A] Subacromial endoscopy showing normal, wispy, interplanar subdeltoid tissue (bursa).

[B] Scar build-up in the subdeltoid area bridges deltoid to rotator cuff, thus limiting motion; this scarring can be resected endoscopically or broken with manipulation (arrow = bridging adhesions, rc = rotator cuff, df = deltoid fascia).

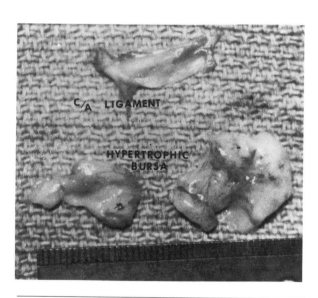

Figure 8.8 Acute swelling and inflammation is extremely rare but was found and resected in a 15-year-old swimmer; symptoms without swelling more commonly arise from erosion into the rotator cuff.

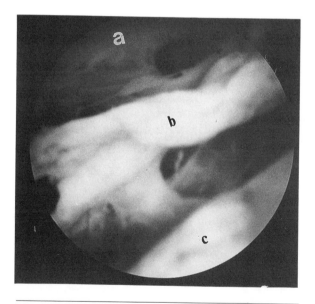

Figure 8.9 Wispy tissue under the acromion wears away early in life; occasionally thick bands remain or are secondary to hemorrhage, causing snapping, friction, and pain (a = acromion, b = bursal band, c = cuff).

Again, what has been described as subacromial bursitis (Figure 8.8) essentially is lesions of the rotator cuff, either partial or full thickness, which may be irritated by subacromial thickenings of tissue or bursal bands (Figure 8.9). Treatment of rotator cuff tendinitis was discussed in chapter 7.

Subscapular Bursitis

Subscapular bursitis, unlike "subacromial bursitis," does exist and is caused by overuse of the scapulothoracic joint to protect one of the other components of the shoulder. It is common after clavicular fracture with or without malunion or after A/C joint trauma with or without arthritis, and is seen with restricted motion of the glenohumeral joint due to arthritis, arthrofibrosis, subluxation, or soft tissue or loose body interposition. Any of these conditions can lead to overuse of the scapulothoracic joint and subsequent breakdown of the associated lubricating bursae. This has been called "washboard syndrome," scapulothoracic bursitis, and subscapular bursitis. It can also occur post-traumatically, as from scapulothoracic compression from a backpack or shoulder contusion when falling in the pit while pole vaulting or high jumping.

The athlete may remember a specific event that led to subscapular crepitation, such as a fall directly onto the scapula, compression to the scapula from athletic equipment such as shoulder pads or a backpack, or being hit in the back by a hammer, a shot, or a ball. More frequently the athlete will not remember the exact event but may remember a preexisting problem of the shoulder that eventually led to subscapular joint overuse.

Diagnostic Imaging

Subscapular bursitis has no particular identifying findings other than rare, small osteochondromas seen on the subscapular surface on the lateral X-ray film (Figure 8.10) or nodular thickening at the superomedial angle or inferior scapular tip (Figure 8.11). In particular, MRIs and CT scans have not been found useful in assessment of this disease.

Classification

Milch (1950) classified subscapular bursitis or snapping scapula in three categories. *Froissemant*

is an asymptomatic, physiologic, frictional sound of subscapular tissue, the result of normal, physiologic, muscular activity. *Froittemant* is a grinding or snapping sound that may or may not be pathologic. *Craquemont*, a loud snapping sound, is most frequently associated with pain and is considered pathologic. Fine crepitation is common, whereas the loud snapping noises are extremely rare.

Differential Diagnosis

The differential diagnosis of snapping scapula includes all types of referred pain. It is not uncommon that a SLAP lesion, labral fraying, or even A/C joint arthritis can produce a snapping in horizontal flexion and hyperabduction that is transmitted through the acromion and scapular spine to the medial or inferior angle of the scapula. Partial rotator cuff tear, subacromial bursal adhesions, and step-off fracture at the greater tuberosity can cause similar findings. Pain posteriorly may not be directly related to the snapping phenomenon, but rather to periscapular and posterior neck muscle spasm from peripheral overuse caused by trying to protect against or avoid use of damaged central structures: glenohumeral joint, acromio-

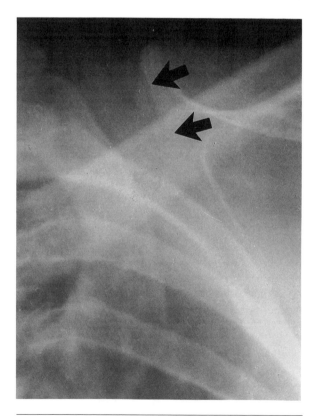

Figure 8.11 Spurs at superomedial or inferior tip of the scapula can cause subscapular irritation.

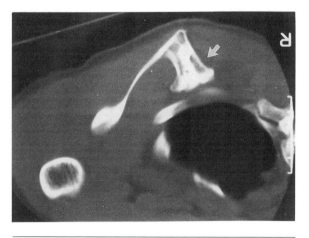

Figure 8.10 Osteochondroma irritating the ribs and causing snapping scapula, seen in radiograph.

clavicular joint, or supraspinatus sliding mechanism. Cervical radiculopathy, thoracic radiculopathy, and scapular tumor must be ruled out.

Management

Treatment of snapping scapula depends on accurate diagnosis. Because so many pathologic conditions about the shoulder can transmit noise to the scapula, the etiology must be sought. Also, breakdown of the subscapular bursae is most commonly a secondary phenomenon occurring with scapulothoracic overuse that develops to protect one of the other joints or mechanisms involved with shoulder motion. The primary cause must be dealt with and eliminated prior to attempted management of the secondary effect, snapping scapula. By eliminating the primary cause, the symptomatic snapping is usually relieved. Gentle mobilization, strengthening of the periscapular muscles, and iontophoresis or phonophoresis to the medial angle of the scapula with the arm behind the back in the "chicken wing position" is usually successful (Table 8.2). A localized injection of pain killer or cortisone is very rarely helpful.

Occasionally a stress or posttraumatic fracture of a rib, or even a fracture of the scapular body (Figure 8.12), may produce a step-off deformity that may need to be resected surgically to remove the snapping phenomenon. If an obvious cause of snapping, such as an osteochondroma (Figure 8.13, a and b), frictional wear (Figure 8.14, a and b), or a dog-eared type of change at the superomedial scapula (Figure 8.15) can be identified, then it can be resected as well.

If snapping continues with no obvious cause, arthroscopic assessment of the glenohumeral joint followed by subscapular endoscopy can be considered (Ciullo, 1986a). Resection of adhesions very similar to the fibrous bands occasionally found in the subacromial bursa can be accomplished endoscopically (Figure 8.16, a-c). Bony spurs and bursal thickening, particularly at the inferior angle, can be resected. Vibrating equipment and repetitive impact in this area should be subsequently avoided. The preoperative physical therapy plan is also followed postoperatively.

Open subperiosteal dissection and debridement of the superomedial or inferior angles of the scapula have been described, but they have limited success when the snapping scapula is secondary to other shoulder pathology.

Subacromial snapping is a real entity but is usually secondary to other shoulder pathology, particularly in the central shoulder: the glenohumeral

Table 8.2 Therapy Program for Subscapular Bursitis

Postural retraining
to bring shoulder blade back

The use of a clavicular strap may be beneficial for both positioning and therapeutic strength training.

Flexibility

Horizontal flexion and hyperabduction stretching to mobilize the A/C joint and to stretch out the posterior capsule and adhesions in order to reemphasize glenohumeral rotation.

Neck and trunk rotational stretching with iontophoresis to the superomedial angle of the scapula or with heat to decrease muscle spasm.

Muscular strengthening

Internal or external rotation strength deficit defined by isokinetic test.

Periscapular muscle strengthening.

Neck and trunk rotational strengthening.

The use of a figure-8 clavicular strap to assist posture or a bite prosthesis may be necessary with temporomandibular joint symptoms.

Neuromuscular retraining

Scapulohumeral rhythm, emphasizing proper use of the glenohumeral joint and deemphasizing periscapular muscles.

Internal and external rotation strengthening continue, keeping shoulder blades back. Teach exercises that must continue following discharge from therapy.

Proprioceptive neuromuscular facilitation exercises; closed and open kinetic chain exercises below horizontal plane progressing toward upper range. Advance to plyometric stretching for throwing activity.

Return to sport

Advance to a home exercise program emphasizing correct posture, normal scapulohumeral rhythm, and strength balancing.

Return to recreational sport or training program once the preceding is accomplished; work with a club pro, trainer, or coach in proper biomechanics of the sport.

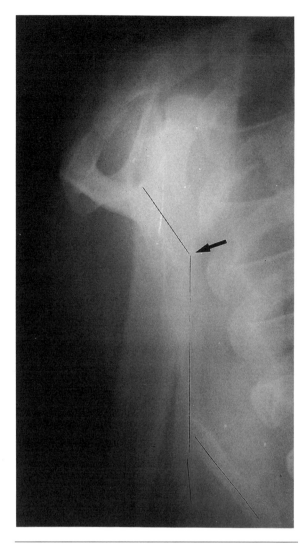

Figure 8.12 Malunion of a scapular fracture sustained in motocross competition led to painful subscapular snapping.

joint, the A/C joint, or the supraspinatus sliding mechanism, all leading to peripheral scapulothoracic overuse. If the underlying cause of the inflammatory or adhesive state can be identified and treated, there is a higher probability of an acceptable result.

Levator Scapulae Syndrome

It is not uncommon that the athlete perceives neck pain as the major problem after a shoulder injury. In actuality, he or she may be avoiding use of the central shoulder: the glenohumeral joint, the acromioclavicular joint, and subacromial sliding mechanism. The surrounding musculature of the scapulothoracic joint is overused to aid in abduction and elevation of the arm. Overuse of the secondary muscles leads to breakdown of these muscles, which are intended to help out rather than act as primary movers. It is not unusual for the athlete to complain of pain from the superomedial angle of the scapula to the base of the neck, and not of shoulder pain at all (Estwanic, 1989).

Physical Examination

Palpation causing pain and identifying muscular spasm along the course of the levator scapulae, most frequently with associated tenderness along the insertion of the rhomboid major and minor, identifies the *levator scapulae syndrome*. Here, the accessary shoulder elevators have been overused, leading to significant pain and even headaches that are usually unilateral and periauricular. Muscle biopsy defines no abnormality. If the condition is left alone, protective decreased use of the central core, leading to further overuse of the accessory periscapular muscles and eventually to pericapsulitis, will accelerate the overall condition.

Even though the athlete may consider the problem to be neck pain, when asked he or she may remember previous trauma to the shoulder. On physical examination, apprehension or impingement findings with tight posterior capsular fibers are not uncommon. Loss of internal rotation and protraction of the scapula with horizontal flexion rather than glenohumeral rotation are exhibited.

Imaging

X-rays of the neck are usually negative; however, X-rays of the shoulder may define osteopenia from disuse, bony avulsion injury due to subluxation, or slight superior migration of the humeral head due to infra-acromial and subdeltoid fibrosis related to rotator cuff pathology. This condition has been called *trigger point phenomenon* and *myofascitis*. Cervical radiculopathy, apical lung tumors, and scapular winging must be ruled out; however, underlying shoulder pathology is often uncovered by physical examination or diagnostic tests such as CT-arthrogram, ultrasound, bone scan, or arthroscopy.

Management

The best way to manage levator scapulae syndrome is by gentle mobilization (i.e., regaining motion first passively then actively), regaining posture, gradually increasing muscular tone, and progressing toward a home maintenance program.

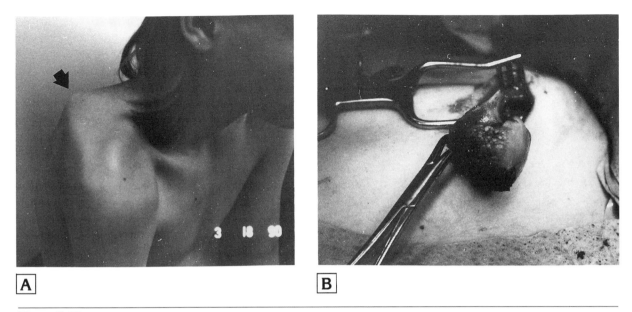

Figure 8.13

[A] Osteochondroma lifting scapula medially, limiting subscapular slide and motion (same patient as in Figure 8.10).

[B] Lesion in same patient removed through 2-cm incision; open procedure takes less times than endoscopic removal.

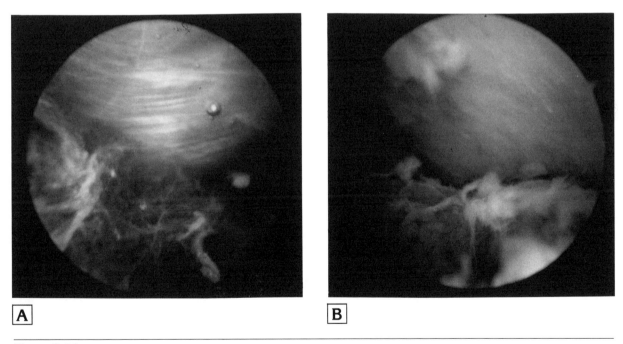

Figure 8.14

[A] Subscapular endoscopy shows normal superomedial angle of periosteum.

[B] Subscapular endoscopy shows worn periosteum and fibrous build-up with subscapular bursitis.

Heavy weights and isokinetic activities like Cybex and Biodex must be avoided. Nonsteroidal anti-inflammatory medication is useful. If sleep disorders occur, a very short course of low-dose Valium, Flexeril, or Elavil may be useful when heat alone is not sufficient to relieve muscle spasm. Ultrasound should be avoided because it can potentially increase fibrosis and make the problem worse. Iontophoresis is often more useful as an adjuvant modality. Increasing aerobic capacity,

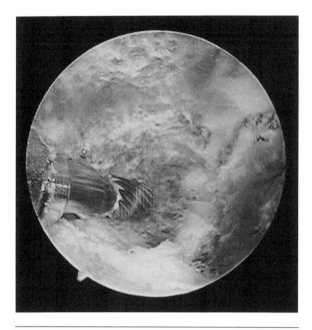

Figure 8.15 Subscapular endoscopic resection of superomedial angle spur.

endurance, and overall fitness helps diminish return of symptoms.

Full mobility, flexibility, and strengthening, along with proper body mechanics, can allow the athlete to return to activity in a relatively short period of time, 2 to 16 weeks. The athlete should not return to sport without having achieved full motion and strength and without having been tutored in proper body mechanics.

Fibrositis

When the athlete has wide-spread muscular spasm about the shoulder and aching with no apparent cause, he or she may have *fibrositis*. This condition has also been labeled fibromyalgia and trigger point phenomenon, among other names. According to the American College of Rheumatology, at least 7 of 14 commonly identified tender points must be identified by palpation (Table 8.3; Smythe, 1981).

History

Pain during sleep is chronic in this condition, and along with almost constant stiffness is a complaint of fatigue on awaking in the morning. Intolerance to cold or to weather change and stress associated with the problem are commonly reported. Morning stiffness is not made better with activity.

Management

X-rays are not useful, and although structural changes may occur about the shoulder, they are less common than in the levator scapulae syndrome because psychological factors play a more dominant role. Elavil, Flexeril, or Dolobid may be of use along with gentle stretching and increased aerobic exercise; however, the patient almost universally requests the use of strong pain medication that should not be prescribed.

Psychological overlay is integral to this syndrome. Pain is well out of proportion to clinical findings, especially in young athletes. Psychological stress caused by pressure from coaches and parents as well as from oneself can modify symptoms. Such stress is not uncommon in high school athletes, particularly females. The young swimmer who has been transported from tournament to tournament by her parents (who believe that *they* have worked hard toward a college swimming scholarship) may have goals considerably different from her parents'. She may be tired of the 7500M work-outs twice a day and would rather spend time on her social life. This leads to an array of complaints that far outweigh physical findings. Relieving stress on the shoulder has little to do with anti-impingement exercises. Family counseling may be more important than orthopedic intervention.

Reflex Sympathetic Dystrophy Syndrome

When the athlete complains that he or she no longer can participate in sport activity because of edema, temperature sensitivity, discoloration or blotchiness, stiffness, burning, or hyperesthesia of an upper extremity, he or she is characterizing *reflex sympathetic dystrophy*. Due to blotchiness and edema, which seem to be related to temperature, it appears as if the muscle tone and vascular flow are out of phase. At this point, the patient may have pain greater than physical findings would seem to warrant. These findings have been labeled as conversion reaction, causalgia, or psychosomatic illness in the past.

The patient may recall an inciting event; however, the event is most often so trivial that it is hard to understand the end-stage results. One jogger lost her running partner and had difficulty coping with her children going off to college. When she later stubbed her toe in a local department

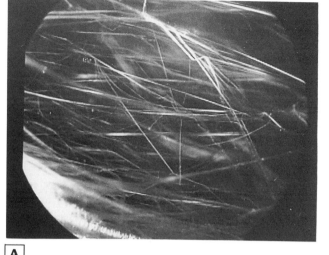

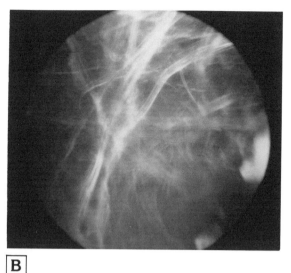

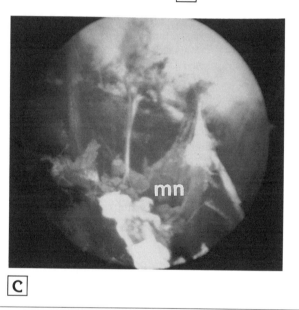

Figure 8.16

[A] Subscapular endoscopy shows normal, wispy, interplanar tissue of subscapular bursa.

[B] Thickened subscapular bands causing crepitation can be resected endoscopically.

[C] Wispy, bursal tissue eroded away and muscle partially eroded due to increased subscapular friction related to postural change; endoscopic resection eliminates crepitation but postural retraining must follow (mn = myonodular necrosis).

store, she developed pain in one leg that was so bad that she eventually requested amputation. The loss of the ability to jog was the basis of her documented reflex sympathetic dystrophy and of her $8 million settlement against the retail shopping chain.

There is no easily identifiable neurologic deficit in reflex sympathetic dystrophy except for increased sympathetic tone, which is not well understood. Laboratory tests are of little value. Thermograms can show significant differences of temperature from side to side, as can temperature probes, which demonstrate a greater than 2° difference in this condition. A triphase bone scan with an early asymmetric flush on one extremity but not the other is pathognomonic of reflex sympathetic dystrophy.

Because pain is related to abnormal blood flow, nonsteroidal anti-inflammatories that inhibit inflammation have little effect. Drugs such as Procardia that increase blood flow can have a dramatic effect. Injection of the sympathetic chain with phenol, alcohol, or guanethidine can diminish

Table 8.3 Fourteen Potential Localized Tender Sites in Fibrositis

Trapezius, midpoint of upper fold	R	1
	L	2
Costochondral junctions, second; maximum just lateral to junctions on upper surface	R	3
	L	4
Lateral epicondyles, "tennis elbow" sites, 1-2 cm distal to epicondyles, within muscle that tenses when long finger is actively extended	R	5
	L	6
Supraspinatus, at origins, above scapular spine near the medial border	R	7
	L	8
Low cervical, anterior aspects of interspinous spaces C4-6		9
Low lumbar, interspinous ligaments L4-S1		10
Gluteus medius, upper outer quadrants of buttocks, in anterior fold of muscle	R	11
	L	12
Medial fat pad, overlying medial collateral ligament of the knee, proximal to the joint line	R	13
	L	14

Note. From "Fibrosis and Other Diffuse Musculoskeletal Syndromes" by H.A. Smythe. In *Text Book of Rheumatology* (p. 487) by W.N. Kelly, E.D. Harris, S. Ruddy, and C.B. Sledge, 1981, Philadelphia: W.B. Saunders. Reprinted by permission.

sympathetic tone and allow circulation to return to normal, either permanently after a single injection, after a set of up to five injections, or only temporarily, which may indicate the need for a surgical sympathectomy to provide relief. Surgery should be managed through a pain clinic where the individuals involved are familiar with the combined team approach of pharmacology, anesthesiology, psychology, and surgery to deal with this problem.

Muscles that have not been used atrophy quickly and will always be weak unless constantly exercised. After the gradual return of passive and active motion, aerobic conditioning and strengthening must follow, but heavy duty exercise with the use of free weights, isokinetic machinery, or heavy guided weight systems must be condemned. Transcutaneous electrical nerve stimulation (TENS) units have been effective in minimizing pain; however, myostimulation units that help bulk up atrophic muscles and secondarily decrease pain have been found to be even more effective. Rest or immobilization is not part of the therapeutic regimen, because they will develop further atrophy and accelerate the condition.

One subset of this syndrome is *shoulder-hand syndrome*, in which a painful shoulder is combined with sausage-like swelling of the digits of the hand on the same extremity. Osteopenia is evident on X-ray, and the blotchy skin changes may develop later. Early mobilization and passive and active motion progressing toward strengthening of all the joints of the extremity must take place simultaneously. With minimal or no therapeutic response, or worsening of symptoms, early sympathetic blocks must be considered.

Be wary when a patient presents with a tight fist that is almost impossible to open and has not been washed for some time. This subset is called *clenched fist syndrome*, which usually means that the patient is mad at someone, occasionally his or her coach or parents but more often a treating physician. This must be handled by a psychologist primarily and an orthopedist secondarily. As in all forms of reflex sympathetic dystrophy syndrome, the psychiatrist, psychologist, or social worker becomes the primary treating medical expert. More can be accomplished in a pain clinic with the use of pharmaceuticals, sympathetic blocks, and physical therapy than by surgical intervention, which can in fact make symptoms worse.

Psychological batteries, such as the Minnesota Multiphasic Personality Index as administered through psychological services, will be useful to help determine whether there is a structural component to the patient's pain. If there is and the psychologist believes that the patient can cope with surgery, eliminating the structural cause of the patient's pain has a higher incidence of success. If there is no structural cause identified by testing or through psychoanalysis, the orthopedist, team doctor, therapist, or trainer may be wasting time in attempting treatment. Even narcotics and anti-inflammatory medication may prove ineffective and are best administered in a pain clinic program.

Summary

Soft tissue injury can lead to pain. Pain can lead to disuse and dysfunction. Inactivity will cause muscle atrophy and fibrosis. With chronicity, symptoms worsen and problems become much more complex.

In dealing with the injuries discussed in this chapter, it is important that inflammatory processes be dealt with early in an effort to avoid late fibrosis and patterns of disuse. As more complex patterns develop, they become harder to treat.

9

Neurovascular Injuries

Neurovascular athletic injuries about the shoulder can be disastrous for the athlete and a diagnostic challenge for the physician.

Nerve injuries can be grouped into three categories. *Neurapraxia* is a mild compression or traction injury to a nerve that recovers in a relatively short period of time, 3 to 12 weeks, necessitating muscular strengthening after this short period of disuse. *Axonotmesis* separates the axonal nerve fiber within its myelin sheath. The neural tube is intact, but because the nerve fiber has to regenerate at about a rate of 1 mm per day, the rate of recovery is correspondingly slower. The end results, however, tend to be excellent. The third category, *neurotmesis*, involves complete destruction of neural elements, and with a severe crush of this sort prognosis is guarded; nerve grafting or resection of the crushed elements and repair of the more normal sections are considered.

Most neurologic traumas from athletic injuries occur with minor crush or traction episodes to nerve; most recover. Unfortunately, some injuries are iatrogenic, such as injury to the musculo-cutaneous nerve during an anterior capsular stabilization or during a Bristow transposition of the coracoid process or subsequent revision, laceration or stretch of the axillary nerve with a capsular shift procedure, and contusion or laceration of the brachial plexus with a misplaced arthroscopic portal. If there is any suggestion of laceration during surgery, surgical reexploration is demanded. Otherwise, postoperative complaints are usually transitory and expectant observation usually yields good results. Iatrogenic stretch of the cephalic vein leading to thrombosis is also possible but managed expectantly and conservatively.

Axillary Nerve Dysfunction

The most commonly injured neurovascular structure in athletic shoulder injuries is the axillary nerve, leading to decreased deltoid function. Most injuries are stretch injuries due to an anterior dislocation pattern and in fact are more common as the individual ages due to decreased pliability of soft structures. Perhaps most are unrecognized and recover spontaneously. Contusion or hematoma to the quadrilateral space also causes injury. Axillary nerve injuries can occur during exposure for a capsular shift or fracture repair. The cause is the same. The course of the axillary nerve (C5, C6) from the brachial plexus and under the front of the inferior glenoid progresses to the quadrilateral space posteriorly with a short medial branch innervating the posterior head of the deltoid and ends in cutaneous distribution over the lateral arm and a longer anterior branch circling the surgical humeral neck, innervating the middle and anterior deltoid heads with a few cutaneous twigs. The anterior branch is most susceptible to fracture or dislocation and to surgical trauma during deltoid muscle exposure of the rotator cuff.

Athletic nerve injuries are most common in collision sports or those sports associated with falling forward; they occur when attempting to stop a fall with an abducted, externally rotated arm with subsequent dislocation. This is the most common nerve injury that occurs with dislocation. If the patient is having considerable difficulty raising the arm a week after dislocation or has numbness over the lateral upper arm, the examiner should be suspicious of axillary nerve palsy, clinically manifested as decreased deltoid function.

No specific X-ray is of any value, and an EMG test is frequently not of any use for the first 3 to 4 weeks but should be done shortly thereafter as a baseline to assess subsequent recovery. EMG may need to be repeated at 3 and 6 months. Following injury there is increased latency and decreased amplitude of response compared to the opposite side, measured from Erb's point. Denervation potential or increased insertional activity is seen in the recovery phase. Because the lateral head of the deltoid is used for elevation with the anterior and posterior heads used for stabilization, the patient should not use the arm in an overhead position until EMG recovery is documented.

When hematoma occurs in the joint, there may be a small rent in the rotator cuff associated with dislocation; lack of deltoid function combined with a negative pressure phenomenon or a hematoma may show an inferior pseudosubluxation on X-ray. This is nothing to be alarmed about if the history is consistent with a dislocation and there is lateral loss of sensation over the proximal arm. Pseudosubluxation is managed in a sling, and at least 95% recover spontaneously in 4 months to 1-1/2 years. Visible atrophy is uncommon but can occur (Figure 9.1). The other 5% become problems over time, and if there is no significant recovery at 12 to 16

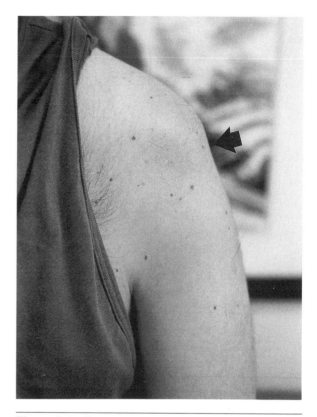

Figure 9.1 Permanent axillary nerve palsy related to shoulder dislocation is rare but persists here in spite of capsular shift procedure that stabilized the joint; deltoid dysfunction limits the ability to position the hand overhead.

weeks after fracture or surgery, surgical exploration may be considered.

EMG changes following dislocation usually show improvement; however, with no evidence of improvement after the first 1-1/2 to 2 years, trapezial transfer, fascial sling techniques, or fusion of the shoulder may be necessary to gain some stability (Figure 9.2).

Early return to sport activity is out of the question when lateral numbness occurs in the upper arm, because deltoid function is jeopardized and the athlete is at particular risk for reinjury. The physician must make the patient aware that this is an unusual but not uncommon problem with shoulder dislocation and that it may take a prolonged period of time for recovery.

Long Thoracic Nerve Palsy

Athletic injury to the long thoracic nerve occurs with activity that causes compression, a direct blow of the scapula against the second rib, or

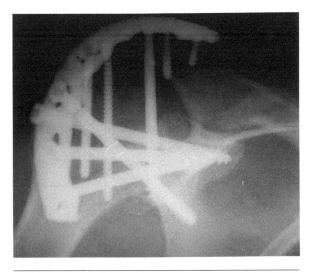

Figure 9.2 Glenohumeral fusion gives a solid base to help in hand positioning in patients with axillary nerve dysfunction.

distracting stretch. Initially the patient may have no pain. The coach or athlete's parent commonly notices the scapular winging, while the patient has only felt fatigue or noticed that he or she was throwing more side-armed. In the athletic population, this injury is common when skateboarding, when wearing a backpack as in mountaineering, or in direct compression as from falling in football or soccer or from resting the barbell asymmetrically on one shoulder in weight lifting (Figure 9.3, a and b). Carrying a duffel bag or tennis racquet, a golf club or tennis racquet coming down on the shoulder, or even just sleeping on the shoulder are common causes of clinical complaints stated in the patient's history.

Other causes of long thoracic nerve palsy that affect serratus anterior function and cause winging of the scapula, which may have nothing to do with the patient's sport, include recent throat infections or viral illness, brachial neuritis, diphtheria, cervical rib resection, lymph node biopsy, and lying on the operating table for general anesthesia. Osteochondroma or Sprengel's congenital deformities, which cause pseudowinging, should be ruled out in the differential diagnosis.

The patient will complain of early fatigue and that the shoulder blade looks unusual. Again, pain may be a late finding related more to muscle spasm of the surrounding musculature, which is being overused to compensate. The winging can be exaggerated by having the patient do fingertip push-ups from the wall (Figure 9.3b). One must make sure that there is no bony prominence or exostosis

radiographically identified on the back of the scapula that must be differentiated and would respond directly to surgery.

EMG is negative for 3 weeks following injury but is useful later in demonstration of recovery. With stimulation at Erb's point along the lateral neck and measurement of the long thoracic nerve (C5, C6, and C7) at the midaxillary line, complete lesions will fail to demonstrate a motor response, whereas incomplete lesions will have prolonged latencies, prolonged polyphasic response, and reduced amplitudes. Increased polyphasic activity will demonstrate early recovery. Measurement of the response of separate digitations of the serratus anterior with distal migration can also demonstrate recovery. Care is taken to avoid pneumo- or hemothorax during this diagnostic procedure.

Long thoracic nerve palsy is usually transient, and most patients recover within a 3-month to 2-year period; nerve regeneration takes place at about a millimeter per day. It is important to keep the periscapular muscles pliable and strong in spite of the weakness and deformity caused by the serratus anterior (Figure 9.4, a and b). A home physical therapy program of flexibility, shoulder shrugs, and heat to decrease muscle spasm is useful to diminish symptoms and maximize function as the electrical input returns. Athletes need not be restricted from sport activity except for swimming, in which the serratus anterior is such an important component; allowing the patient to swim without the strength of this muscle can lead to scapulohumeral dysfunction and impingement syndrome.

There is nothing that can be done to accelerate the rate of recovery; luckily most of these injuries recover on their own following neuropraxic stretch in 3 to 24 months. If not, the patient has the choice of living with the problem or having a complex surgical reconstruction, including fusion of the scapula to the rib cage with hardware or non-absorbable suture or transfer of the pectoralis minor and a fascial graft. These techniques, however, do not have consistently good results, nor can they offer the ability to return to normal athletic function.

Spinal Accessory Nerve Injury

Considerable pain when lifting the arm can occur after a contusion or traction injury to the neck. The spinal accessory nerve (CN XI), which supplies the trapezius, passes obliquely through the sternocleidomastoid after leaving the jugular foramen at

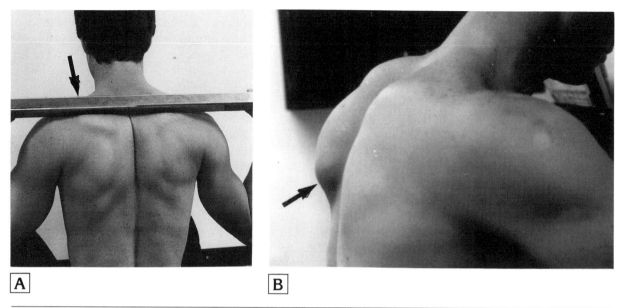

Figure 9.3

[A] Long thoracic nerve palsy associated with compression from barbell bar in body building.

[B] Resultant scapular winging from long thoracic nerve palsy. Upward and medial displacement of the scapula with external rotation of the scapular body and inferior tip is due to unopposed levator scapulae and rhomboid function that will lead to neck pain or spasm of the overused muscles.

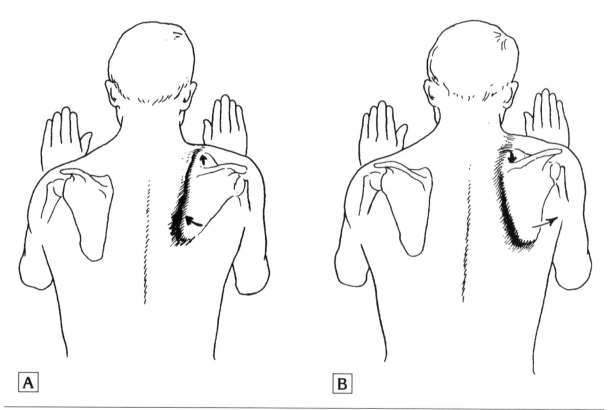

Figure 9.4 Scapular winging.

[A] With long thoracic nerve palsy, the inferior scapula rotates inward and protrudes, migrating superiorly due to loss of stability related to serratus anterior dysfunction.

[B] Spinal accessory palsy leads to outward rotation of the lower scapula and inferior migration due to paralysis of the trapezial fibers.

the base of the skull. It crosses the posterior triangle of the neck to innervate the trapezius. Contusion to this area, as seen in boxing, karate, and football, can lead both to significant discomfort in attempting to raise the arm in abduction and to paralysis of the trapezius, leading to a variation of scapular winging in which the inferior scapula is displaced laterally and the body of the scapula shifts inferiorly (Figure 9.4b). Most such injuries resolve on their own as work-up for suspected rotator cuff injury or shoulder subluxation progresses.

The author has had three cases of individuals who fell backward on their shoulder blades or who suffered blunt trauma to the posterior neck while playing football that were referred in for posterior subluxation of the shoulder. Subluxation was made possible by the scapular winging secondary to long thoracic or spinal accessory palsy (Figure 9.5, a and b). When the nerve injury recovered, as documented by EMG and clinical exam, posterior subluxation was no longer evident, and the patients returned to full athletic activity.

Stimulating the posterior triangle and assessing the trapezius muscle evoked motor response with EMG can indicate a latency which can be rechecked every 6 weeks to assess recovery. However, if the atrophy in the trapezius progresses and there is no clinical or EMG evidence of recovery at 3 months, exploration of the nerve should be considered to free up adhesions. Laceration of the nerve requiring surgical reattachment is extremely rare in athletes.

Brachial Plexopathy

Brachial plexus traction injuries—"stingers," "zingers," or "burners"—are frequently diagnosed in sport injuries; however, they are not really that common. A fall onto the neck and head pushing away from the affected shoulder can stretch the brachial plexus. This occurs less commonly than abducted externally rotated jarring of the shoulder, which leads to a stretch of the joint capsule and of the medial cord of the brachial plexus, causing tingling in the two ulnar digits or the arm "going dead." Most of these diagnosed injuries are in fact associated with "dead arm" phenomenon (Rowe & Zarins, 1981) or shoulder subluxation, and no significant damage to the brachial plexus actually occurs.

Although uncommon, traumatic crush or traction plexus injuries can occur with or without

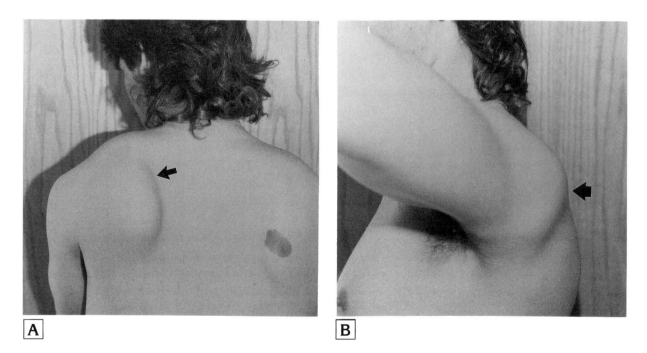

Figure 9.5 Long thoracic palsy associated with scapular winging.

   [A] Upward and lateral displacement of the scapula and internal rotation at the inferior tip.

   [B] Abnormal scapular rotation may be associated with posterior shoulder dislocation when attempting to elevate the arm; this usually resolves as serratus function and normal scapular dynamics recover.

shoulder dislocations or fractures about the shoulder joint. Brachial plexus stretch should be suspected if the mechanism of injury determined by observation or history indicates that the shoulder was depressed in one direction while the head and neck were stretched in the opposite direction. This is most common in football and motorcycling.

A mild stretch may recover in a few days but may even take a few months to resolve. Nerve root avulsion is not recoverable and may be involved with cervical spine injury. If avulsion occurs at the supraclavicular fossa, then nerve grafting may be required to restore function. Fracture or stress injuries commonly injure the trunks of the brachial plexus, whereas an open penetration may injure the cords. Injury of the nerve roots at the cervical spine must be differentiated because these are not amenable to surgical repair. EMG will help define the pathology.

Unless there is an open injury, the athlete will most likely be treated conservatively at first; EMG at 6 weeks and then at 3 to 4 months postinjury is mandatory to help delineate a nerve root injury, which has no potential for recovery, from a distal nerve injury, which does. If there is no clinical improvement 8 months following injury, the outlook is dismal. The patient usually does not return to his or her previous sport if upper extremity linkage is a significant component.

Although nerve root avulsion is not recoverable, tearing within the brachial plexus may respond to surgery, and a temporary stretch associated with subluxation or dislocation should recover. *Idiopathic brachial neuropathy*, a syndrome of acute pain with no apparent reason, can affect the shoulder. It occurs in individuals in the 20- to 30-year age range and therefore potentially can be seen in a large segment of the athletic population. It may extend from the scapula down to the hand or rarely may involve both shoulders at the same time. It has been labeled as reflex sympathetic dystrophy or crossover reflex sympathetic dystrophy and can affect any part of the brachial plexus together or separately. The suprascapular, the long thoracic, and the axillary nerves are commonly affected either together or with spotty distribution. The cause is thought to be associated with viral illness, autoimmune disease, or recent immunization (Tsairis, Dyck, & Mulder, 1972). There is an 80% recovery by 2 years and 90% by 3 years, and consultation at a pain clinic for pain management is mandatory. Steroids, anti-inflammatories, and other medications have no significant role; the patient and physician must wait this out.

Electrodiagnosis is useful in assessing brachial plexopathy, specifically to rule out nerve root avulsion and to determine the anatomic components of the lesion, its severity, and the prognosis for recovery. An experienced electromyographist can document an absent somatosensory evoked potential with normal compound peripheral sensory nerve action potentials; this is evidence of nerve avulsion. If this is apparent early on, myelography can document the cause. Normal somatosensory evoked potential and absent compound peripheral sensory nerve action potential would show continuity of at least some axons. Independent stimulation of the medial, ulnar, musculocutaneous, and radial nerves in an effort to elicit a somatosensory evoked potential can help map out the segmental involvement of a plexus injury. Nerve conduction studies and brachial neuritis are usually normal. Low cervical paraspinal fibrillations may be useful to differentiate a C5-C6 radiculopathy from brachial plexopathy. *Cervical radiculopathy* should also be differentiated from brachial plexopathy.

Radial Nerve Injury

With a distal third humerus fracture the radial nerve is often compressed or traumatized in the area of the spiral groove before it turns forward to pierce the lateral intramuscular septum and then traverse distally down the arm. About the shoulder and upper arm, the nerve can be compressed in the axilla by a crutch or rifle sling or by a blunt contusion, such as falling on a hurdle. This leads to temporary triceps paralysis and loss of sensation in the posterior cutaneous nerve distribution.

Near the deltoid insertion, crush injury may lead to hematoma or periosteal build-up, commonly called a *helmet exostosis* (Figure 9.6), because the nerve is relatively uncovered and unprotected. This may affect the radially supplied muscles beyond the triceps. Nerve contusion association with helmet exostosis usually recovers within 4 to 6 weeks; periosteal build-up may need operative resection if insertional activity documented by EMG remains compromised in the distal radially supplied muscles.

The most common cause of radial nerve injury is fracture to the distal third of the humerus where the nerve may become entrapped. Extensor muscle function of the hand may be compromised. With an open fracture, exploration of the nerve should be done, and laceration, if demonstrated, should be repaired. Open reduction should be done at that

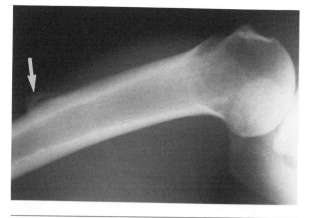

Figure 9.6 Helmet exostosis, commonly seen in football. Blunt contusion may lead to hematoma or periosteal new bone, usually temporarily irritating the radial or axillary nerve.

time. With a closed injury, diagnosis of the fracture should be evident on X-ray, and it is worthwhile to wait for the EMG result over the next 3 to 4 weeks to see if recovery is progressing prior to nerve exploration. It may take 6 to 7 months for full recovery and one should wait before undertaking nerve exploration. If the palsy develops after humeral stabilization surgery, reexploration with repair and release of the nerve from the fracture fragments is mandatory (Figure 9.7, a and b). If manipulation was necessary to get proper positioning and the palsy developed after this closed procedure, then exploration is again necessary.

Most of the palsies associated with fracture resolve if not iatrogenically induced. Most associated fractures managed in the sugar-tong splint and sling recover in 6 or 7 months. If there is no improvement noted by EMG in the first 6 to 8 weeks, explorative surgery may be indicated. With no recovery or limited recovery, tendon transfer to compensate for lost extensor function of the hand should be considered.

Effort Thrombosis

Subclavian or axillary vein thrombosis as an acute variant of thoracic outlet syndrome has been labeled *effort thrombosis* due to the associated muscular activity that seems to trigger this phenomenon (Dunant, 1981; Nuber, McCarthy, Yao, Schafer, & Suker, 1990). It is most common in weight lifting but can occur in any upper extremity muscular effort, including swimming and pitching. It has even occurred in a female runner due to use of hand weights (Haber & Storey, 1990).

Diagnosis

The affected athlete characteristically complains of acute pain and edema of the affected arm after a period of vigorous activity. Compression to the venous system deep within the chest wall leads to thrombosis and superficial venous dilation with up to a 1-in. increase in the circumference of the upper arm. If thrombosis is found acutely, the patient could be considered for thrombolysis therapy with streptokinase. The patient is then placed on I.V. heparin followed up with warfarin protocol for thrombosis in an effort to prevent pulmonary embolism.

Unfortunately, the patient susceptible to this injury does not usually present to the physician acutely. After the thrombus sets up and collateral circulation is poor, the patient will complain of swelling in the extremity with use or disuse and of a diffuse aching in the arm related to activity. A venogram is useful to define either the acute or chronic case; however, there is no good method of symptomatic relief with chronicity. Resection of the first rib or the costocoracoid ligament has been suggested. Posttraumatic syndrome of continued swelling and pain occurs in 90% of cases treated conservatively.

Differential Diagnosis

One must rule out use of oral contraceptives or other patient factors that can lead to a hypercoagulable state. Infection, drug abuse, sarcoidosis, tumor, dehydration, cardiomyopathy, and kidney disease must be considered in differential diagnosis, and anabolic steroid use in body building may be a cause as well. Acute management most likely would result in better response; but, again, these patients usually do not present acutely.

Dorsoscapular Nerve Compression

The dorsoscapular nerve is a motor nerve originating from C5 and supplying the levator scapulae, rhomboid minor, and rhomboid major muscles. It enters the scalenus medias muscle, which is subject to compression or hypertrophy. Injury can occur with weight training and contact sports such as rugby, football, and basketball.

With compression, the athlete complains of a toothache-like pain along the course of the levator scapulae and rhomboid muscles with diffuse radiation of pain in the lateral upper arm and lateral

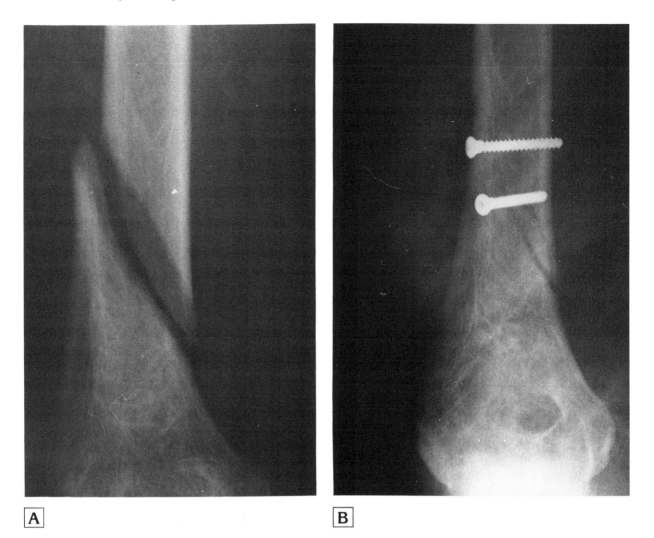

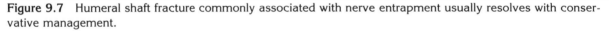

Figure 9.7 Humeral shaft fracture commonly associated with nerve entrapment usually resolves with conservative management.

[A] With obvious nerve entrapment or symptoms following manipulation or open reduction, surgical exploration is warranted to assess nerve status.

[B] With exploration, the fracture is fixed.

dorsal forearm. Due to discomfort the patient may position the arm so that scapular winging is suspected; this pseudowinging may have no neurologic basis. The examiner may press on the nerve at the back of the neck to reproduce the pain. Characteristically, the patient can relieve tension on the scalenus medias muscle by placing the hand on top of the head. This condition is often misdiagnosed as levator scapulae syndrome, fibromyositis, poor posture, or trigger point phenomenon (Kopell & Thompson, 1959).

Treatment includes therapeutic massage, cervical traction, spray and stretch technique, anti-inflammatory medication, and muscle relaxants. When this fails, surgical release of the scalenus medias posteriorly will relieve tension on the

dorsoscapular nerve and allow the athlete to return to sport activity within a few weeks.

Quadrilateral Space Syndrome

The teres minor superiorly, the humeral shaft laterally, the teres major inferiorly, and the long head of the triceps medially define the quadrilateral space through which the posterohumeral circumflex artery and axillary nerve pass (Cahill & Palmer, 1983). Compression of these structures leads to occasional paresthesia in a spotty distribution over the entire upper extremity that is made worse with abducted external rotation. This is most commonly found in throwing activity such as baseball and will interfere with performance. The athlete also complains of night pain when sleeping either on his or her back or in a prone position with the arm elevated above the head. The pain pattern is spotty and frequently cannot be reproduced on subsequent examinations. There may be tenderness in the front of the side of the shoulder, particularly over the quadrilateral space. Paresthesias in the upper extremity will be atypical and can be reproduced with an apprehension maneuver in abducted external rotation. This same maneuver can diminish the pulse, as it does normally in 80% of individuals, so that thoracic outlet syndrome is frequently misdiagnosed (Wood, Twitto, & Verska, 1988). Night pain also may lead to misdiagnosis as a rotator cuff tear. Pain with pitching activity implicates impingement syndrome in the differential diagnosis.

A subclavian arteriogram visualizing the posterohumeral circumflex artery as it passes through the quadrilateral space is used to make the diagnosis. In this study, the artery will be patent with the arm at the side, but in abducted external rotation it will become partially or totally occluded. EMG studies and other diagnostic studies have not been found helpful.

Treatment consists of periscapular muscle strengthening, biomechanical analysis of the patient's throwing technique to correct irregularities, and selective steroid injections with rest. If this fails and the athlete elects further intervention, treatment is posterior decompression of the neurovascular structures of the quadrilateral space by releasing the teres minor tendon inferior to the deltoid, along with neurolysis and mobilization of the bundle. During surgery the arm must be placed in abducted external rotation to make sure that the pulse is relieved. Early range of motion and exercise are mandatory, and physical therapy for strengthening is initiated at 2 to 3 weeks. Return to pitching activity can occur when motion and strength are full and pain is gone.

Suprascapular Nerve Entrapment

The suprascapular nerve originating from C5 and C6 is usually fixed within a fibro-osseous tunnel through the suprascapular notch and covered by a transverse scapular ligament where it innervates the supraspinatus muscle and gives off sensory fibers to the glenohumeral capsule and the acromioclavicular joint. The nerve continues, passing around the base of the acromion to innervate the infraspinatus. Injury to this nerve commonly occurs near the transverse scapular ligament (Hirayama & Takemitsu, 1981) or around the base of the acromion and is associated with traction injury, weight training, repetitive throwing (such as pitching or volleyball), or contusion (such as that caused by the use of a backpack or participation in rugby, football, and gymnastics). With trauma, both the supraspinatus and infraspinatus may be involved, but isolated involvement of the infraspinatus with entrapment near the spinoglenoid notch can occur with weight training, pitching, and serving in tennis.

Depending on the level of entrapment, both the supraspinatus and infraspinatus or the infraspinatus alone may be involved. There is loss of strength of the short external rotators in abduction and external rotation. X-ray may show a small suprascapular notch and MRI can disclose an adjacent dilation of the nerve. EMG crossing Erb's point may define pathology.

Rest, anti-inflammatory medication, therapeutic massage, periscapular muscle strengthening, and spray and stretch modalities may relieve symptoms. A very aggressive therapeutic program should be instituted, particularly with isolated infraspinatus atrophy, because late surgical decompression is rarely successful. Early decompression of the suprascapular notch tends to be more successful, and if muscle power returns after such decompression, the patient may return to athletics. Myostimulation may be helpful to help prepare the muscle for reinnervation. Because the infraspinatus is a major depressor of the humeral head, without its strength, posterior capsulitis, posterior glenoid erosion, subluxation, and superior migration of the humeral head leading to subcoracoid or subacromial impingement syndromes can occur. Without the return of infraspinatus function, competitive return to sport is unlikely. Subacromial bursoscopy with subdeltoid adhesion resection behind the A/C joint may be useful to decompress the suprascapular nerve without difficult open dissection.

Thoracic Outlet Syndrome

Compression of the nerves and blood vessels of the upper extremity as they pass into the axilla through the interval between the first rib and the scalene muscles is called *thoracic outlet syndrome*. It has been called cervical rib syndrome, droopy shoulder syndrome, and ptosis of the scapula and may overlap with dead arm syndrome (Leffert & Gumley, 1987).

Epidemiology

There is no specific sport that causes thoracic outlet syndrome, although blunt contusion to the scalene muscles can lead to the fibrosis associated with this syndrome, and therefore it is more common in contact sports. If the patient is prone to develop this syndrome, he or she would be most symptomatic in overhead activity, particularly throwing sports and some gymnastic events.

Etiology

Roos (1979) described nine different types of structural abnormalities that lead to compression of the plexus and the brachial artery and vein. An abnormally long transverse process at C7 and cervical ribs can cause compression of the thoracic outlet. Poor posture, pendulant breasts in jogging, and carrying heavy loads as in backpacking are common causes, leading to pain or numbness experienced at the end of the small and ring fingers with overhead activity or throwing.

Natural History

If left untreated, either athletic performance is seriously hampered, symptoms may remain with overhead activity, or progressive atrophy specifically of the fine motor ulnar musculature of the hand can occur.

Diagnosis

The athlete may complain of pain radiating from the neck down the arm into the medial aspect of the forearm and to the ring and small finger while participating in overhead activity. This may progress to night pain as well.

The patient may present with symptoms that are spotty or may be entirely arterial, venous, or neurologic. There may be a drop in arterial pulse with abducted external rotation (the *Wright maneuver*), a phenomenon that occurs in at least 80% of healthy individuals (Wood et al., 1988). Decreased pulse with the arm at the side or abducted up to 40° while the athlete turns his or her hyperextended neck to the affected side (*Adson test*) is rarely positive. One of the best tests was described by Roos (1979): With both shoulders placed at 90° of abduction and hands overhead, the athlete opens and closes the hands slowly for 3 minutes. When the athlete is unable to keep the arms above the head due to ischemic pain, thoracic outlet syndrome is inferred. A *Spurling sign* of pain with direct pressure over the brachial plexus or the interval between the clavicle and scapular spine is also a valuable test. Local tenderness directly under the midclavicle can be found. Neurologic clinical changes may be isolated to painless, partial thenar atrophy.

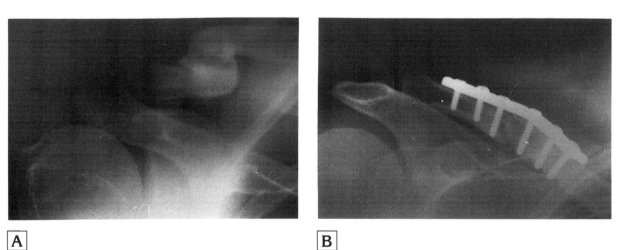

Figure 9.8

[A] Thoracic outlet syndrome related to malunion of midclavicle bony protrusion inferiorly.

[B] Symptoms relieved with bone resection, clavicular lengthening, and corrective open reduction internal fixation.

Imaging

X-rays are not very useful in this syndrome except for demonstrating associated cervical ribs, abnormally long processes of C7, and malunion or nonunion of midclavicular fractures (Figure 9.8, a and b). MRI studies have not been found to be of use, and an arteriogram to demonstrate decreased blood flow may be found positive in only about 20% of individuals, so it is a relatively poor diagnostic tool. EMG may be of use when a double crush phenomenon occurs, that is, when sensitivity of the median and ulnar nerve elsewhere in the arm, which may present as a cubital tunnel or carpal tunnel syndrome, amplifies symptoms in the shoulder and thus produces the "double crush" (Osterman, 1988). EMG evidence of partial chronic denervation of C8 and T1 may substantiate neurologic involvement.

Differential Diagnosis

Medial and ulnar nerve compression syndromes without the double crush phenomenon must first be ruled out. Apical lung tumors, such as pancoast tumors, metastatic tumors, and adenocarcinoma, as well as cervical radiculopathy must enter the differential diagnosis. Shoulder instability and postoperative fibrosis about the shoulder can also decrease space in the thoracic outlet and lead to symptoms that are best treated first with therapy and mobilization rather than rib resection or other surgery that can increase scar tissue and thus make symptoms worse. Postural changes must be assessed.

Management

If a diagnosis of thoracic outlet syndrome is made, conservative management must be stressed (Table 9.1). The fibrotic process that initiates compression can be made worse by further surgery. Shoulder shrug exercises, gentle manipulation progressing toward strengthening, and posture improvement, including the use of a clavicular strap to bring the shoulders back, are often successful. If not, surgical rib resection or lysis of adhesions in the scalene muscles followed by secondary rehabilitation can be considered but should be done by someone very familiar with such procedures.

Complications

Vascular compression can lead to blanching of the hand or even to occlusion due to embolization of a subclavian arterial thrombus. When this is

Table 9.1 Conservative Rehabilitation Program for Thoracic Outlet Syndrome

---

Restriction of activity

No purses, heavy coats, or backpack straps on affected shoulder.

No carrying heavy suitcases, briefcases, or bookbags with affected arm.

No significant overhead activity or hand above clavicular level. This includes sport activity and work activity, and even while driving the elbow should not rest out the car window or on the upper part of the steering wheel.

With continuous pain that is not responding to exercise, consider weight loss or breast reduction surgery.

Exercise (Use of clavicular strap may facilitate postural component)

Postural exercise to keep shoulders back; isometric strengthening to position shoulder.

Abduction strengthening and wall push-offs.

Neck strengthening: lateral, rotational, extension, and flexion. Strong emphasis on shoulder shrug exercises.

Supine bench exercise, light weights (1-5 lb, 0.45-2.25 kg) with small roll between shoulder blades.

> With elbows bent 15° and arms behind body, bring up to body level.

> Bring weights from body level forward to touch overhead, again with elbows bent 15°, then return to starting neutral position.

Prone bench exercises

With weights on floor and elbows bent 15°, lift up to level of bench (neutral position). Repeat 5-8 times as tolerated.

From neutral position, bring weight to side of bench and then straight upward behind back. Repeat 5-8 times.

With arms in neutral position, elbows bent 15°, raise weight overhead and then back to neutral position. Repeat 5-8 times.

Return to regular activity, emphasizing proper posture, proper biomechanics, and continued strengthening and stretching.

---

suspected, angiography must be done. Atypical pain patterns can lead to the initiation of reflex sympathetic dystrophy. Lack of treatment may lead to muscle atrophy about the hand and a considerable inability to participate in athletic endeavors. Surgical intervention can lead to increased fibrosis and worsening of the condition.

Prognosis

Females with poor posture tend to have these neurologic symptoms and tend to improve with shoulder shrug exercises, temporary clavicular straps, and postural training. Rehabilitation may take from 2 to 12 weeks. If excessive breast tissue has initiated symptoms, the use of a jogging bra or even reduction mammoplasty can return the athlete to training within a few weeks. With progressive disability, further atrophy that may not be reversible occurs in the hand. It is important to treat the condition as soon as possible so that secondary changes, such as overuse spasm of the trapezius, levator scapulae, and rhomboid muscles, do not occur and hamper rehabilitation.

Summary

Neurovascular injuries about the athlete's shoulder present a clinical challenge. Clinical examination is most important here, and electrical analysis often helps to identify the neurologic problem and gives some prognosis toward recovery. The roles of the clinician and athlete demand patience in many of these injuries. The predicted recovery of neurologic injuries depends on the actual structural damage, the type of nerve involved, and the nerve length. Muscle rebalancing can occur as neurovascular reinnervation progresses.

10

Fractures

Injuries to the capsular extensions that hold bones together and create joints, sprain injuries, have been discussed in chapter 6. Damage to the musculotendinous units that move the shoulder have been discussed in chapter 7. Athletic trauma also occurs to the bones that affect the shoulder's athletic performance and will be discussed in this chapter.

Clavicle

Clavicular fracture is the most common shoulder fracture associated with athletics. Overall, 1 in 20 youth fractures of the entire skeleton is a clavicular fracture. The most common mechanism of clavicular fracture is transmission of force indirectly or falling onto an outstretched hand or onto the point of the shoulder, as is common in hockey, football, wrestling, soccer, and ice skating. Direct force to the clavicle is the less common form of injury but is seen in karate, kick boxing, or jousting or with contact by a puck, stick, or ball as in hockey, lacrosse, or baseball.

Natural History

Most clavicular fractures heal; less than 2% proceed to nonunion. Healing may be affected by whether the fracture is open or closed or by the location of the fracture. Fractures of the proximal clavicle, usually at an earlier age, are mostly epiphyseal and are very difficult to visualize on X-ray. Fractures of the distal clavicle may occur into the A/C joint or near the coracoclavicular ligaments, leading to unstable support patterns that affect healing.

Generally, even if the clavicular fracture is untreated, it will heal. There most likely will be some overlap or step-off and abundant callus formation that will affect cosmesis but have little effect on short-term function. There is some concern that long-term changes can occur in association with altered mechanics due to angulation or malunion at the fracture site. These include scapulothoracic bursitis, A/C joint arthritis, and subsequent erosion or impingement into the rotator cuff. Overall, long-term complaints are uncommon.

Diagnosis

The athlete with an injured clavicle may remember an audible snap and immediate pain at the time of injury as well as an immediate deformity or swelling surrounding the clavicle. These are important factors in the history. Nevertheless, because of plasticity of bone, the young athlete may in fact have a greenstick fracture, and a snap may not have been heard. Because the proximal apophysis of the clavicle may not close until age 35 and because the cartilage of the distal clavicle may work as a growth plate, many injuries to the ends of the clavicle may in fact be growth plate injuries. A/C joint separation is unusual before age 16 in an athlete where it most likely represents a growth plate fracture or periosteal stripping at the distal clavicle.

Physical Examination. Physical examination reveals a painful deformity associated with acute fracture injury of the clavicle, with crepitation felt with pressure over this area. The athlete most likely will be holding the elbow to support the depressed distal fragment and upper arm. He or she will not want to abduct or forward flex the arm, because either of these actions will put stress on the clavicular strut. If assessment is delayed, hematoma formation may mask what earlier or later may be an obvious clinical deformity. The patient may complain of numbness or neurovascular changes in the hand, which indicate an ominous prognosis. It is important to look for associated abnormalities, because brachial plexus trauma and

even vascular injury leading to death have been associated with midclavicular injuries. Respiratory embarrassment and dysphasia have been associated with posterior subluxation of a displaced proximal clavicular shaft.

Imaging. The clavicle is not often seen well on standard shoulder X-rays. At least two views are important to assess the fracture. An AP film and a film angled up 15°, including the shoulder and apical chest, are the most important views for most clavicular fractures (Figure 10.1, a and b). One-third normal radiation is necessary so that soft tissue detail is obtained and overpenetration avoided. The inclusion of the shoulder and apical chest may help avoid overlooking evidence of associated injury, such as pneumothorax, coracoid fracture, or glenohumeral injury. A second X-ray at an angle different from the preceding but also in the AP plane will help define anterior or posterior displacement at the fracture site.

Proximal clavicular fractures are not well defined on routine X-rays. Because the majority of these in the athletic population are associated with injury to the proximal growth plate (sternoclavicular sprain, considered in chapter 6), the radiographic assessment of choice is the CT scan. If there is acute swelling or neurologic changes associated with deformity, then a venogram or arteriogram may be indicated to rule out thrombosis or vascular laceration and to see if immediate neurovascular exploration and repair are indicated.

Classification. Clavicular fractures are commonly classified into three groups, ranging from

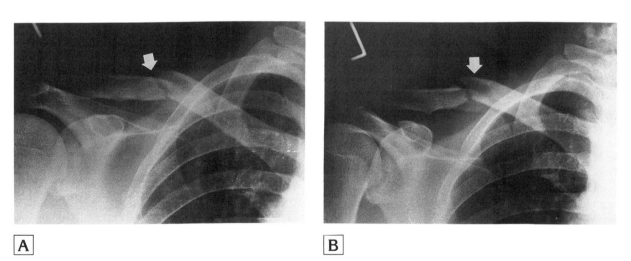

A

B

Figure 10.1 The clavicle is an S-shaped bone, and as in all skeletal analysis, assessment from two angles is necessary:

[A] Standard AP view;

[B] 15°-upward-angled view.

Zone 1, midshaft fractures, which are most common, to Zone 3, proximal third fractures, which are the least common (Figure 10.2).

Zone 1. Zone 1 fractures in the middle third constitute 80% of clavicular fractures. As the sternocleidomastoid pulls proximally and the weight of the arm and the pectoralis major pull distally, the proximal fragment is elevated and the distal fragment is correspondingly depressed (Type I). This fracture may be comminuted or may have an intrafragmental vertical component (Type II). The inferior spike or subsequent healing callus may interfere with neurovascular function. Revising the bump to accommodate straps utilized in motor racing or parachuting is not uncommon (Figure 10.3, a-c). Symptoms of hypertrophic nonunions of the midshaft along with thoracic outlet syndrome usually resolve following open reduction and internal fixation of the fracture and debridement of the bump.

Zone 2. Zone 2 fractures, occurring in the distal third, constitute 15% of clavicular fractures. Within this group are five subclassifications, which can be further divided. Type I is an interligamentous injury between the acromioclavicular capsular ligaments and the coracoclavicular ligaments. These tend to remain non- or minimally displaced and heal well, except in hockey, in which repetitive trauma may lead to nonunion (Figure 10.4).

Type II injuries have a subtype A, in which the fracture line is medial to intact coracoclavicular ligaments, and a subtype B, in which the fracture occurs between the coracoclavicular ligaments with trauma propagated through the trapezoid ligament and with the conoid remaining intact. Type III injury involves propagation of a fracture into the distal articular surface. There may be no displacement, but these microfractures may stimulate an absorptive phase that may mimic or actually be the cause of osteolysis of the distal clavicle or that may lead to A/C joint arthritis in the healing process, or both. Rarely, a fragment may be extruded, leading to a painful subcutaneous prominence.

Children have a propensity toward Type IV injury, in which the distal clavicle slips out of the periosteal sleeve with the ligaments attached to this sleeve. A new clavicle may form within that sleeve, leading to a widened clavicle or a bifid deformity (Figure 10.5). In adults, Type V injury

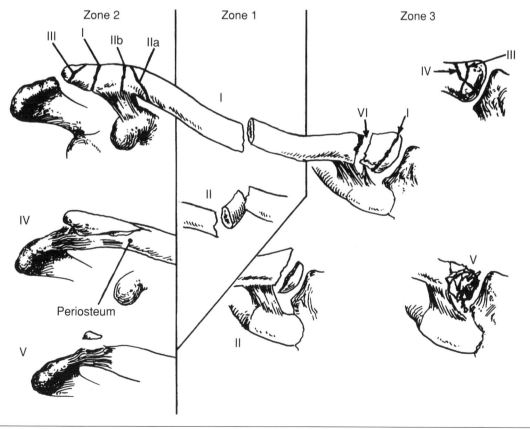

Figure 10.2 Clavicular fracture patterns.

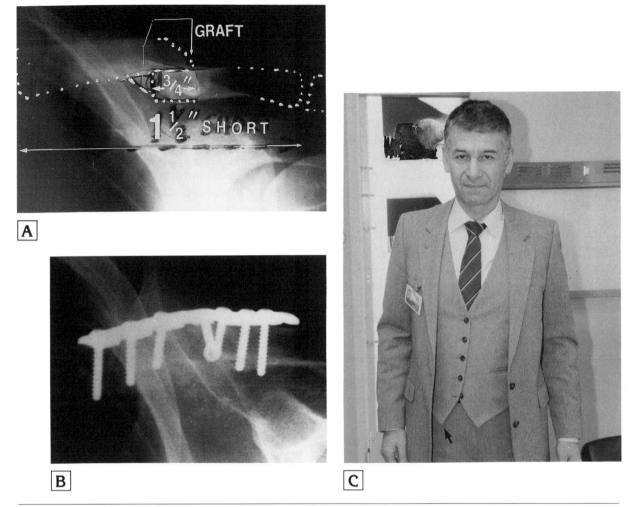

Figure 10.3

[A] Malunion of midshaft clavicular fracture leaves shortening of 1-1/2 in. compared to the opposite side (lengthening osteotomy planned).

[B] Lengthening osteotomy implemented, and clavicle is brought out to length with lag screw and plate fixation.

[C] Shortening of the clavicle will throw off the linkage system. Here, after bringing the clavicle out to length, in the same patient as in [A] and [B], the vest custom fitted prior to osteotomy no longer hangs as it did preoperatively.

can occur when the A/C capsular ligaments and coracoclavicular ligaments remain attached to an inferior fragment, and significant instability develops, leading to deformity, pain, and A/C symptoms.

Zone 3. Zone 3 clavicular injuries of the proximal one third constitute approximately 5% of clavicular injuries. These are mostly physeal injuries in young athletes. In the older age group there is less chance of a physeal injury; however, classification remains the same. In Type I there is minimal displacement, and in Type II there is considerable displacement because the ligaments surrounding the sternoclavicular joint are disrupted. Type III

injury is a fracture into the physeal separation that can occur even up to age 35. Type IV is an intra-articular fracture, usually occurring in adults, and it tends to be the most symptomatic when subsequent arthritis is evident; it is very difficult to treat. Type V is extremely comminuted and has a high tendency toward subsequent late arthritis of the sternoclavicular joint.

Subclassification. Clavicular fractures, regardless of zone, are further subdivided into groups: A, less than 100% displacement at the fracture site; B, more than 100% displacement; and C, fracture with concomitant neurovascular compromise. *Open* fractures penetrate the skin; *closed* fractures do not.

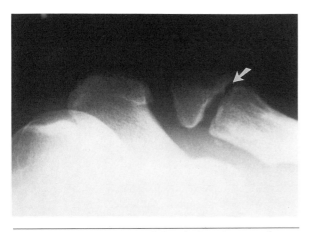

Figure 10.4 Nonunion of distal clavicle in professional hockey player who complained of pain for 8 years; no previous X-ray had been taken.

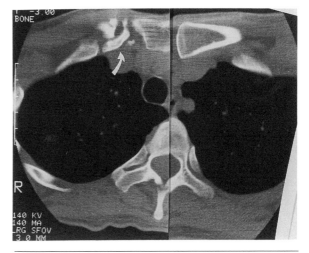

Figure 10.6 Proximal clavicular fracture. Sternoclavicular joint looked normal on routine AP X-ray, and swelling was assumed to be due to early degenerative joint disease. Comminuted fracture is easily assessed by CT study.

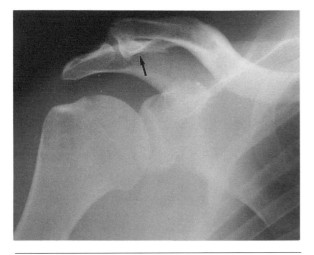

Figure 10.5 The bifid clavicle resulting from youth A/C joint injury and periosteal stripping.

Differential Diagnosis

Differential diagnosis includes A/C joint separation, which can occur concurrently with clavicular fracture. Comparative X-ray of the opposite side or a CT scan will help define the situation. Sternoclavicular separation must be ruled out. Again, CT is the radiographic tool of choice at the proximal end of the clavicle (Figure 10.6).

Congenital pseudarthrosis may become clinically symptomatic after trauma; however, painless heterotopic nonunion is more characteristic with the proximal fragment tilting up and forward and the distal fragment pointing up and backward. Cleidocranial dysostosis has a larger gap between the bone ends, and although the distal clavicle may be palpable, it is usually much smaller than

normal. If minimal trauma leads to clavicular fracture, tumor or metastatic disease must be ruled out.

Management

Management of clavicular fractures is usually conservative; a sling or clavicular strap is generally satisfactory. If there is no evidence of healing of a fracture near the A/C joint within 4 to 6 weeks or earlier if coracoclavicular ligament injury is apparent, then open repair may be considered (Figure 10.7).

If an open fracture of the clavicle presents acutely, it needs to be irrigated and debrided to minimize risk of osteomyelitis. Open reduction and internal fixation are justified at this time. If there is concurrent evidence of neurovascular injury, including numbness or extreme swelling near the fracture site implicating arterial injury or swelling of the ipsilateral upper extremity implicating venous compression, then surgical exploration and repair of the neurovascular structures with concurrent open reduction and internal fixation of the fracture would be appropriate. The open reduction should be done to prevent disruption of the neurovascular repair as well as to take advantage of the skin incision.

Complications

Complications include infection or osteomyelitis (if the fracture is open), neurovascular compromise, and the fact that more serious injury might be overlooked. A significant amount of energy is

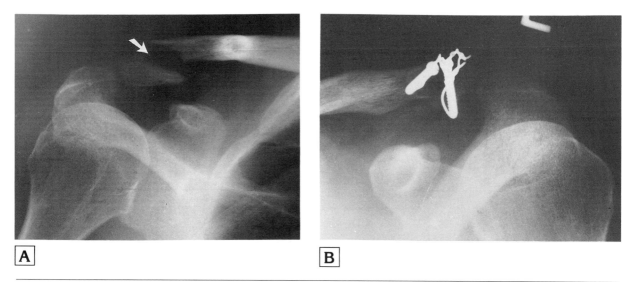

Figure 10.7

[A] Problem fracture lateral to ligaments with coracoclavicular ligament rupture.

[B] Lateral fragment too small for plate fixed with cannulated screws and figure-8 tension band.

necessary to break a bone. The bone may rupture the pleura, and pneumothorax may be a complication. Clavicular fracture may have occurred with trauma to the glenohumeral joint, coracoid process, or brachial plexus, or even may include nerve root avulsion in the neck. Shortening of the clavicle, malunion, or exuberant callus formation may develop with conservative management. The callus may in fact cause neurovascular symptoms, including thoracic outlet syndrome. Clavicular shortening may throw off dynamic function of the shoulder. Vascular intimal tears and thrombosis can also occur with clavicular injury.

In treatment, open reduction has a 5% incidence of nonunion, but conservative management only 1%. This does not necessarily mean that there is a higher incidence of nonunion with surgery than without surgery, but rather reflects that the most serious injuries are operated on. Nonunion may be associated with the severity of trauma or inadequate immobilization or fixation. Pin fixation can lead to pin migration. Osteomyelitis or infection can be associated with an open reduction, and a secondary painful scar can occur where bone graft is harvested. Malunion can occur and may lead to subscapular bursitis or A/C joint arthritis and subacromial impingement symptoms. Fractures into the joint obviously can lead to degenerative arthritis.

Prognosis

The individual can return to sport activity after there is a painless full range of motion and strength is near normal. This takes from 12 weeks to 1 year. Even after 12 weeks when there is no point tenderness and motion is full, it is important to avoid contact sports and to avoid falling on this extremity for at least 1 year. There is vascular change because the intraosseous blood supply has been disrupted. Bone is remodeling, and there is definitely a tendency toward refracture. If there is a significant prominence in this area, adequate padding should be utilized. Long-term problems will probably become more frequent because athletes are continuing in recreational sports and performing over a longer period of time than they did in the past. Slight irregularities or malunions at the A/C joint will be reflected in altered shoulder mechanics, particularly involving the A/C joint, subscapular space, and rotator cuff.

Cost Containment

For cost containment the most important factor is not to go overboard with treatment and assessment of proximal clavicular injury in young athletes. As the fastest area of bone healing, it has the most tendency to remodel; most injuries at the end of the bone are physeal. Unless a severe or progressing clinical deformity is noted in this area, serial X-rays will not alter the course of management.

Patient Education

The athlete should be informed that surgery is an option but that the major problem, abundant callus, particularly at the most common midshaft fracture, is considered to be cosmetic. Surgery in effect trades a bump for a scar. Plating the fracture will increase its healing time; however, open reduction and internal fixation theoretically will restore the bone length and give the most normal mechanical usage of the shoulder afterward.

Strenuous activity may lead to a stress riser and to the potential to fracture at the end of the plate (Figure 10.8). The plate may need to be removed later on. It is important to keep the muscles strong so that there will be less tendency to refracture. The athlete should not go back to activity until the area is painless, there is a full range of motion, and strength is near normal. Otherwise there is a high tendency toward reinjury.

Prevention

As with most fractures, there are no adequate preventative measures to avoid clavicular injury. Most athletic injuries occur in competition or when the patient is caught off guard. A well-maintained athletic field may prevent falling during training. Coordination and training may minimize the possibility of being caught off guard and are the best preventative measures.

Scapula

The scapula is well covered with muscle. Other than the glenoid socket fractures that occur with dislocation, most scapular fractures imply significant trauma. For this reason, they are associated with high falls, as in pole vaulting, or high energy, as in auto racing, motocross racing, and snow-mobiling. Fractures or nonunions through acromial growth plates can occur in young athletes, and avulsion of the coracoid tip or superior aspect of the scapular spine has been associated with baseball pitching in adolescents.

The most common etiology of scapular fractures in athletes occurs with subluxation or dislocation of the humeral head. Most frequently, impaction on dislocation or at the time of reduction will break off a fragment at the anteroinferior glenoid (Figure 10.9); rarely a fragment is broken off with posterior subluxation. The capsule may pull off a small fragment of the posterior rim at time of anterior dislocation.

Superior subluxation can cause injury to the acromion or coracoid, and impaction of an adducted upper arm (falling laterally on the shoulder) can cause an impaction or starburst type of fracture into the glenoid. This may propagate across the scapula or cause an isolated fracture across the scapular neck (Figure 10.10).

Impingement may occur if the neck fragment heals in varus or in a superior position. Falling on one's back as in judo and aikido has been known to cause scapular body fractures, but these are more common in high-impact sport injuries, as occur in snowmobiling and motor vehicle racing. In such multitrauma cases, however, there is so much energy involved that the scapular injury frequently is overlooked initially as more important problems, such as abdominal injury, associated rib fractures, and pneumothorax, must be dealt with primarily.

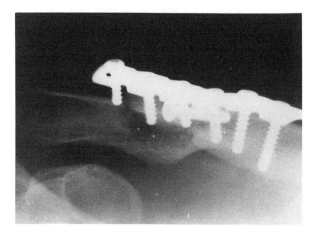

Figure 10.8 Refracture of the clavicle at the proximal plate through a screw hole stress riser 1 week following open reduction and internal fixation and premature return to sport activity.

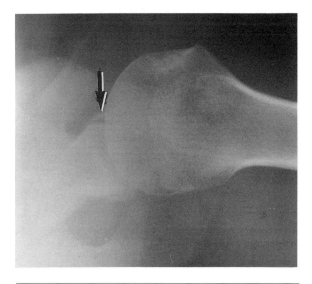

Figure 10.9 Anterior glenoid rim fracture associated with anterior dislocation.

Natural History

Assuming that associated injuries such as pneumothorax, pelvic injuries, or abdominal injuries are taken care of properly, the untreated scapular fracture generally does quite well (Figure 10.11). The muscle envelope allows rapid healing in most cases, and unless a major fragment at the gleno-humeral joint goes on to nonunion or malunion and instability, there is usually no great problem. Occasionally the scapular body malunion or fibrous union may lead to subscapular symptoms and crepitation; this is not usually disabling in everyday activity but can interfere with athletic performance. Luckily, the injuries that affect scapulothoracic rhythm are uncommon.

Diagnosis

Although the motorcyclist, auto racer, or runner hit by a vehicle may not be able to give a history, bruising about the scapula must make one suspicious of a scapular fracture and associated injuries such as rib fracture and pneumothorax (Figure 10.12). A football player who was tackled while trying to push himself off the ground can relate the cause of acute injury. This type of high energy impact must also cause suspicion of a scapular fracture, although this fracture would more likely be at the glenoid rim, and associated injuries would be much less life threatening.

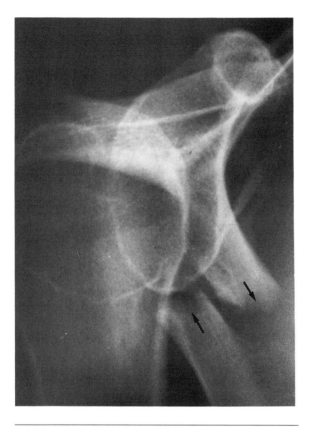

Figure 10.10 Fracture at scapular neck.

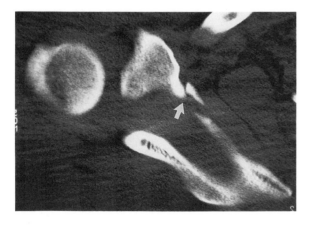

Figure 10.11 Scapular fractures may have minimal displacement due to muscular envelope. Glenoid fragment remains aligned with scapular body in spite of intervening fracture at neck.

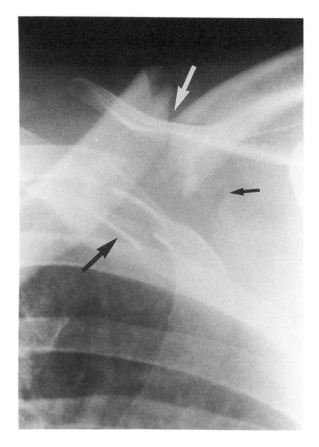

Figure 10.12 Scapular body fracture (small black arrow) associated with rib fracture (large black arrow) and midshaft clavicular fracture (white arrow).

Physical Examination. Evidence of contusion to the back, top, or lateral aspect of the shoulder are associated with scapular fractures. Inability to lift one's arm, clavicular fractures, evidence of brachial plexus injury, and vascular trauma under the clavicle have significant correlation with scapular fractures.

Imaging and Lab Analysis. X-rays of the scapula are not very well defined, and lesions can be missed. If the distance from the medial scapular border to the spine is different from one shoulder to the other, or if by chance a fracture is noted on the scapular body, radiographic evidence of scapular trauma can incidently be detected. Axillary X-rays done in a supine or a prone position, even angled down 45° from either of these positions, can give evidence of fracture of the scapular spine and the base of the coracoid. The axillary X-ray, lateral scapular view, and 15°-downward-angled AP Grashey view done tangentially at the glenohumeral joint can give evidence of avulsion fractures around the glenoid rim. A CT scan or three-dimensional reconstruction CT scan can help in surgical reconstruction and is warranted in complex fracture patterns.

Anyone with significant contusion to the back or point of the shoulder should have arterial blood gases checked, not only to rule out scapular injury itself, but to help assess concurrent injury to the lung. A chest X-ray is warranted, as well as the standard office four-view X-ray series.

Classification. Injuries to the scapula can be graded as Type A, acromial; Type B, body; Type C, coracoid; and Type D, injuries involving the scapular neck and glenoid fossa (Figure 10.13).

Type A. Type A injury involves the scapular spine or acromion, which was a late evolutionary development and exists to help contain the humeral head. Because of the acromion's late development, it has multiple epiphyseal centers, and stress prior to fusion may lead to nonunion or fibrous union in between centers of ossification, which in turn leads to instability and wear into the rotator cuff. The scapular spine is particularly prone to blunt trauma with minimal displacement or even to stress fracture after impaction from a baseball or from martial arts weapons or after falling on the point of the shoulder.

Type C. Type C injuries occur at the other end of the containment spectrum, that is, the coracoid. The coracoid is the anterior prominence of the scapula and is connected to the acromion by the coracoacromial ligament and a number of suspen-

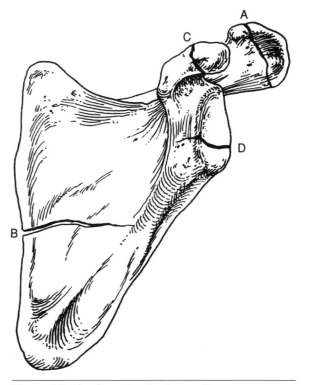

Figure 10.13 Scapular fracture patterns.

sory ligaments and to the clavicle and the humerus, maintaining the superior integrity of the glenohumeral joint. Fracture or subluxation in a superior direction can fracture the coracoid as well, or because of coracohumeral attachment, inferoanterior displacement may pull off the coracoid (Figure 10.14, a and b). Skeet shooting or the use of a rifle may fracture the base of the coracoid.

Type B fractures, or fractures into the body of the scapula, occur with the highest energy injuries. These fractures are well enveloped in muscle and in most cases do not require surgical intervention (Figure 10.15).

Type D. Type D injuries, or injuries into the scapular neck or glenoid fossa, are the most common injuries found in athletics (Figure 10.16). Type D1, or fracture at the base of the scapular neck, is usually stable if the clavicle and superior mechanisms remain intact. If there is an A/C joint separation or clavicular fracture, a Type D fracture can be quite unstable, and fixation of the A/C joint or clavicle is required to afford some stability.

D2 injuries are glenoid rim fractures that commonly occur with dislocation. Posteriorly, these fractures are usually due to avulsion within the capsule, and anteriorly they can be due to impaction at the time of dislocation or reduction.

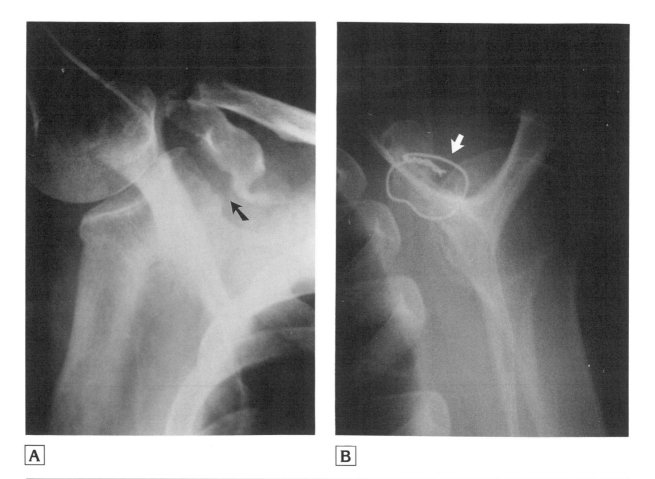

Figure 10.14

[A] Coracoid avulsion fracture.

[B] Postoperative reduction of coracoid with tension band; associated SLAP lesion was repaired arthroscopically.

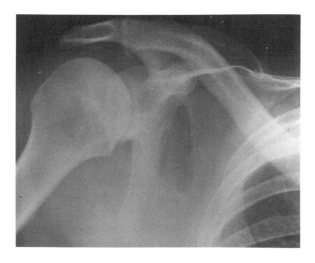

Figure 10.15 Scapular body fracture healed well due to surrounding muscular envelope, which maintained peripheral muscular attachment.

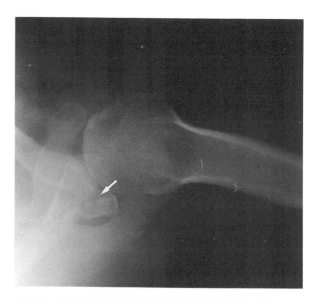

Figure 10.16 Impaction of humeral head causes glenoid fracture at scapular neck, which remains stable postinjury.

Large inferoanterior rim fractures, which frequently take up to 20% to 30% of the joint, are associated with persistent instability and require open reduction and internal fixation or capsular reattachment to the residual socket (Figure 10.17). Absorbable Vicryl pins or cannulated screws are useful if the athlete is extremely muscular, when positioning of more substantial hardware is next to impossible.

When Type D2 injuries are not treated acutely, the arthritic loose fragment is usually not salvageable, and the capsule must be attached to the remaining rim. The type of injury that breaks off 25% to 30% of the surface may drag the superior mechanism apart as well, so that superior glenohumeral ligament reanchoring to the glenoid and coracoglenoid ligament, as well as closure of an interval defect, tightening of the coracohumeral ligament, or repair of the SLAP lesion may be indicated to give the stability necessary to return to athletics.

Type D3 injury occurs with an abducted impaction injury, as in falling laterally on one's elbow, in which a horizontal or an oblique fracture into the glenoid surface skives an inferior fragment that includes part of the glenoid neck. This fragment usually remains with the humeral head, implies a superior mechanism disruption, and needs operative repair, which is difficult and often requires anchoring through the base of the coracoid with lag screw fixation.

Type D4 injury occurs transversely through the glenoid. This fracture propagates through the scapular neck and often includes the base of the

coracoid, because it occurs when lateral force on a slightly abducted arm pushes the humeral head upward to the curved upper glenoid (Figure 10.18). Injury through the rotator cuff or with associated A/C joint injury is not uncommon. One must look for injury to the brachial plexus, axillary nerve, musculocutaneous nerve, and suprascapular nerve with this type of injury. With luck these nerve injuries are transitory and should be serially assessed.

Type D5 injury develops with propagation of energy through the humeral head and into the scapula (Figure 10.19). This separates the upper and lower glenoid fossa, but because of muscle tissue surrounding the scapula, significant displacement is not the rule. In this case, after a short period of immobilization, active motion can be started.

Type D6 injury also occurs with axial loading in line with the plane of the scapula, which may lead

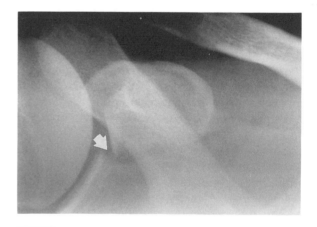

Figure 10.18 Type D4 glenoid and coracoid fracture with displacement at the glenoid.

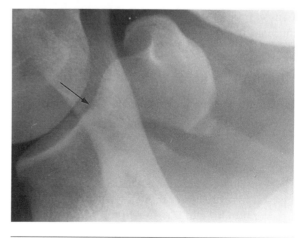

Figure 10.19 Type D5 glenoid and coracoid fracture into relatively undisplaced glenoid surface.

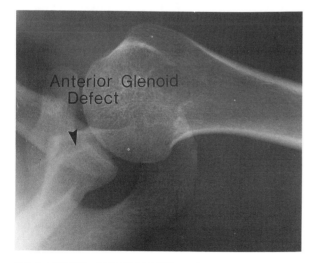

Figure 10.17 Erosion of the anterior glenoid rim due to recurrent dislocation may necessitate capsular reattachment to the deficient rim to afford stability.

to a starburst fracture pattern of the glenoid or to propagation into the scapula neck and beyond into the body, which in turn leads to fragmentation of the superior and inferior glenoid aspects. Open reduction and internal fixation can be attempted, but luckily these fractures do amazingly well without surgery, because the surgical exposure itself might lead to potential dysfunction.

Differential Diagnosis

Because of the rim fractures commonly associated with subluxation and dislocation at the glenohumeral joint, as well as the amount of trauma necessary to develop coracoid base or intrascapular fractures, differential diagnosis is limited. The most common confusion is with apophyseal and epiphyseal lines. Because the acromion is an evolutionary afterthought, there are many physeal lines that fuse late. In fact, trauma prior to the time of fusion or even after time of fusion may leave these physeal lines susceptible to fibrous union or stress fracture. In the young athlete this may be confused with an acute fracture. The older athlete who is susceptible to injury from high-energy impact and trauma may have an open growth plate. For example, the mesoacromion–meta-acromion junction commonly does not fuse until age 27, and a fracture may be missed. An axillary lateral X-ray and a comparison view of the opposite side is important to help avoid mismanagement. An unfused apophysis is believed to exist in 2% of the adult male population. It is 60% bilateral, but radiographic symmetry does not rule out injury on one of the sides. The best method to assess an unfused apophyseal injury is digital pressure to see if pain is produced. The base of the coracoid and the superior angle of the scapula may pull off in a growth plate injury in adolescent throwers. X-ray comparison with the opposite side will avoid confusion with normal apophyseal growth plate patterns.

Management

Management depends on the severity of the injury. Obviously, multitrauma must be handled appropriately, and the scapular fracture often is of the least concern. Associated rib fractures, pneumothorax, and hemothorax take precedence, as does treatment of abdominal injuries or other extremity injuries. In acute injury there is no rush for surgical intervention for rim fractures or glenoid extension fractures, unless there is significant mechanical instability, such as the inferior fragment and the humeral head moving together as a unit separate from the scapula. In scapular fracture a period of rest of 2 to 4 weeks followed by a gradual return of strength, especially of the humeral head depressors, may allow the athlete to return to full capacity within 6 to 12 weeks. Surgery is not indicated unless the injury recurs. Strengthening through physical therapy preoperatively acquaints the patient with postoperative exercises and hopefully will accelerate his or her progress.

The types of sports in which scapular body fractures occur, such as race car driving, motocross racing, or snowmobiling, may not require full function at the glenohumeral joint, and, other than minor complaints of scapulothoracic crepitation, the athlete may return to his or her sport with minimal discomfort. Most of these injuries can be managed conservatively, that is, by placing the patient in a sling until comfortable, usually 7 to 10 days, starting passive and active elevation, and then progressing toward strengthening exercises. Because of the muscular envelope around the scapular body, most fractures heal rapidly.

Complications

The main complications of scapular fractures are glenohumeral instability and subscapular crepitation. If after 3 weeks there is still some indication that the humeral head moves with an inferior fragment of glenoid, open reduction and internal fixation are mandatory for stability. If motion at the fracture site decreases, surgery can be avoided.

With open fracture, internal fixation and stability should help the healing process. The problem with leaving the injury alone is that stretch or laceration of neurovascular structures can progress and the injury can increase in severity. Potential complications of open treatment include osteomyelitis, nonunion, or worsening of overall mobility, because these fractures are very difficult to stabilize. The recent development of pelvic reduction plates and malleable thin hardware has led to better treatment of these fractures; however, the surgeon must be aware of neurovascular planes and normal anatomy in addressing these fractures.

Fractures involving the scapular body can lead to scapulothoracic bursitis, which may be merely annoying or may considerably limit motion. Involvement of the glenoid socket can lead to degenerative arthritis, necessitating prosthetic replacement, which would eliminate subsequent aggressive athletic activity.

Patient Education

The physician should tell the patient who has had scapular glenoid involvement that loose bodies and the need for subsequent reconstructive surgery might be anticipated. This may necessitate removal of loose fragments arthroscopically or as an open procedure and may require different types of surgical correction, including bone block and capsular stabilization that might limit motion. The physician should tell the patient that the injury is serious if the scapular body has been involved and that there is significant risk of neurovascular injury, painful nonunion, or arthritis with attempted operative correction.

Prevention

There is no way to prevent this type of injury other than learning proper falling techniques and increasing strength in internal and external rotation to keep the humeral head depressed and to allow muscles to work as shock absorbers. Nevertheless, the age of the patient, the density of the bone, and the energy of impaction dramatically alter the injury pattern sustained.

Humerus

Fractures about the shoulder and upper arm are not unusual in athletics. The injury sustained depends on the age of the athlete, the thickness of his or her bone, the energy pattern sustained in injury, and the mechanics of overuse. The range of injury encompasses stress fracture to displaced fracture.

Epidemiology

Humeral shaft fracture occurs in young pitchers and arm wrestlers. Such injury also occurs in athletes who either attempt to stop a fall or sustain blunt trauma to the upper arm, as in football, karate, and boxing.

Etiology

The etiology of injury varies significantly. Direct force can cause a humeral shaft oblique or straight fracture, whereas rotational force or twisting can cause a spiral fracture. Stress fracture or separation through the proximal humeral physis can occur with a single throwing episode or with repetitive throwing episodes. Fracture of the humeral head can occur with direct force, impaction, or dislocation. Trauma is the major cause of fractures of the proximal or midhumerus in younger individuals, whereas thinning of bone is correlated more highly with fracture in the older athlete. Obviously, fracture through a growth plate is more common in youth, whereas comminuted fractures may be more common with osteopenia and older age.

Natural History

The humeral shaft or epiphyseal injury in a young individual is much less disabling than malunion and intra-articular component injuries in an older individual, primarily because of the remodeling that can occur in youth. In the younger individual remodeling is the major factor in healing, and it compensates well. In the older individual, fractures in the joint or near the joint are more common and less forgiving; there is essentially no remodeling, and avascular necrosis and arthritis are more of a handicap.

Diagnosis

There is no historical factor that is of any significance other than the athlete reporting having heard a "snap" or "pop" at time of injury and significant pain afterwards. Contrary to most sport injuries about the shoulder, fractures of the proximal humerus and shaft rely on X-ray more than history for proper diagnosis. Clinical examination may demonstrate extreme swelling or ecchymosis and that the athlete holds the affected extremity closely with the other arm.

Imaging. If a humeral shaft fracture is suspected, a coaptation splint may make AP and lateral X-rays more comfortable (Figure 10.20). It is perhaps more important to keep the arm as it lies, because internal and external rotation views of the humeral shaft or proximal humerus may merely rotate the lower fragment while the upper fragment stays in place. To assess the proximal humeral head and neck, the four-view office series should be done. If it is too painful to abduct the arm for the supine axillary film, merely elevating the elbow on foam pads will give significant detail. The humeral head and neck will be well detailed. There may be considerable radiographic torsion of the shaft, but this is of little significance (Ciullo, Koniuch, Teitge, & May, 1982). In the pediatric and adolescent athlete, primarily because of slow closure of growth plates about the shoulder, comparison views of the opposite shoulder must be taken to help assess fracture patterns.

Classification. Grading of the fracture varies by age group and is important in considering conservative versus surgical management. The classification systems are not all-inclusive. Obviously, fractures can occur with dislocation, such as fracture

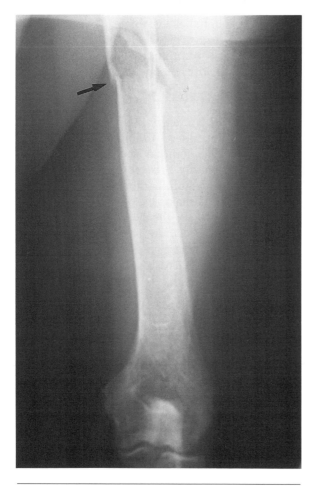

Figure 10.20 This 89-year-old roller blader fell and sustained a midshaft humeral fracture and radial palsy, assumed to be associated with hematoma. Symptoms resolved in 4 weeks using an external functional brace.

of the glenoid, coracoid, or acromion, and these are considered elsewhere in this book.

Growth Plate Injury. Utilizing the Salter-Harris classification (Salter & Harris, 1963; Figure 10.21), Type I is rarely seen in athletics except in young pitchers who have "Little League shoulder," or a stress fracture at the physeal line, and who continue to pitch with pain (Adams, 1966); displacement can occur (Figure 10.22). Displacement is managed surgically by closed reduction and percutaneous fixation under image intensification, using K-wires that are bent to prevent migration into the joint or preferably the newer cannulated AO 3.5 or 4.0 screws with large heads that will not migrate and can be percutaneously removed.

Type II Salter-Harris fractures through the growth plate propagating into the metaphysis posteromedially are the most common physeal

shoulder injuries to occur in young athletes. These occur from direct trauma, such as a kick or a fall directly on the shoulder as in soccer and football, or from indirect trauma, such as falling on the elbow or an arm outstretched behind the back or in front of the body, which most commonly occurs when sliding into base in baseball. These injuries occur primarily in the 12- to 17-year-old age group. The younger the patient is, the more displacement is allowed in management. Even 50% opposition of the fracture fragments and 40° angulation would be acceptable with 1 year of growth remaining.

In an acute injury, reducing the fracture under anesthesia should be attempted, which can be done by injection into the fracture hematoma, preferably in the operating room with an image intensifier. The arm is reduced in functional elevation (between strict abduction and strict forward flexion) in line with the plane of the scapula if the shaft is anterolateral and the bone spike into the metaphysis is posteromedial. The examiner can use his or her fingertips to maintain position of the humeral head fragment, spin the shaft into place by abducting and forward flexing the arm, and then bring it down to the side. In most cases reduction remains stable, and the patient can be placed in a Velpeau sling. There may be a slight loss of reduction over the next few days, but with remodeling this is generally of no significance. When the fragments do not lock into place, this usually means that the biceps tendon, periosteum, or other soft tissue is interposed.

Some orthopedists prefer a salute position, placing the patient in a spica cast with the arm abducted and forward flexed away from the body. However, there is a tendency toward development of brachial plexopathy in this position. More preferable is the use of a percutaneous pin into the proximal fragment, rotation of the shaft, and slight distraction of the fracture using the pin as a joy stick to release any soft tissue. This may allow the fragments to lock into place, at which point removal of the pin is possible. Otherwise, if there is a tendency toward redisplacement and instability, the pin can be driven across the growth plate into the head fragment and held in place with a number of small screws (preferably the cannulated type or a pin-screw device) placed percutaneously under image intensification control.

Type III physeal fracture, that is, an intra-articular extension of a physeal injury, is extremely rare and can occur with a dislocation, which would implicate significant trauma in a young athlete. It necessitates open surgery to replace the fragment and pin it in place.

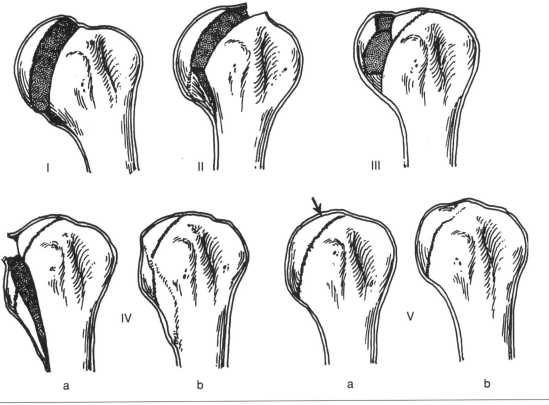

Figure 10.21 Youth growth plate fracture patterns.

Adapted from "Injuries Involving the Epiphyseal Plate" by R.B. Salter and W.R. Harris, 1963, *Journal of Bone and Joint Surgery*, **45A**, pp. 587-622.

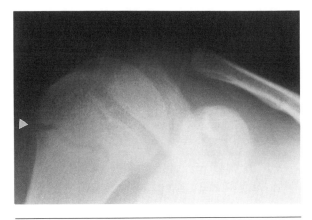

Figure 10.22 Little League shoulder, stress fracture at growth plate. Note widening of physis and lateral calcification (Adams, 1966).

Type IV injury similarly requires open reduction and internal fixation, but the pinning is through the metaphyseal fragment. Considerable degenerative changes are expected if Type III and IV physeal injuries are not reduced properly.

Type V injury implies longitudinal impaction of the humeral head to only a segment of the physeal plate, which leads to partial closure of the plate and growth arrest. This cannot be radiographically detected initially and mandates radiographic follow-up until growth is complete if an impaction type of injury has occurred and pain develops.

Shaft Fracture. Rotational and straight trauma to the upper arm in pitching and arm wrestling and direct contusion in karate, boxing, skiing, and football have led to humeral shaft injuries in both young athletes and adults. These are handled with a coaptation splint or a sugar-tong splint wrapped around the inside of the arm, around the elbow, and around the upper arm. The splint is used in conjunction with a sling and can be discarded at 3 weeks for a young athlete and at 6 weeks for an adult.

Lower-third humeral shaft fractures are associated with neurologic trauma to the radial nerve as it wraps around the back posteromedially to anterolaterally; absence of radial nerve function with this injury is commonly observed for the first 3 to 4 weeks. If nerve function does not return, exploration and fixation of the fracture might be considered. Most radial nerve palsies associated with this fracture resolve on their own. The exception to this is nerve palsy following primary operative intervention or closed reduction. If palsy developed after either of these, exploration and removal of the radial nerve from the fracture area with operative fixation of the bone is indicated.

Humeral Head Fracture. In active high school, college, and professional athletes, humeral head fractures commonly occur in association with dislocation of the glenohumeral joint. In older athletes and masters level professionals, a fall of as few as 3 feet or a direct impaction into the shoulder may be enough to fragment the humeral head into multiple pieces. The extent of fracture injury is therefore related to age, activity, the energy of trauma involved, and the condition of bone.

Compaction injuries commonly related to subluxation may range from mere abrasions seen arthroscopically but not radiographically to large indentations that are a mechanical cause for instability (Figure 10.23, a and b). Although Hill-Sachs lesions (Hill & Sachs, 1940) were originally described as impaction injuries in the posterolateral humeral head with anterior laxity, such impaction can occur at any point of the humeral head, indicating the line of energy transmission or type of dislocation. Inferior subluxation may cause abrasion or impaction at the top of the humeral head. Posterior dislocation can cause a reverse Hill-Sachs lesion at the anterior humeral articular surface.

Such abrasions or impactions are graded as Type A, abrasion; Type B, less than 20% impaction; Type C, 20% to 45% impaction; and Type D, greater than 45% impaction (Figure 10.24a). This indicates the extent of humeral head involvement, not the depth of the impaction.

Codman (1934) must be credited with the development of a fracture classification system for the humeral head. He described the four major fracture fragments: A, greater tuberosity; B, lesser tuberosity; C, articular head; and D, shaft (Figure 10.24b). Neer (1970) expanded this system to emphasize displacement needing surgical reduction to avoid avascular necrosis. Neer stated that segments displaced over 1 cm or angulated greater than 45° would be considered displaced and that displacement needs surgical reduction. The system is simple in that the number of displaced fragments are essentially as Codman originally described them, and if the articular segment is devoid of blood supply, it necessitates open reduction or even artificial shoulder joint replacement. Fracture dislocation occurs with this type of injury, as does rotator cuff tearing; concurrent repair must be considered.

With humeral head displaced fracture, avascular necrosis is a common complication, leading to degenerative changes within the joint, progressive wear of the rotator cuff, and loss of function of the shoulder. Jakob, Kristiansen, Mayo, Ganz, and Müller (1984) and the AO Group have amplified

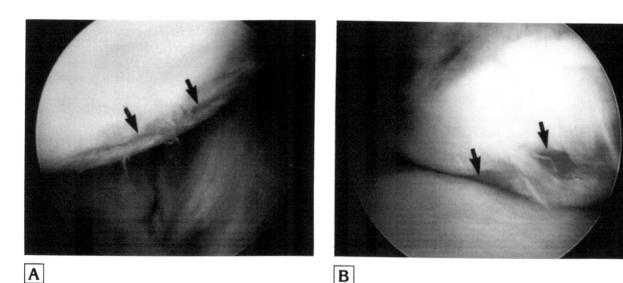

[A]

[B]

Figure 10.23 Hill-Sachs lesion, or impaction of posterior humeral head against anterior glenoid rim with anterior glenohumeral dislocation or subluxation, varies from

[A] minor abrasion to

[B] impaction fracture contributing to mechanical instability.

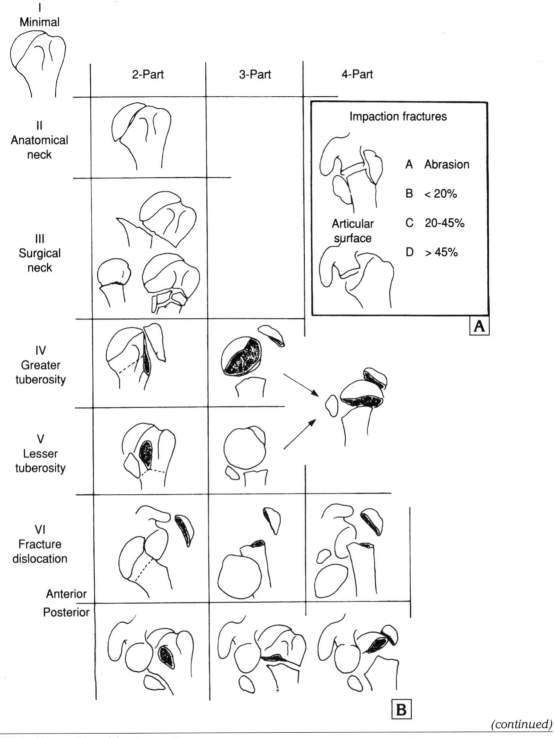

(continued)

Figure 10.24 Humeral head fracture patterns.

[A] Impaction fractures.

[B] Neer (1970) modification of Codman's (1934) classification system.

Adapted from "Displaced Proximal Humeral Fractures" by C.S. Neer, 1970, *Journal of Bone and Joint Surgery*, **52A**, pp. 1077-1089.

222 • Shoulder Injuries in Sport

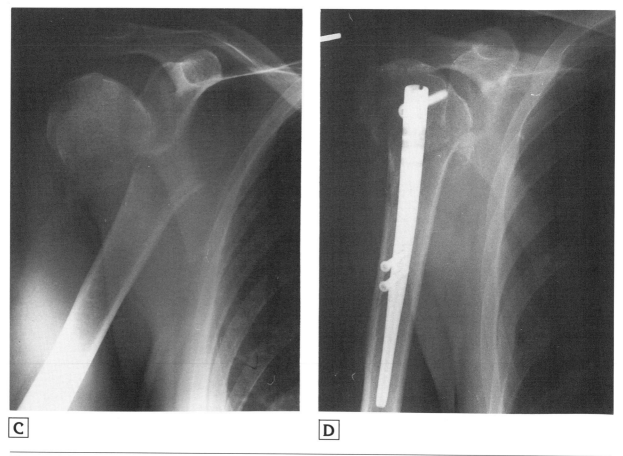

C   D

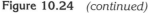

Figure 10.24   *(continued)*

  [C] Wheelchair athlete with limited lower extremity strength fell while attempting wheelchair transfer, sustaining four-part hand fracture of minimally displaced tuberosities and displaced humeral shaft.

  [D] Patient in [C] had displaced shaft fixed with locking Polarus rod (Acumed, Inc., Beaverton, OR). The minimally displaced tuberosities were only sutured, patient returning to wheelchair transfer in 3 weeks.

Dr. Neer's concepts. Type A in the AO classification occurs when there is no isolation of the articular segment from a vascular supply, that is, if it is extra-articular and still attached to the greater or lesser tuberosity. Type B has higher risk of avascular necrosis with intracapsular involvement. Even though three or four segments are involved, displacement is minimized. Their Type C injury has the highest rate of avascular necrosis, being intracapsular and having all four segments involved. Obviously, the greater the articular displacement and the less blood supply, the more chance for avascular necrosis. Preserving the blood supply in operative internal fixation is mandatory, and overzealous exposure can strip vascular supply and can lead to avascular necrosis, infection, or osteomyelitis of involved segments. There is now a tendency to use limited internal fixation (Figure 10.25, a and b).

Differential Diagnosis

Differential diagnosis is extremely limited because diagnosis is primarily radiographic. The fracture could be associated with a pathologic condition, such as aneurysmal bone cyst in a young individual or metastatic cancer in an older individual. The amount of bleeding, ecchymosis, and swelling would be the same. Inability to lift the arm may confuse this condition with rotator cuff tear, dislocation, calcific tendinitis, hemorrhage into a bursa, acromioclavicular sprain, adhesive capsulitis, or even impingement syndrome. These are easily differentiated by X-ray.

Management

If the fracture is stable, that is, minimally displaced with no motion noted in examination or in different X-ray positions, the arm should be kept still in

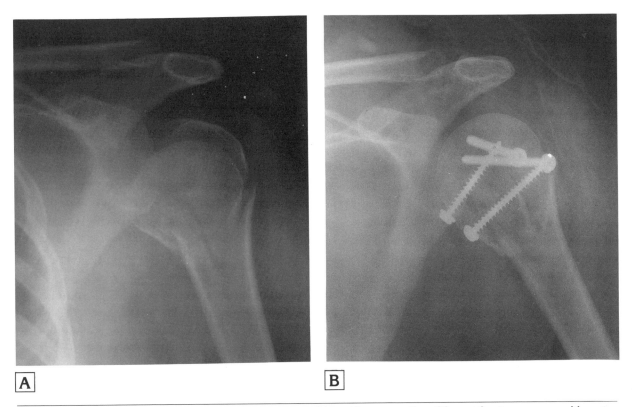

Figure 10.25 39-year-old competitive cross-country skier with a more than 20-part fracture managed by reconstruction of bicipital groove with limited fixation of AO screws and absorbable Vicryl pins.

[A] Preoperative multifragment fracture in osteopenic bone (previous salpingo-oophorectomy).

[B] Postoperative reduction with minimal fixation, returning to full function.

a sling for 2 to 3 days, and then early Codman exercises (in the sling) by bending forward at the waist can be initiated. If the fracture is not stable as seen by fluoroscopy at the time of percutaneous pinning or by the feeling of insufficient fixation at the time of operative repair, then the shoulder should be kept still in the sling for 3 weeks prior to initiating early passive exercises. When there is no pain with palpation and no significant discomfort with passive motion, usually at week 4 through 8, then active motion can be initiated.

A young athlete should have no pain in the area, full motion, and full return of strength prior to returning to activity, which may take 12 to 16 weeks. The older athlete must emphasize early motion and also regain full motion and strength as well as excellent healing noted by X-ray prior to returning to activity; otherwise he or she risks reinjury. Recovery may take up to a year in this older group.

In younger individuals conservative management is most likely the best treatment, because there is considerable remodeling. In older individuals for whom remodeling is not a factor surgical intervention is more necessary to reposition fragments, and early mobilization is mandatory to prevent postoperative stiffness.

Complications

A physeal injury, or injury to the growth plate, can lead to premature closure of the area. Partial closure may change the version of the glenoid neck, specifically to a varus or valgus attitude. Complete closure may lead to growth arrests such that this extremity becomes shorter than the other. A common complication of humeral shaft fracture is radial nerve trauma. The humeral head exhibits the widest range of potential complication. Malunion, fibrous union (Figure 10.26), and nonunion (Figure 10.27, a and b) may lead to poor cosmesis, decreased function, and significant pain.

More complex problems occur with neurovascular trauma, avascular necrosis, adhesive capsulitis, inadequate fixation, or hardware problems (Figure 10.28). Although it is commonly believed that operative intervention can cause the worst results, it must be remembered that patients with the highest degree of malpositioning or complicating factors

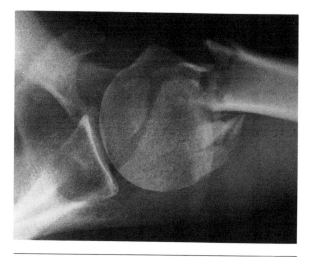

Figure 10.26 Painful fibrous union at surgical humeral neck with slight cosmetic dissymmetry and almost normal function.

such as biceps interposition and head splitting fractures are the most readily considered for operative intervention. They would predictably have had poorer results such as avascular necrosis or limited function anyway. Avascular necrosis or poor function may require hemiarthroplasty or total joint replacement, particularly in an older individual.

Prognosis

The goal is to return to activity as soon as possible, particularly for the older athlete. Factors such as osteoporosis may have been involved in the humeral head fracture, and activity is the best method of maintaining or regaining bone density. Stiffness is sure to develop if mobility is not established quickly. The young athlete in whom a stress fracture has displaced the growth plate must avoid pitching until pain is gone, full motion is established, and there is radiographic evidence of healing. This may take 1 year or longer, because pain can continue until the growth plate closes.

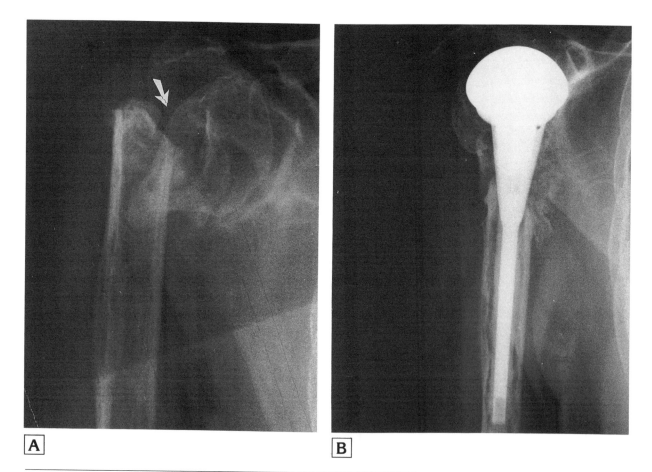

Figure 10.27

[A] Nonunion with humeral head fracture.

[B] ''Shish kebab'' cement-in fixation utilizing muscular attachments eliminated pain and increased function.

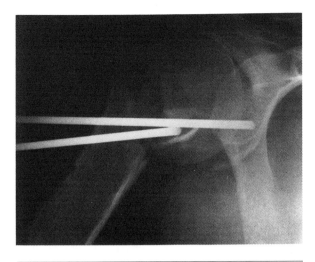

Figure 10.28 Attempted reduction of humeral neck fracture by pin fixation led to penetration of hardware into joint and nonunion of humeral neck.

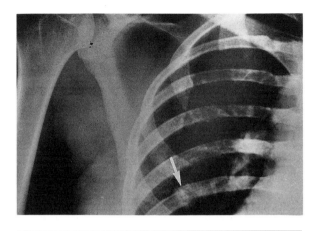

Figure 10.29 Rib stress fracture in college rower.

The long-term problem with humeral shaft injuries is nerve palsy, which may be permanent and may require muscle transfer to compensate for a radial nerve problem. Proximally, avascular necrosis and degenerative arthritis of the humeral head may be problematic. Malalignment may require osteotomy, which has a tendency to cause avascular necrosis and stiffness; manipulation under anesthesia or joint arthroplasty may become necessary. A fracture dislocation in an older athlete has a high correlation with rotator cuff pathology. Because older patients are already susceptible to fracture due to osteopenia, a prolonged period of disuse is a further disadvantage. Increased motion and shoulder utilization are important, and weight training may become a part of the older individual's regimen for injury prevention.

Patient Education and Prevention

The patient must be well rehabilitated prior to returning to activity. Otherwise, reinjury or a more complicated injury can occur. The athlete must have full range of motion, must have been taught a flexibility and strengthening program, must have full strength, and must go over the fundamentals with his or her coach or club pro prior to returning to sport in an effort to prevent reinjury or more serious injury.

Stress Reaction

Stress fractures can occur from chronic overuse. They most commonly develop in areas of growing bones, such as apophyseal lines and physeal plates, where injury has been referred to as "growing pain."

Epidemiology

Injuries in growing area of bone most commonly occur when muscles are not strong enough to work as shock absorbers, so that bone takes the stress. In youth athletes this occurs with weight training and repetitive throwing.

Pathology

In long bones, cyclic loading can lead to microfracture build-up. About the shoulder this most commonly occurs in the rib and has been seen in activities like weight training and rowing (Figure 10.29). Widening of the *proximal humeral physis* has been labeled as "Little League shoulder" by Adams (1966) and tends to occur in the zone of hypertrophy near the area of provisional calcification of the growth plate. There are also a number of scapular apophyses that may not fuse due to stress. Most commonly the two to five ossification centers of the acromion, which usually fuse by age 22, may be affected by stress, primarily subluxation, leading to what has been called *os acromiale* (Kohler & Zimmer, 1988; Liberson, 1937).

The physician must be aware of apophyseal lines, especially because contusion in youth contact sports such as basketball, football, skate boarding, and baseball may lead to misdiagnosis when X-ray identifies an apophyseal line. Many of the so-called mesoacromial deformities or os acromiale are in fact related to superior subluxation or impaction: The instability of the glenohumeral joint is transmitted across to the acromion, leading to increased motion at the apophyseal line and failure to heal or to development of a stress reaction (Figure 10.30, a-c). This in turn propagates an impingement phenomenon and makes the situation worse. Many patients who are found with an os acromiale or mesoacromial deformity later in life remember an athletic injury from their youth such as blunt contusion, impingement symptoms, or falling on an outstretched arm that forced the humeral head upward.

Natural History

If there is point tenderness about an apophysis or growth plate, it is important to stop the inciting activity. Otherwise, there can be slippage in areas such as the proximal humeral physis such that malunion and deformity can occur. If apophyseal nonunion or mesoacromial deformity is in fact due to a chronic stress reaction, early treatment may avoid later rotator cuff and subluxation symptoms (Figure 10.31, a-d).

Diagnosis

A young athlete may not be able to recall an exact injury that caused pain at a growth plate, at an apophysis, or in a long bone related to a stress

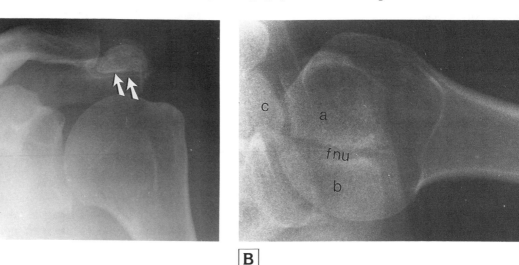

[A]

[B]

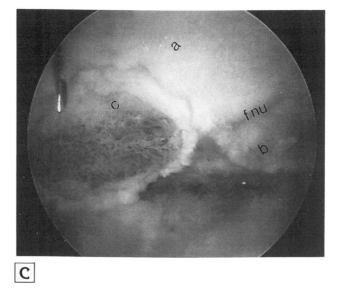

[C]

Figure 10.30 Mesoacromial deformity may be a stress fracture due to superior motion of humeral head.

[A] Double-rim sign on AP film pathognomonic of mesoacromial deformity.

[B] Mesoacromial deformity is best seen on axillary view.

[C] Corresponding arthroscopic view of loose anterior fragment (a) and acromial base (b) in relation to distal clavicle (c). Fibrous nonunion (fnu) is apparent following subacromial decompression, acromioplasty, and claviculoplasty. Note marking needle through A/C joint.

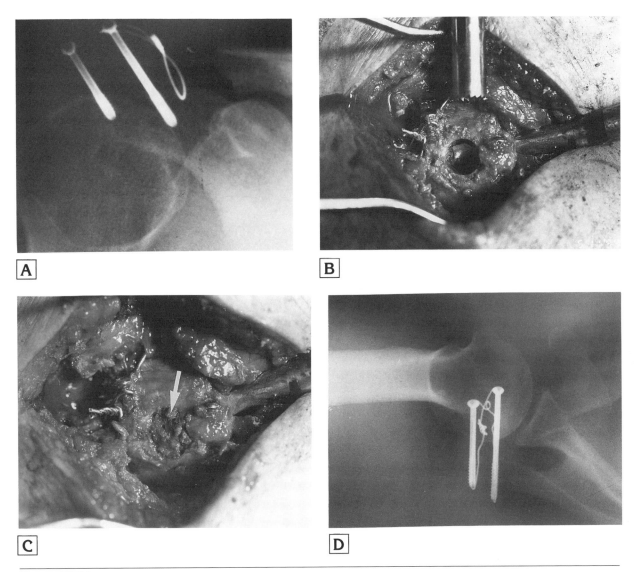

Figure 10.31

[A] Open reduction and internal fixation of a nonunion mesoacromial fracture utilizes lag screw fixation, resection of nonunion site, and distal clavicle bone graft with a tension band following endoscopic subacromial decompression so that the deltoid is not taken down, and therefore earlier rehabilitation can be initiated.

[B] Circle plug excision of the nonunion area can allow rotational osteotomy or bone graft from another area.

[C] Bone graft from distal clavicle resection shown in place with compression screw fixation and tension band to allow early motion exercises; the hardware does not need to be removed unless late subacromial symptoms or subcutaneous pain are implicated.

[D] Alternately cannulated screw, figure-8 wire fixation with bone graft gives excellent stability.

fracture unless blunt contusion was involved. Frequently the blunt contusion is merely aggravating a preexisting condition and brings that condition to the forefront. Once the symptoms develop, however, the patient can point to a specific area that hurts during everyday and athletic activity. Point tenderness near a growth plate or apophysis in a young athlete is assumed to be a stress fracture until proven otherwise. Bone scan will be useful in defining stress injuries, particularly early on when the sclerosis that occurs in healing is not yet evident. Routine X-rays are important, but if stress reactions are suspected, it is important to take a plain X-ray of the opposite side for comparison (Figure 10.32, a-c).

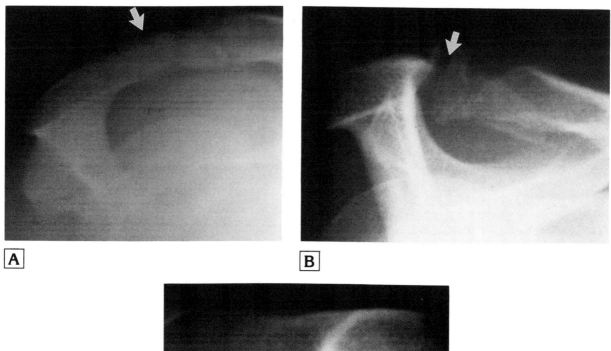

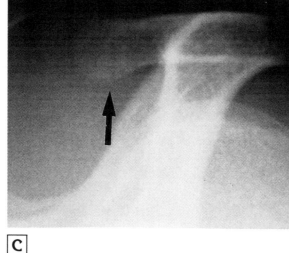

Figure 10.32

[A] Acute overuse acromial stress fracture in a 16-year-old swimmer, which went on to heal with a decreased training regimen; opposite shoulder was normal.

[B] A fracture similar to that above went on to nonunion, because continued overuse leading to impingement symptoms from a loose anterior fragment.

[C] Stress fracture may develop into fibrous union and moderate impingement. Alternately, it may heal, leading to a central projecting bulge into the supraspinatus outlet—a type IV acromion.

Differential Diagnosis

Most stress reactions occur in young athletes, but tumors and bone cysts must be ruled out as well. Snapping under the scapula may be misdiagnosed as subscapular bursal adhesions, and the possibility of rib fracture must be assessed carefully.

Management

The treatment of bone breakdown related to cyclic loading is to stop the inciting activity and give the bone a chance to heal. In young athletes this healing is rapid. Modifying activity can also decrease the incidence of occurrence. The advent of T-ball has markedly diminished the incidence of proximal humeral growth plate widening in Little League pitchers. New Little League rules that reduce the number of innings that a young athlete may pitch have also markedly diminished the incidence of this entity. Unless the physis falls off over the growth plate, there is no cause to consider surgery. Rest, that is, avoiding throwing,

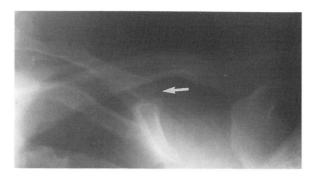

Figure 10.33 Cervical rib stress fracture in body builder led to thoracic outlet complaints.

can eliminate symptoms of Little League shoulder in 4 to 6 weeks. If sclerosis or widening of an apophyseal line such as in the acromion demonstrates a difference between the symptomatic and nonsymptomatic shoulders, overhead activity must be curtailed and humeral head depressing exercises of the infraspinatus and subscapularis initiated. Stress fractures about the rib (Figure 10.33), unusual before the age of 18, are usually treated with rest; however, if periosteal callus is excessive, surgical decompression or correction may be necessary.

Prognosis

The young athlete can return to activity when symptoms are essentially gone. There should be no pain in palpation over the injured area and no pain with activity. The athlete should gradually phase into regaining motion and strength and then into activity. Gradual return to activity must be stressed to the coach as well so that reinjury does not occur. Training the surrounding musculature allows the development of shock absorbers to take stress and helps to avoid reinjury. Proper body mechanics and linkage of all involved parts will help diminish the incidence of reinjury.

Summary

Skeletal injury about the shoulder can seriously hamper athletic performance. Acute injury leads to the need for immobilization or surgery, both of which lead to muscle atrophy and imbalance.

Clavicular fractures often do not warrant operative intervention and do well with a short period of immobilization. Scapular body fractures likewise do well if treated conservatively due to the soft tissue envelope that aids in alignment and healing. Displacement near the humeral neck that throws off the pull of rotator cuff, deltoid, and chest musculature more commonly needs surgical intervention to ensure athletic function.

Children have the highest potential for remodeling and rarely need surgery for injuries about the shoulder's growth plates; rest and immobilization are often enough to manage slight or moderate displacement. The adult athlete, however, does not have that potential for remodeling or adaption, and treatment more commonly necessitates a greater degree of operative intervention. Anatomic alignment of bony fragments about the shoulder is the goal. This will allow the most favorable return of muscle balance, strength, and coordination following osseous injury.

11

Osteoarthropathy: Arthritis and Arthrosis

Mechanical dysfunction due to wear or inflammation will seriously hamper the normal gliding motion at articular surfaces. Such changes will restrict the shoulder's athletic performance. Because the shoulder joints are functionally linked together, a problem at the glenohumeral joint, acromioclavicular joint, or sternoclavicular joint will lead to abnormal mechanics and muscle imbalance as other structures attempt to compensate for the damaged joint.

Because of the interrelationship of these joints, the common clinical patterns of osteoarthropathy will be described first, and specific problems and treatment modalities discussed afterwards.

General Overview

Osteoarthropathy is most commonly divided into osteoarthritis, an early phase of inflammation, and osteoarthrosis, the burnt-out stage of the disease.

Osteoarthritis may occur as thinning or loss of buffering articular cartilage about the shoulder at the acromioclavicular, glenohumeral, and sternoclavicular joints. This may lead to *osteoarthrosis*, a process of enchondral ossification of cartilage, complete loss of cartilage, or bony hypertrophy at the joint surface that distributes load across a wider area; the end result is bone-on-bone contact at the joint. *Heterotopic osteoarthropathy* is a third type of bone change at the joint due to metaplastic development of fibrous tissue into bony tissue; the frictional result can also lead to pain (Berg & Ciullo, 1995) (Figures 11.1, a-d and 11.2).

Epidemiology

A/C joint bony breakdown can be associated with almost every sport. Sternoclavicular arthritis occurs more commonly with contact sports such as football, rugby, and lacrosse. Glenohumeral arthropathy can be seen as an end stage of rotator

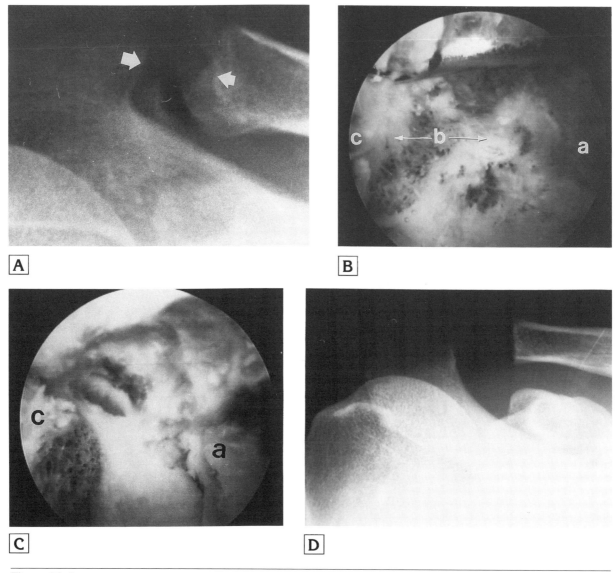

Figure 11.1

[A] Heterotopic osteoarthropathy of the A/C joint following arthroscopic A/C joint resection. Joint reforms within 4 weeks, leading to symptoms similar to the preoperative status. This condition is seen following endoscopic or open resection in patients with obesity, pulmonary problems (emphysema, COPD, tumor), polycythemia, Pickwickian syndrome, or asthma and in chronic smokers; decreased oxygen tension may lead to fibroblastic metaplasia of bone in the healing process (Berg & Ciullo, 1995).

[B] Bridging heterotopic bone seen arthroscopically (a = acromion, b = bone bridging Mumford gap, c = clavicle).

[C] Repeat endoscopic resection leaves parallel gap. Indomethacin and refraining from smoking are successful in preventing recurrence of bony bridging.

[D] X-ray following repeat resection.

cuff impingement or may be due to lack of stability associated with recurrent dislocation or subluxation. End-stage impingement leading to glenohumeral arthrosis is most common in swimming and weight training. Degenerative glenohumeral arthritis associated with recurrent dislocation is more common in the contact sports previously listed, but most common with hockey (Figure 11.3). Instability leading to glenohumeral subluxation can also wear out the articular surface during sports such as handball and racquetball. Avascular necrosis leading to degenerative glenohumeral arthritis has been associated with iatrogenic dose-pack cortisone medication, use of antiasthmatic medication, and exposure to high pressure changes such as in scuba diving.

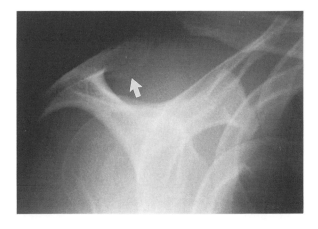

Figure 11.2 Build-up of bone under the acromion following acromioplasty may interfere with normal joint-like sliding of the supraspinatus against the acromion.

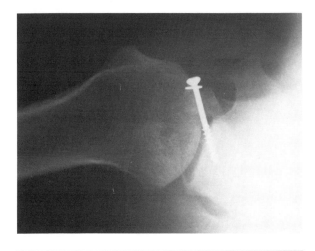

Figure 11.3 Glenohumeral arthritis continues in spite of attempted stabilization with coracoid transfer of bone in this professional hockey player.

Pathology

The hallmarks of osteoarthrosis are the same in the acromioclavicular, glenohumeral, and sterno-clavicular joints. After the initial inflammatory phase, there is joint space narrowing, formation of peripheral osteophytes, subchondral sclerosis, cyst formation, and surrounding osteopenia (Figure 11.4, a and b).

In addition, there may be central breakdown of the articular disk in the A/C joint and breakdown of the labral capsular complex in the glenohumeral joint. Progressive stretching of the capsule due to arthritic effusion in the sternoclavicular joint can accelerate arthritis. Although arthritic spurs form as the body's defense to instability, their formation

can lead to further erosion and stretching of the surrounding soft tissue.

Differential Diagnosis

When X-ray changes are seen there is a high correlation with clinical findings of arthritis. X-rays lag behind the actual pathology in that chondral thinning may not be well appreciated. Arthrotomy or arthroscopy usually demonstrates more pathology than is evident on X-ray. It must be remembered that degenerative changes can occur without symptoms, or variance in pain tolerance can alter the clinical significance of degenerative change.

The examiner must correlate radiographic change to the history and clinical findings. Pain in the extremes of motion, horizontal flexion, attempted hyperabduction, and reverse extension is seen not only in A/C joint arthritis, but also in rotator cuff pathology, initiation of capsulitis, and scar build-up between the deltoid and rotator cuff. Accurate clinical examination is critical.

Pain over any of these joints can be due to septic arthritis, rheumatoid arthritis, neuropathic changes, or metastasis, especially in the older athlete. Neuropathic joints about the shoulder may be painful, including Charcot joints where pain is common in wheelchair athletes affected with syringomyelia (Figure 11.5, a and b). Cervical radiculopathy can present as pain about the shoulder joints as well, and examination of the cervical spine with EMG when indicated is important. MRI, computer tomography, and plain X-rays are valuable in assessing neoplasia or subchondral cysts, especially with osteopenia that occurs in older age groups.

Management

Initial management of arthritis consists of anti-inflammatory medication, gentle mobilization exercises, stretching, and strengthening. Muscles must be built up to work as shock absorbers to unload the affected joint. Increased motion can decrease fibrosis about the joint, which in some cases can be demonstrated on plain X-ray to open an A/C joint that has been essentially closed due to degenerative change (Figure 11.6, a and b).

Naprosyn and aspirin tend to work well to diminish synovial inflammation associated with early arthritis. Once the inflammatory phase is diminished and there has been a loss of articular cartilage or disk material, then medications such as Voltaren and Ansaid are more effective. The A/C joint responds well to Indomethacin in single unit dosage every morning. Fibrosis in itself is

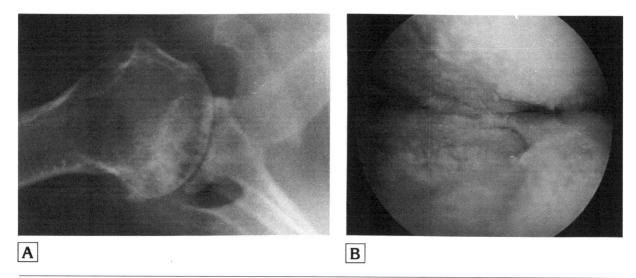

Figure 11.4 Inflammatory breakdown may lead to cystic absorption and sclerotic reformation of bone at a joint.

[A] Widening at the articular interface by bony build-up will help distribute the force over a larger distance.

[B] Nevertheless, arthritic symptoms continue due to loss of frictionless surface.

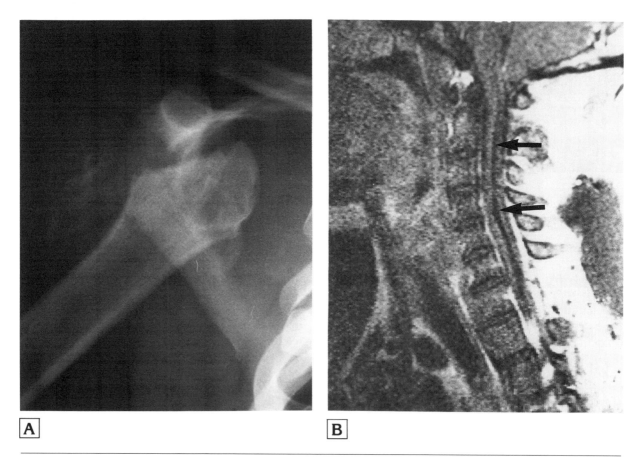

Figure 11.5 Fluid build-up and arthrosis may lead to painless breakdown or even dislocation, as in this Charcot joint related to syringomyelia in a former wheelchair athlete with spina bifida.

[A] X-ray of painless chronic dislocation.

[B] MRI showing expanding syrinx in cervical cord.

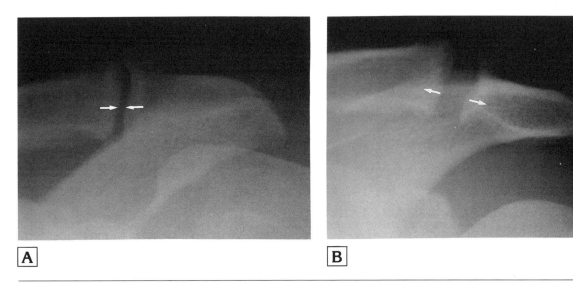

Figure 11.6

[A] Bone-on-bone grinding and relative lack of motion in acromioclavicular joint arthritis may lead to pain with direct pressure or to compensating periscapular muscle spasm related to scapulothoracic overuse.

[B] Horizontal flexion and hyperabduction stretching may unlock the joint and even allow some fibrous ingrowth, eliminating symptoms in as little as 4 weeks of physical therapy or home exercise.

painful, and mobilization can markedly diminish pain. Physical therapy should be considered when there has been no response to a home management program and anti-inflammatory medication.

When conservative methods fail, surgical intervention can be considered, primarily for the acromioclavicular and glenohumeral joints. Surgery does not work well on the sternoclavicular joint because of this joint's anchoring function for the entire extremity, and it is rarely necessary. Sternoclavicular surgery is considered a salvage procedure. A small shift in orientation or decrease in motion due to arthritic change, stiffness, or pain can be immediately obvious and affect performance.

Prognosis

If anti-inflammatory medication in conjunction with mobilization and strengthening is successful in limiting arthritic pain, the patient can return to athletic performance. This may take from 2 weeks to 6 months. Assuming that the athlete seeks medical attention as soon as symptoms develop, the time needed to return to the previous level of activity should approach the lesser end of the spectrum.

Patient Education

The athlete must be advised against the "no pain, no gain" philosophy. When pain develops, medical attention should be sought. Early mobilization and strengthening, along with anti-inflammatory

medication, can markedly change the course of degenerative arthritis. Once degeneration progresses to an end stage of instability problems or muscular degeneration, then management becomes a salvage situation (Figure 11.7, a and b).

If conservative measures diminish symptoms, it is mandatory that the athlete continue the strengthening and stretching program on a lifetime basis in an effort to maintain the ability to perform athletically. The athletic activity itself will not be enough to minimize symptoms, and specific exercises and stretching must augment the normal training program in order to allow participation to continue more comfortably.

Prevention

There is no guaranteed way to prevent arthritis. Microtrauma and even fracture into the joint from athletic activity with luck can be compensated for by keeping muscles strong so that they work like shock absorbers to decelerate arthritis. Proper mechanics in athletic performance, flexibility, and strength can all diminish the microtrauma that will lead to degenerative change and must be stressed before arthritis develops.

Acromioclavicular Arthropathy

The A/C joint is the most commonly affected of the three shoulder articulations. Its inherent stability and relative lack of motion make it the most

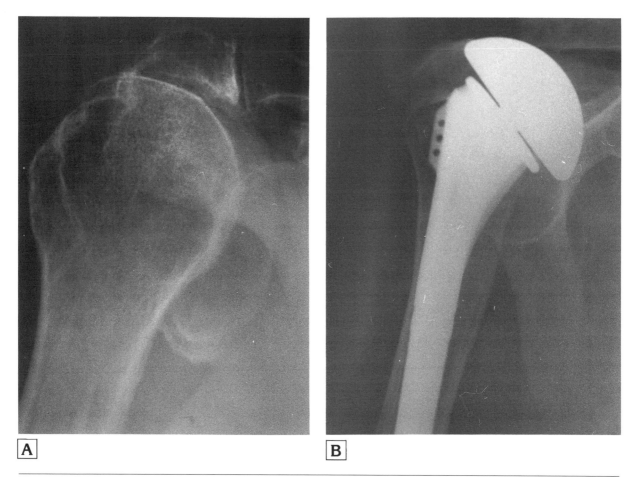

A   **B**

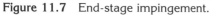

Figure 11.7   End-stage impingement.

  [A] Humeral head contact against the acromion through a massive hole in the rotator cuff leads to bony glenohumeral breakdown, inferior acromial spurs, and progression of A/C joint arthritis.

  [B] Stuffing the joint with an oversized prosthesis allows contact of both the acromion and humeral head. This salvage procedure allows a return to activity such as swimming, golf, and occasionally tennis.

susceptible to micromotion build-up and degenerative change. Energy transmitted through a subluxating humeral head irritates the undersurface of the acromion, leading secondarily to degenerative change at the A/C joint. Micromotion of a meso-acromial fibrous union or nonunion similarly causes breakdown at the A/C joint and degenerative change.

Pathogenesis

The distal cartilage of the clavicle acts as a growth plate and is responsible for longitudinal growth. The unossified end clavicular cartilage, or disk, buffers motion between the two bones. With calcification, this cushioning effect is lost, and the bone-on-bone contact causes pain. The articular cartilage undergoes a process of enchondral ossification to obtain length; the end stage, however, is degenerative arthritis (Figure 11.8).

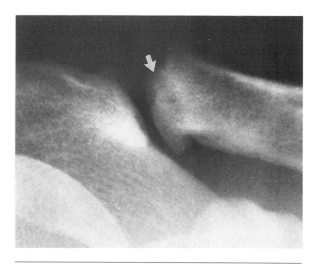

Figure 11.8   Echondral ossification at the distal clavicle may allow clavicular growth in youth but is the common basis of degenerative arthritis, especially with aging.

Fractures into the A/C joint, which can be seen either radiographically or by arthroscope, lead to bleeding in this area that subsequently can ossify the articular disk of the clavicular cartilage (Figure 11.9).

The S-shaped clavicle and the C-shaped articular disk allow energy transmission through the joint when they are working in concert. However, decreased motion, increased irritation in energy transmission to the joint, and repetitive trauma can lead to atypical ossification patterns and breakdown within this joint such that its normal AP vertical orientation becomes more angular on AP X-ray (Figure 11.10, a and b). A C-shaped or cup shaped change is another possibility (Figure 11.11). These changes will allow for dissipation of energy along a longer surface, usually paralleling the direction of the coracoacromial ligament.

C-shaped, cup-shaped, or other variations are due to stress forces possibly related to utilization patterns and posture. These variations do not allow normal motion, so that grinding is produced in overhead activity, accelerating the arthritic process. Jamming the rough surfaces together, as when sleeping on the shoulder, will cause pain. Hyperabduction, horizontal flexion, and reverse extension—the normal motions through the joint—will become progressively limited and painful. Because similar findings can occur with sprain injury and because there is some overlap with fibrotic changes in rotator cuff disease and adhesive capsulitis, the X-ray is critical to aid in diagnosis.

If the rotator cuff has a hole in it that the humeral head can buttonhole into, energy is transmitted directly to the acromion and then secondarily to the A/C joint, leading to further breakdown and inflammatory changes about the A/C joint and also accelerating degeneration. A SLAP lesion or labral interposition may wedge the humeral head upward into the A/C joint. An acromioclavicular sprain injury, which may or may not be associated

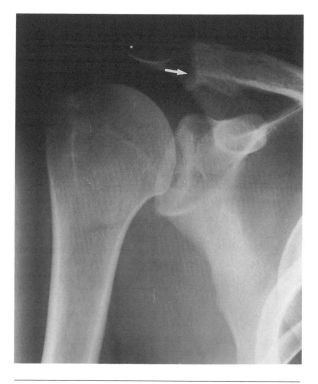

Figure 11.9 Fracture or microfracture into the A/C joint may introduce a blood supply and ossify the clavicular end cartilage or disk, leading to arthrosis.

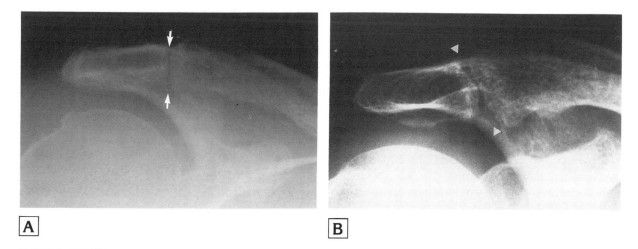

Figure 11.10 Change in orientation of the A/C joint (seen on AP X-ray).

[A] Normal superior-to-inferior straight joint.

[B] Angulation at the A/C joint may be secondary to stress remodeling caused by forces parallel to the coracoacromial ligament; this increases grinding at the joint in overhead motion.

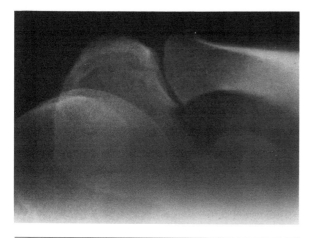

Figure 11.11 Stress remodeling or congenital difference may be the basis of a cup-shaped or a C-shaped A/C joint; this must be taken into account to produce a parallel gap at resection.

with a small capsular avulsion fracture, also leads to degenerative arthritis or the formation of peripheral spurring to help stabilize the joint.

Natural History

A/C joint arthritis, if untreated, can get progressively worse. It is not unusual, however, that the athlete may change the demands on this joint; that is, the athlete may decrease participation in certain sports and elect less stressful sport activity as he or she gets older. As demands decrease, so might the symptoms. Arthritic changes at the A/C joint, however, can also contribute to the impingement process, accelerating rotator cuff disease.

Diagnosis

A/C joint arthritis may be symptomatic during athletic activity but also may be annoying with simple actions such as reaching backward in reverse extension to slip on a shirt sleeve, with overhead activity such as weight lifting, or with activity across the front of the body such as pulley work or narrow-gripped weight activity. The athlete may have activity pain or night pain that is made worse by sleeping on the shoulder, which compresses the arthritic surfaces together.

Physical Examination. The A/C joint may be prominent due to osteophytes, and there may be tenderness with palpation. Pain at this joint, if arthritic, will be made worse with horizontal flexion, hyperabduction, and reverse extension (Figure 11.12).

There may be anteroposterior instability causing pain and grinding. Superior displacement associated with previous separation is also common, particularly if the separation was only partial or if there was a fracture into the joint or inferior periosteal stripping associated with that separation (Figure 11.13). Such a change may be clinically suspected and radiographically verified.

Imaging. X-rays may disclose spurring of the A/C joint, which may be unilateral (even just under the clavicle) and which lead to impingement problems. Bone scans are equivocal. They may disclose significant pathology, although they can be falsely negative if the degenerative arthritis is burnt out or has spread the force over a distance, decreasing inflammation. One must treat the symptoms and rely on clinical examination rather than bone scan.

Differential Diagnosis of Osteolysis

There is no strict grading system for A/C joint arthritis; however, presentation varies. Osteolysis, or focal absorption of the distal end of the clavicle, is a common presentation in athletics (Figure 11.14, a and b). Osteolysis occurs in males and females, specifically with weighted activity.

In 1983, when Wayne State University's football coach initiated an aggressive weight training program, eight individuals on the team developed osteolysis at the same time. This is a self-limiting problem, and all of these individuals resolved symptoms with anti-inflammatory medication, mobilization exercises, and refraining from weight training over an 8- to 16-week period. The distal clavicle reossified, no arthritis occurred, and all players returned to full activity.

Development of arthritis in the healing phase is not uncommon. If arthritis develops, distal clavicle resection can be considered. Alternatively, a primary A/C joint cyst unrelated to rotator cuff pathology may form (Figure 11.15, a and b).

Management

The A/C joint itself with its V-shaped, posteriorly based orientation is set up to develop arthritis. A sprain or fracture into this joint or energy transmission up through the acromion from the humeral head due to subluxation or functional interposition can cause breakdown. Attempted mobilization with horizontal flexion and hyperabduction stretching exercises along with anti-inflammatory medication, specifically Indomethacin, can manage this conservatively.

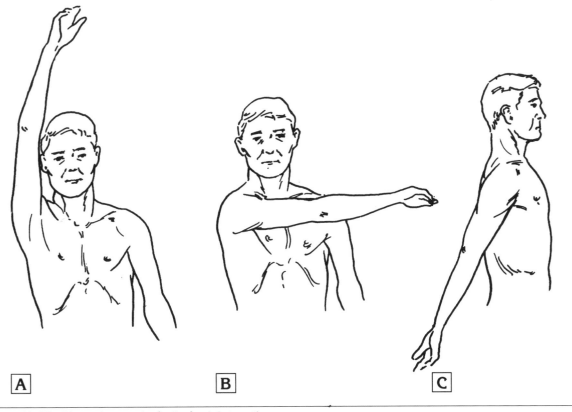

Figure 11.12 Normal acromioclavicular joint motion—

[A] hyperabduction

[B] horizontal

[C] reverse

—is painful with arthritis or acute sprain.

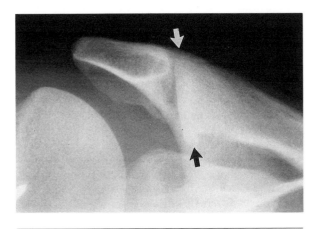

Figure 11.13 Widening of the distal end of the clavicle, increasing surface area, may follow A/C joint sprain, fracture into the joint, or separation associated with inferior periosteal stripping.

When conservative management fails, then surgical debridement of the joint can be considered. Surgical debridement involves resecting the distal end of the clavicle and infra-acromial and clavicular spurs when the joint is vertical in orientation or resection of the inferior triangle of the medial acromion and the superior triangle of lateral clavicle to give a parallel 1-cm gap when there is an oblique orientation to the joint (Figure 11.16). This can be accomplished either with open surgery or arthroscopically.

Dome decompression or resection of the osteophytes on the inferior surface by endoscopic means may eliminate symptoms if A/C joint motion can be restored (Figure 11.17, a-c). Endoscopic subacromial debridement or resection of the distal clavicle by an experienced surgeon does not take longer than an open procedure, but rehabilitation is generally quicker, because the deltoid is not taken down and therefore does not have to heal prior to the initiation of motion (Table 11.1).

Degeneration of the A/C joint, caused either by trauma or by abnormal stresses across the joint,

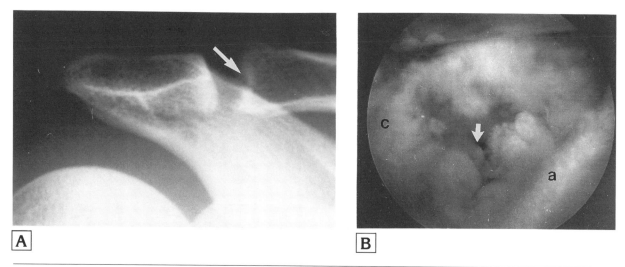

Figure 11.14

[A] Osteolysis at the distal end of the clavicle. Inflammatory absorption may resolve on its own, leading to re-creation of joint or arthritic changes.

[B] Arthroscopic equivalent. Note granulomatous tissue and bony erosion (arrow) at lateral clavicle (c) abutting medial acromion (a).

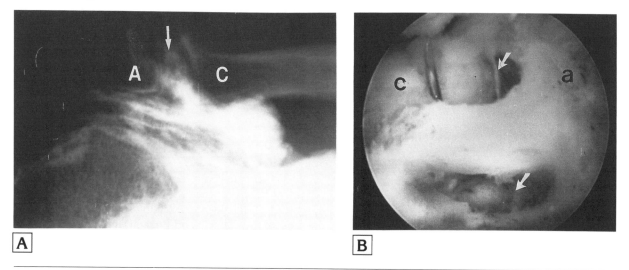

Figure 11.15

[A] Geyser sign on CT-arthrogram usually indicates glenohumeral fluid leakage through a hole in the rotator cuff with a secondary synovial cyst developing in the A/C joint. Iatrogenic injection of contrast dye into the subacromial space is seen here. At surgical lateral clavicectomy, no hole was found in the rotator cuff. This was a primary A/C joint cyst.

[B] Subacromial endoscopic view of the opening of the synovial cyst at A/C joint in the same patient.

can seriously hamper athletic performance. The patient will tend to throw more side-armed or have difficulty in weight training. If osteolysis develops, weight training should be temporarily halted. Although the A/C joint does not have a significant amount of motion, osteophytic locking of its limited motion leads to overuse of the sterno-clavicular, glenohumeral, and scapulothoracic joints. Symptoms of subscapular bursitis are not uncommon following degeneration of the A/C joint. Once spurring develops under the clavicle or acromion, wearing into the rotator cuff (impingement) occurs and leads to erosion of the superior suspensory mechanism, muscle thinning, and superior migration of the humeral head; this increases force against the acromion and

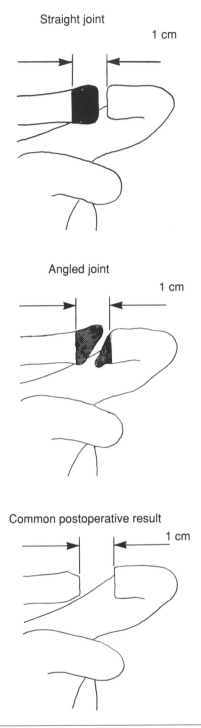

Straight joint

1 cm

Angled joint

1 cm

Common postoperative result

1 cm

Figure 11.16 Regardless of arthritic or stress remodeling of the joint, the end result must be a parallel resection accomplished either arthroscopically or in open surgery.

accelerates A/C arthritis. Thus develops a self-perpetuating problem leading to end-stage triad degeneration.

In treatment with stretching and strengthening, pain may not decrease or may worsen, and opera-

tive intervention may be necessary. Occasionally, after surgical debridement of the joint, heterotopic bone formation may develop, related to either premature activity, previous injury and related A/C laxity, or a pulmonary osteoarthropathic problem in recreational athletes who are somewhat barrel-chested, who have symptoms of emphysema or polycythemia, or who have a significant history of either smoking or asthma. Although this is not a common situation, when it does occur with associated instability, stabilization of the A/C joint with a temporary transfixion Simmon's pin or a clavicular coracoid temporary screw can help redevelop normal mechanics in this area.

When there is no obvious coracoclavicular ligament problem or A/C instability, re-resection with adjuvant Indomethacin therapy or, rarely, radiation therapy in resistant cases can be considered. Re-resection with medication is most often successful. Occasionally, when the deltoid is taken down for distal clavicular resection, it may be avulsed with premature activity; loss of deltoid strength results. Immobilization after open decompressive surgery for at least 4 weeks is necessary to help prevent this complication.

When pain continues following distal clavicle resection, especially when associated with a grinding or click in the shoulder with overhead activity, a SLAP lesion that most likely was related to the original symptoms should be suspected. The proximity of the two joints (Figure 11.18a) means that functional interposition within the glenohumeral joint can be transmitted and can cause symptoms at the acromioclavicular joint. A needle placed through the A/C joint passes through the rotator cuff (Figure 11.18b) then directly into the SLAP lesion if one is present (Figure 11.18c) and demonstrates the correlation.

When pain near the A/C joint persists following distal clavicle resection, it is rarely associated with arthritis of the coracoclavicular joint. This joint is present instead of coracoclavicular ligaments in 1% of the population (Figure 11.19).

Glenohumeral Arthropathy

The athlete with glenohumeral arthritis usually presents late. He or she can no longer rotate the arm well in swimming, has difficulty serving overhead in tennis, or has a constant ache in the shoulder that is accompanied by loss of motion.

Epidemiology

Glenohumeral arthritis can result from direct trauma such as energy transfer through the joint

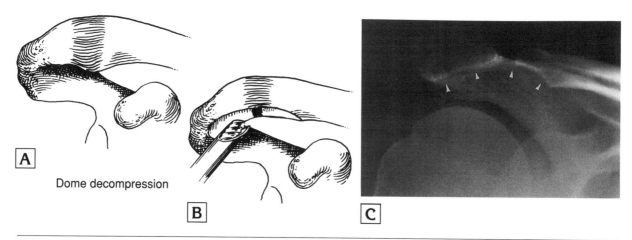

Figure 11.17 Dome decompression of the A/C joint may unlock the joint, restoring motion merely by resecting inferior osteophytes endoscopically.

[A] Preoperative appearance.

[B] Endoscopic technique.

[C] Radiographic result.

on impact loading as in playing handball (Figure 11.20, a and b) or stopping sideways momentum by an arm outstretched in functional abduction. The shoulder is not designed to be a weight-bearing joint. Sport activity such as body building, weight training, or gymnastics may place an unnatural load on the shoulder, which can lead to the development of arthritis.

Pathogenesis

Dislocation can lead to Hill-Sachs posterolateral humeral fractures or anteroinferior glenoid rim fractures, which in themselves can release chondral debris; loose bodies within the joint can scrape the surface and potentiate arthritis (Figure 11.21). Fragmentation of the glenoid rim or posterior humeral head can release small particles of bone or chondral surface that the synovial lining will attempt to absorb. In the process of absorption, lysosomal enzymes are released, which secondarily affect the joint surface and may cause progressive cartilage thinning. This may be the origin of chondolysis as well.

A hole in the rotator cuff will diminish the normal hydrostatic fit of this joint as the humeral head migrates upward due to deltoid action, lack of pull, and humeral head static depression by the thinning supraspinatus. Subscapularis muscle stretching, also associated with the subluxation and dislocation phenomenon, diminishes the humeral head depressing effect; the up-riding of the humeral head further erodes the rotator cuff,

which allows this cyclic change to continue. Other factors can contribute.

Avascular necrosis is occasionally associated with steroid usage, such as in the treatment of asthma, which is often treated in swimmers and cross-country runners, as well as in dose-pack treatment for athletic injury. The condition is rare but it does occur. In avascular necrosis, formation of subchondral cysts will cause bone to collapse under the articular surface, and without proper pressure, which allows for elimination of waste products and absorption of nutrients, articular cartilage degeneration occurs. Trabecular breakdown of dead bone or revascularization in the healing process may cause pain associated with vascular congestion. Core decompression or removing a central plug of bone may relieve this vascular congestion and minimize pain. A bone strut or graft placed in this area may minimize the potential for collapse, which does not occur as often in the shoulder as it does in the hip, because, again, the shoulder is not a weight-bearing joint. Before collapse, symptoms are treated conservatively, that is, with anti-inflammatory medication and avoidance of weight bearing on the extremity. The course of the disease is followed by X-ray or MRI (Figure 11.22, a and b). After subchondral collapse and secondary loss of a smooth joint surface, hemi-arthroplasty becomes the treatment of choice.

Synovial inflammation increases circulation, which can cause some ossification of the chondral surface, but also is associated with the formation of a synovial pannus that can grow across the articular surface, interpose into the joint, and interfere with normal nutrition of articular cartilage.

Table 11.1 Postoperative A/C Joint Program Following Arthroscopic Debridement

Stage 0   Preoperative education
(To decrease symptoms in an effort
to avoid surgery, add Indomethacin)

Pendulum, Codman, and wall-climbing exercises.

Horizontal and hyperabduction stretching.

Internal and external rotation strengthening with arm at side; progress toward abduction.

Stage 1   Postoperative

In sling overnight. Ice or ice cuff in recovery.

Remove sling at day 1; can shower but otherwise avoid heat for 3 days.

When motion is tolerated with arm at side, do fine manipulation with the hand free from immobilizer. Avoid overhead activity or heavy lifting. Increase activity as comfort dictates.

Stage 2
Progressive mobilization and strengthening

If manipulation or subdeltoid scar debridement was done concurrently, start physical therapy by day 4 for passive forward flexion and external rotation at side, and progress toward passive horizontal flexion, hyperabduction, and reverse extension.

At day 4, internal and external rotation elastic tubing exercises; continue pendulum and wall climbing.

Stage 3   Return to activity

Return to work or school, but avoid lifting more than 5 lb (2.25 kg) and overhead activity for 3-4 weeks.

With return of full strength and motion, can return to recreational sports at 4-10 weeks or to competitive sports at 8-16 weeks as comfort dictates.

Home program emphasizing continued flexibility and strengthening.

Note. With concurrent arthroscopic capsular stabilization or SLAP lesion repair remain in sling for 4 weeks and delay mobilization, then follow Table 6.3 in chapter 6. With open debridement of A/C joint add 6 weeks to allow deltoid to heal before initiating this program. Maximum medical recovery may take 6 months.

Glenohumeral joint laxity allows transmission of force through the cuff to the acromion. The acromion responds by thickening an anterior meniscal rim, which will ossify over time or merely work as a brake to help prevent further subluxation. In the process, this thickened tissue can increase erosion of the cuff, or repetitive stress across this anterior rim will hamper fusion of the mesoacromial apophysis or lead to stress breakdown of this bone, possibly yielding the mesoacromial variation seen on axillary X-ray (Figure 11.23). Loose bone in the front of the acromion further erodes into the rotator cuff or transmits energy across the A/C joint, developing further arthritis.

A thinned cuff can lead to superior migration of the humeral head, decreasing congruity of the glenohumeral joint, and therefore increasing arthritis (Figure 11.24a). With arthritis and even an absent superior cuff, superior migration may be avoided by the development of a calcific block

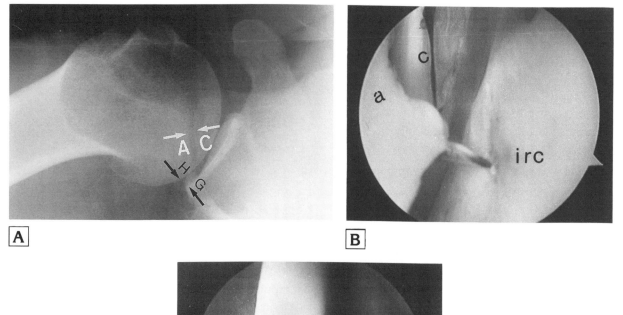

Figure 11.18 Underlying SLAP lesion may lead to continued pain after distal clavicle resection.

[A] Proximity of acromioclavicular (AC) and glenohumeral (GH) joints seen on axillary view.

[B] A needle placed through A/C joint first contacts rotator cuff in an area showing the blush of early impingement (a = acromion, c = clavicle, irc = impingement rotator cuff).

[C] Pushed further through the rotator cuff, the needle exits under SLAP lesion; tissue caught within glenohumeral joint can transmit symptoms or snapping up through A/C joint and may continue even after A/C joint resection (sla = superior labral avulsion, b = biceps).

due to an acromial spur and calcification of the coracoacromial ligament (Figure 11.24b). This may be due to continued integrity of the subscapularis and infraspinatus head depressors. A medial osteophyte may form in the joint in response to loss of cartilage to make up for lost articular distance (Figure 11.24c); however, this osteophyte decreases smooth gliding motion, and the body will utilize periscapular muscles and scapulothoracic motion to compensate, leading to overuse or breakdown of these structures as well. Central migration of the humerus into the glenoid socket can also occur (Figure 11.24d).

The athlete or former athlete with glenohumeral arthritis usually presents late. At this point athletic endeavors have been seriously challenged by breakdown of articular cartilage. Associated scar, loss of articular surface, muscle atrophy, imbalance, or wear places treatment in the salvage category, for relief of pain rather than for the purpose of returning to athletic endeavors.

Diagnosis

The presenting complaints are characteristic. The athlete complains that he or she can no longer participate in his or her particular sport, at least

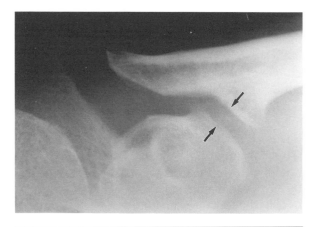

Figure 11.19 Continued aching and grinding following A/C joint resection may be due to coracoclavicular arthritis; 1% of individuals have a joint (which may become arthritic) rather than ligaments in the coracoclavicular space.

not to the level of previous activity. There is a complaint of loss of motion, stiffness, and constant aching from the front to the back of the joint. Initially, pain is worse on awakening but may decrease as the shoulder loosens up with activity.

Physical Examination. Glenohumeral arthritis will demonstrate pain in palm-up or palm-down abduction and may have grinding, particularly along the scapular plane. There may be grinding transmitted to the skin or the undersurface of the acromion or scapula with rotational testing, or a visible shift with motion. Inability to lift the arm comfortably can lead to adhesive capsulitis, loss of internal or external rotation, limitation at the extremes of motion, or even hiking of the shoulder in attempted abduction of the arm, mimicking rotator cuff disease. With advanced disease, horizontal flexion is primarily scapulothoracic, and periscapular overuse pain may occur.

Imaging. A bone scan will be positive with glenohumeral arthritis and plain X-rays on axillary

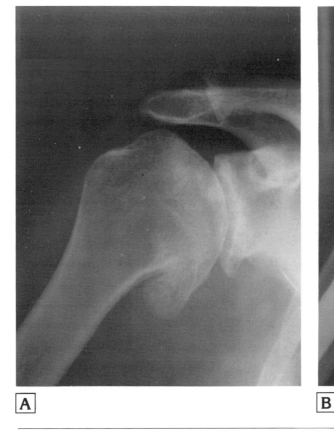

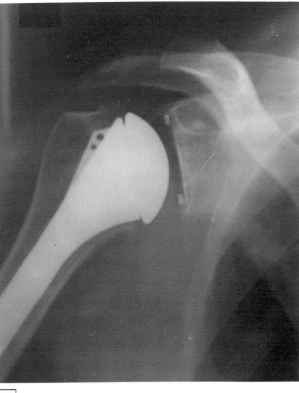

[A]

[B]

Figure 11.20 Glenohumeral arthritis in a 29-year-old handball player.

[A] Impact loading may turn a mobile joint into a weight-bearing joint, leading to articular breakdown and spread of force through a larger contact area.

[B] Endoscopic A/C joint resection and open glenohumeral "total" joint replacement may relieve symptoms of constant pain, but return to handball activity would not be medically recommended.

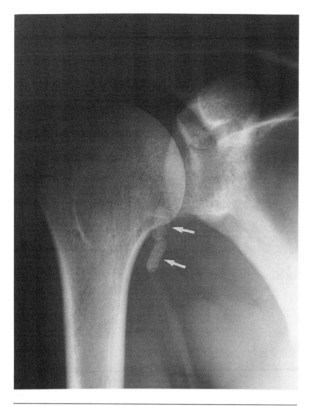

Figure 11.21 Chondral debris following dislocation or injury can lead to loose bodies that work like gravel within the joint and accelerate arthritis, particularly with an underlying instability.

film show the abnormal migration of the humeral head, subchondral cysts and sclerosis, and peripheral osteophytes, particularly around the edge of articular cartilage that extends the weight-bearing surface to distribute stress over a larger interval (Figure 11.25, a and b).

Eccentric glenoid erosion tends to be posterior (Figure 11.26). Posterior erosion can be verified on CT. CT-arthrogram can show labral pathology or rotator cuff degeneration associated with this arthritic phenomenon and also may demonstrate defects in the articular chondral surface. MRI works well to disclose osteonecrosis and vascular changes associated with degeneration. Sed rate will be positive, and if there is a coexistent rheumatoid disease, even in an athlete, then the rheumatologic panels may be appropriate.

Classification. Grading arthritic deformity of the glenohumeral joint is the same as articular cartilage grading throughout the body. Type 1 arthritis is blistering or softening of the articular surface. Type 2 change consists of "bacon stripping," shag, or early shedding of articular cartilage. Type 3 is irregularity of the surface with fissuring down to subchondral bone or significant thinning, usually associated with a yellowish tinge to the cartilage. Type 4 arthritis is almost complete loss of surface with small chondral islands usually remaining.

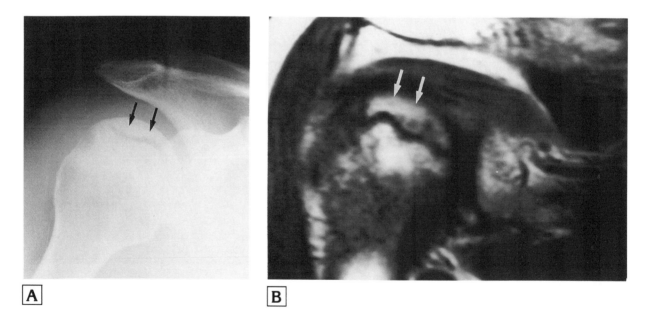

Figure 11.22 Avascular necrosis in a 41-year-old elite swimmer with a history of steroid use for asthma.

[A] Pain may exist even without subchondral collapse in the early stage, here documented on X-ray with a crescent sign.

[B] Area of dead bone is more easily demonstrated on MRI.

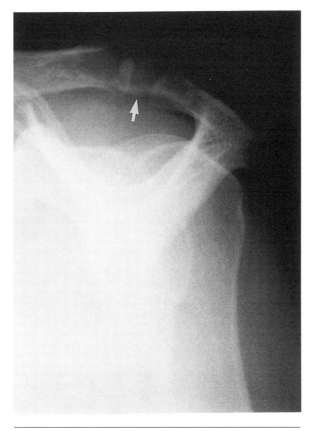

Figure 11.23 Mesoacromial loose anterior edge may accelerate wear into the rotator cuff, leading to instability and degeneration of the glenohumeral joint.

Management

Chondrolysis in the athlete's shoulder is rare. This is an extreme form of arthritis in which impaction of the joint surfaces may lead to fragmentation of cartilage and to a lysosomal reabsorption of cartilage, which looks like an autoimmune response. If the patient complains of severe pain after impact injury and has initially normal X-rays that quickly change over the next few months to show extreme inflammatory reabsorption of the joint surfaces, this condition must be suspected (Figure 11.27). This may be a process such as sternoclavicular hyperostosis or acromioclavicular osteolysis. Treatment is initially conservative but rapidly requires surgery. Aspirin and Naproxen may increase chemical bonding of articular cartilage and decelerate the rapid loss of cartilage. Therapy must be done as well to help prevent stiffness and keep the cartilage as healthy as possible. If this fails, however, hemiarthroplasty is the only alternative for a stiff, painful shoulder.

In *avascular necrosis*, subchondral breakdown will lead to collapse of the articular surface and subsequent loss of cartilage. Prior to chondral collapse, the process may be arrested with core decompression. Pain may be related to the vascular engorgement associated with revascularization and reossification. Radiographically, bony regrowth over dead bone is seen as sclerosis or creeping substitution. Decompression may relieve associated pain. With slight initial collapse, a bone graft to strut the avascular segment may help avoid further collapse.

Primary glenohumeral arthritis rarely is the result of athletic performance itself, except in activities like handball and racquetball in which impact loading can lead to the arthritic condition. Instability as produced in swimming and tennis can lead to secondary early wear and tear of the joint as well. The shoulder is essentially a non-weight-bearing joint. Even with arthritis of the glenohumeral joint, as long as mobility and surrounding strength (allowing muscles to work as shock absorbers) can be maintained, surgery can usually be avoided. The sliding coefficient of friction, which increases when the articular surface becomes shaggy, can be modified by arthroscopic debridement; resection of frayed cuff, biceps, labrum, synovium, and bony spurs with chondral shaping can decrease symptoms significantly (Figure 11.28, a and b).

When strengthening, stretching, or arthroscopic debridement fails to provide significant relief in an older athlete or after posttraumatic change, such as athletically produced fracture into the joint, hemiarthroplasty or a total shoulder replacement procedure is indicated. This is a salvage technique for end-stage disease, and it is not advisable to have the patient return to athletic performance after joint replacement, although some older athletes do (Table 11.2).

Osteophytic change at the glenohumeral joint can lead to progressive surface erosion, blockage of motion, surrounding muscle atrophy, and wear into the surrounding rotator cuff muscle tissue by the osteophytes themselves. Pitting erosion of the top of the humerus related to a SLAP lesion can also wear into the rotator cuff. Avascular necrosis leading to chondral collapse provides an irregular humeral surface that can erode superiorly into the cuff, causing thinning; humeral head replacement may be useful to both eliminate pain and decelerate further cuff erosion (Figure 11.29, a and b).

When motion is limited at the glenohumeral joint and energy transmission is brought up through the A/C joint, osteophyte formation on both sides of the rotator cuff rapidly accelerates

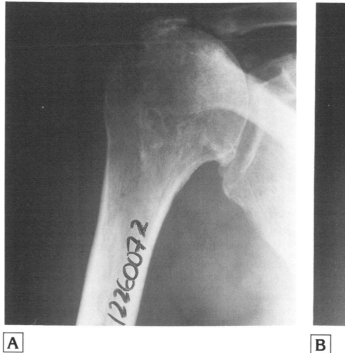

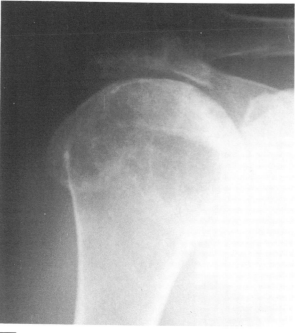

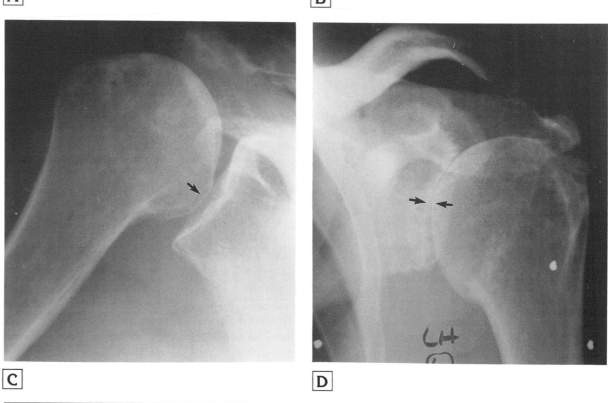

Figure 11.24 Glenohumeral responses to cartilage loss.

[A] Symmetrical wear and superior migration associated with loss of cuff material, with motion stopped by the A/C joint. Occasionally, subacromial ossification will prevent superior migration.

[B] Subacromial osteophyte and calcification of coracoacromial ligament may block superior migration even with complete loss of the supraspinatus, as in this 81-year-old swimmer, who now swims 1 mile a day breaststroke and is no longer able to swim freestyle.

[C] Medial osteophyte as a spacer.

[D] Progressive medial migration into the glenoid, base of coracoid, and A/C joint.

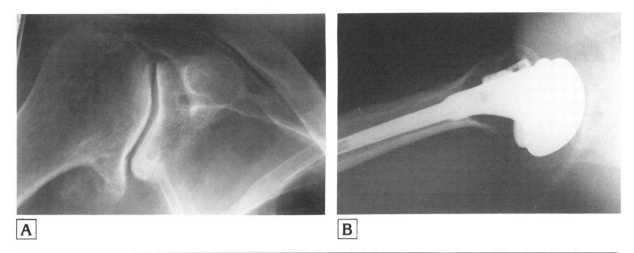

Figure 11.25 Glenohumeral degenerative arthritis.

[A] Flattening of humerus and development of peripheral osteophytes will distribute force over a greater distance when cartilage is no longer present to shield stress.

[B] Artificial joint replacement will decrease friction and pain and potentially increase motion at the joint, depending on residual muscle function.

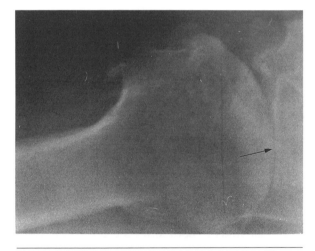

Figure 11.26 Eccentric wearing of the glenoid tends to be posterior, probably associated with posterior subdeltoid adhesions and muscle imbalance.

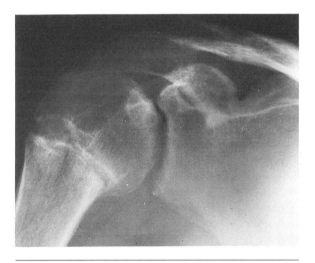

Figure 11.27 Chondrolysis in a 28-year-old recreational scuba diver. The glenohumeral joint was the only joint involved. Severe pain with initially normal X-ray was followed 3 months later by complete collapse of cartilage and stress fracture, or Looser line across the humeral neck to initiate a new motion plane because of severe friction at the glenohumeral joint. There was no response to anti-inflammatory medication, physical therapy, or even attempted manipulation at the time of hemiarthroplasty, which was done to salvage the joint.

disease, leading to superior migration of the humeral head and an end-stage impingement phenomenon in which ultimately there is no cuff to buffer the humeral head from the acromion. This is a very difficult situation to manage; total joint arthroplasty as a salvage procedure for an old athletic problem does not work well without cuff tissue. Of course, there could be breakdown of the artificial joint, specifically if activities like swimming, tennis, golf, and weight training continue after surgery. Hemiarthroplasty with an oversized humeral head to contact both the acromion and

glenoid may prevent further erosion or migration, causing decreased wearing and therefore decreased symptoms, and may allow return to activities like golf, swimming, and occasionally tennis (Figure 11.30, a-c).

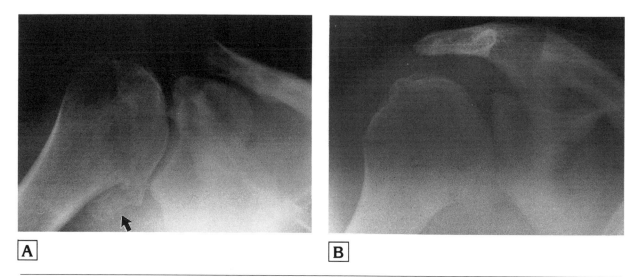

Figure 11.28 Degenerative arthritis in anabolic steroid–abusing body builder, age 31.

[A] Slight available motion provided a sliding sensation of rough surfaces within the joint, eliminating ability to weight train.

[B] Arthroscopic debridement allowed return to weight training and almost full pain-free range of motion.

Sternoclavicular Arthropathy

The sternoclavicular joint can become arthritic, with fracture into the joint leading to small step-off deformities. Instability due to capsular sprain and injury to the costoclavicular ligaments also leads to degenerative change. Arthritic changes occurring at the A/C joint limit motion of that joint and subsequently increase demand on the sternoclavicular joint and lead to its breakdown as well. Sternoclavicular joint arthritis is difficult to manage clinically, and as arthritis progresses, so does the clinical challenge. Management tends to be quite frustrating.

Epidemiology

Sternoclavicular arthritis may initiate with a fall on an outstretched or a reverse-extended arm, or with energy transmission down the clavicle to the sternoclavicular joint. Direct trauma to the front of the clavicle similarly can sprain costoclavicular ligaments or the capsular ligaments about the sternoclavicular joint, leading to early wear and tear and progressive arthritic degeneration.

Diagnosis

A history of capsular sprain or subluxation with slight deformity at this joint in the past is relevant; it may take many years for arthritic symptoms to develop.

Physical Examination. A slightly anteriorly displaced prominent sternoclavicular joint is the usual presentation in arthritis. There is pain with horizontal flexion, when lifting, when using the arm at chest level, or even when turning a steering wheel or doorknob.

Imaging. Plain X-rays are usually not valuable in assessing the sternoclavicular joint, although the *serendipity view* may show some relative step-off or arthritic change. An *inspirational view* angled toward the opposite shoulder at 45° through the S/C joint while allowing the patient to breathe will obscure rib detail and highlight the joint (Figure 11.31). Obviously, both sides are taken for comparison.

Bone scan is equivocal, just as in the A/C joint, but can be very definitive. CT scan is the diagnostic technique of choice, which may show fracture into the joint or narrowing, cysts, avascular necrosis, or osteophyte formation (Figure 11.32, a and b).

Differential Diagnosis

Swelling of the sternoclavicular joint may not always be due to athletic traumatic osteoarthritis but could be due to inflammatory conditions such as rheumatoid arthritis, scleroderma, psoriasis, idiopathic chondrolysis, gout, and so on, which can make athletic performance difficult. Conditions such as condensing osteitis, sternocostoclavicular hyperostosis, and postmenopausal osteoarthritis, as well as metastatic carcinoma, can affect this joint

Table 11.2 Rehabilitation Protocol Following Glenohumeral Arthroplasty

---

Stage 0   Preoperative education

Pendulum and wall-climbing mobilization exercises.

Internal rotation stretching with towel behind the back; external rotation strengthening with cane at the side.

Internal and external rotation strengthening with elastic tubing.

Stage 1   Postoperative day 1

Passive forward flexion to 90° and external rotation to 20°, or as comfort dictates, done by surgeon.

Physical therapy to administer and teach external rotation and passive elevation exercises.

Overhead pulley to assist in passive elevation with utilization taught by therapist.

Pendulum exercises at least four times a day.

Sling off in chair or in bed, but on for ambulation purposes.

Occupational therapist consulted for activities of daily living, such as feeding and dental hygiene.

Patient to advance to 120° assisted forward flexion and 25° external rotation at the side (or the extent of motion at surgery, if less) prior to discharge (postponed four weeks with repair of large rotator cuff tear).

Stage 2   At 2-3 week follow-up

Remove stitches.

Check motion; reinforce home exercise program. Add more stretching if necessary.

Supine forward elevation with assistance of other hand and external rotation with arm at side more often.

Stage 3   6-8 weeks postoperative

Increase internal and external rotation strengthening.

Periscapular muscle strengthening and posture to be emphasized; use therapist if losing motion.

Advance to wall push-up exercise and activity as tolerated.

Return to activity.

   Competitive overhead activity is to be discouraged.

   Golf, swimming, and other recreational activity as tolerated can be done, but stretching and strengthening are to continue nevertheless.

---

in the athletic population. What has been labeled as *postmenopausal arthritis* is an almost painless lump that develops in postmenopausal females and occasionally is associated with pregnancy in the younger age groups. This is self-limiting and is treated conservatively with anti-inflammatory medication. *Condensing osteitis* and *sternoclavicular hyperostosis* appear to be a continuum of disease associated with joint swelling, slight expansion of the medial third of the clavicle, and sclerosis (Figure 11.33). Sclerotic changes may occur in the medial clavicle or the inferior medial clavicle or may be a progressive problem also involving the first rib, the sternum, and ossification of the ligaments in between (Figure 11.34). Pain due to inflammation or fusion in this area will affect athletic performance. At this point, resectional arthroplasty with stabilization may be considered as a

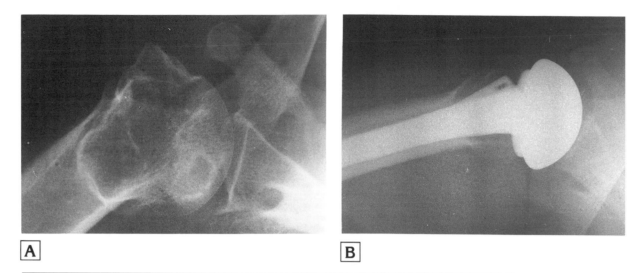

Figure 11.29 Avascular necrosis in elderly swimmer taking steroids for asthma.

[A] Subchondral cyst and sclerotic creeping substitution will lead to collapse of cartilage surface.

[B] Replacement hemiarthroplasty allowed return to swimming, golf, and tennis with no complaints.

salvage technique for pain relief, not for return to aggressive sport activity.

Management

When laxity and related arthritis occur at the sternoclavicular joint, athletic activity at chest level and above, particularly in a loaded condition as in weight training, is almost impossible due to discomfort. This tends to change the type of recreational sport or aerobic training that the athlete participates in. If strengthening of surrounding muscles and anti-inflammatory medication are successful, then the athlete can return to more normal activity. If not, then surgery is definitely a salvage situation.

Resecting the proximal end of the clavicle to remove the arthritic condition is not very successful. If shortening of the sternoclavicular space occurs, symptoms recur, and stabilization with soft tissue interposition and reconstruction of costoclavicular ligaments are salvage procedures to get the patient back to more comfortable daily activities but not to the rigors of most athletic competition (Figure 11.35, a and b). If instability in this area was the origin of arthritis, then soft tissue

reconstruction must also include reconstruction of the costoclavicular ligament.

Summary

Articular cartilage works as a shock absorber and allows for a smooth motion in athletic performance. Loss of a frictionless surface seriously hampers athletic efficiency. Introduction of a blood supply to the articular surface or progressive wear due to repetitive impact and overuse can initiate arthritis.

Muscle strengthening to absorb shock and awareness of proper mechanics may help eliminate the causes of arthritis. Once pain develops and muscular imbalance occurs, progression of arthritis may be rapid. Salvage surgery remains an attempt to minimize pain, but return to peak athletic performance is not expected. Isolated A/C joint arthritis without the involvement of erosion into the rotator cuff may be the exception, but it is rare. Earlier intervention ideally would lead to more satisfactory results. When presentation is late, salvage rather than complete return of function becomes the goal.

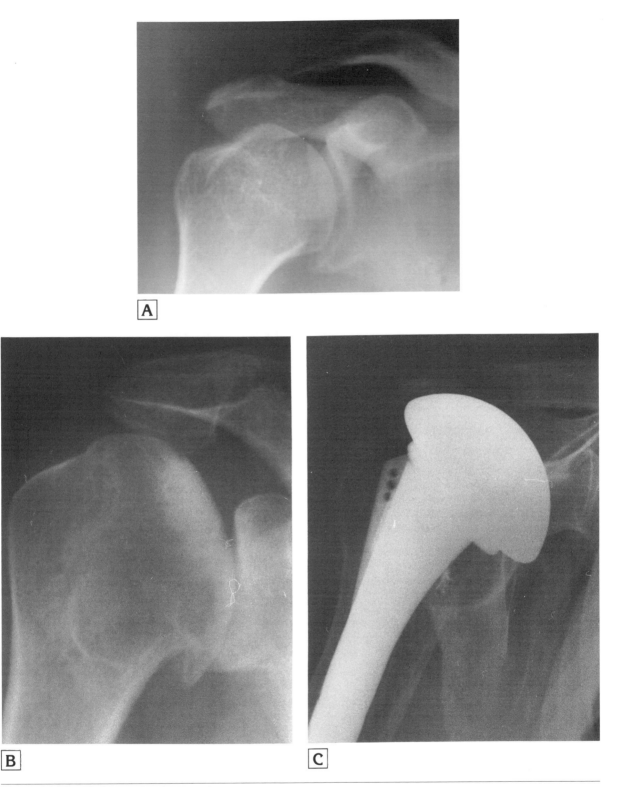

Figure 11.30 End-stage impingement.

[A] Superior humeral head osteophyte contributes to wear of rotator cuff.

[B] Progressive superior migration and medial osteophyte replacement of cartilage loss in same patient 10 years later.

[C] Oversized humeral head replacement contacts acromion and glenoid to prevent further migration and erosion, restoring variable but improved lateral rotation with abduction; this is a salvage technique done for pain relief, not for return to overhead sport.

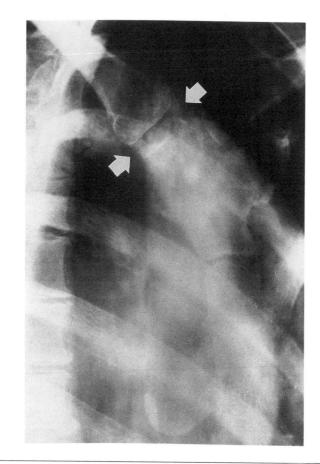

Figure 11.31 Inspirational view X-ray. Bony overlap often obscures detail at the sternoclavicular joint. Angling an AP X-ray 45° toward the side opposite that being investigated, aiming at the sternoclavicular joint, and asking the patient to breathe normally (rather than holding his or her breath) will obscure rib detail and give good detail at the sternoclavicular joint; obviously, each side is taken independently and compared (a technique developed by our radiology technician, Julia Jubran).

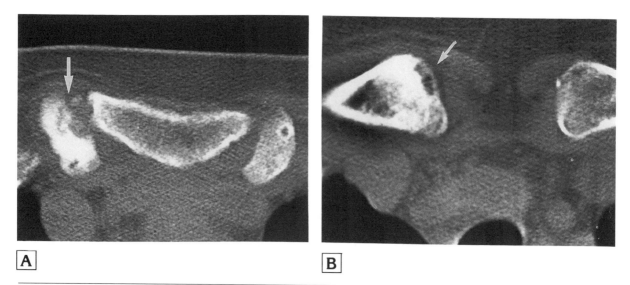

Figure 11.32 Sternoclavicular joint is best assessed by CT scan or MRI.

[A] Degenerative arthritis.

[B] Avascular necrosis in proximal clavicle leading to pain at sternoclavicular joint.

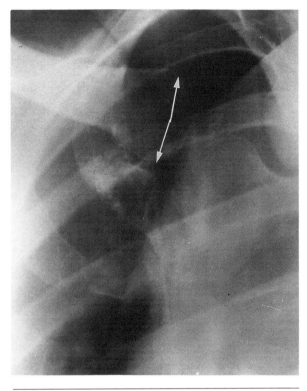

Figure 11.33 Initially painless swelling ("post-menopausal arthritis") may become painful or calcific (compared to normal side, Figure 11.31).

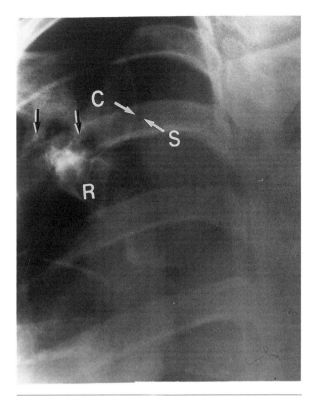

Figure 11.34 A 32-year-old golfer initially diagnosed with condensing osteitis and thoracic outlet syndrome progressed to what appeared to be chondrocalcinosis and sternoclavicular hyperostosis. She was treated successfully with weight loss and nonsteroidal anti-inflammatory medication, allowing her to return to golf painlessly. Thoracic outlet symptoms were due to swelling in this area (C = clavicle, S = sternum, R = rib, black arrows = calcified costoclavicular ligaments).

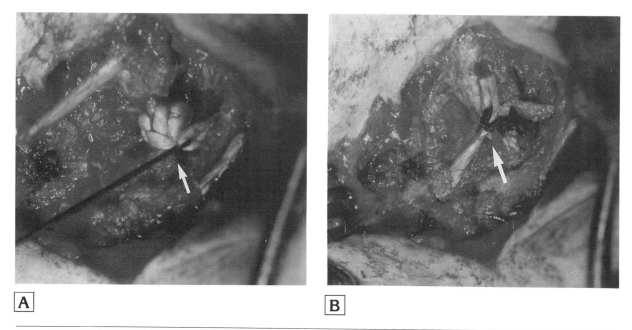

Figure 11.35 Resection of the proximal clavicle for arthritis leads to considerable lack of power and continued pain.

[A] Following proximal clavicle resection, a knotted palmaris longus tendon spacer passed through drill holes in the sternum and clavicle can restore stability to the shoulder for elevation.

[B] The ends are tied over on themselves; excess length can be used to reconstruct costoclavicular ligament if necessary.

Part III

Principles of Shoulder Rehabilitation

Treatment of the athlete's injured shoulder does not end with an accurate diagnosis. The goal of making that diagnosis is to guide the rehabilitation effort. Motion must be preserved, and strength follows. After achieving motion and strength, coordination becomes the next goal.

Even surgical intervention for severe structural damage is not the end point. Again, this merely prepares the athlete to be better involved with the rehabilitation effort. The physician is most often responsible for making the initial diagnosis. The trainer and therapist work together in the rehabilitation phase to regain a useful shoulder that will be ready for performance.

12

Accurate Diagnosis and Staging Therapy

The key to rehabilitation in shoulder injury is proper diagnosis. Treating an athlete for suspicion of impingement by external rotation strengthening of the supraspinatus and infraspinatus can in fact make him or her feel worse and become more symptomatic if the underlying cause of the impingement is actually antero-inferior subluxation and a tight posterior joint capsule. In this case it is not unusual for the athlete to complain that he or she feels worse in physical therapy. This most often can be attributed to improper diagnosis.

The patient tells the examiner what is wrong. It is important to listen to the history and tie in physical examination of specific motion deficits and positive clinical signs to arrive at the proper diagnosis. An understanding of structural problems that can occur with certain athletic activities will suggest the proper course of treatment to the examining physician.

The goals of a therapeutic program are first to achieve painless and full range of motion, to achieve flexibility, and *then* to work on strength and endurance. It is a mistake to emphasize strength first before range of motion, because muscles need to be exercised through their full ranges to achieve maximum potential and to avoid imbalance. As more motion is obtained, more muscle fibers become available to exercise. Overzealous strengthening efforts prior to the return of motion can lead to overuse within that limited motion or to further imbalance. Premature effort toward strengthening is a major cause of failure in physical therapy after surgical reconstruction, because tissue healing must occur first. Guiding the direction of fibroblast orientation and avoiding maturation of unnecessary adhesions are the goals of initial passive mobilization.

Surgery is never considered the "cure" for shoulder disorder, but instead is done to yield mechanical stability so that exercise and training become more feasible. It is in fact the athlete's, not the physician's, responsibility to effect a cure. This does not occur by itself, especially after a considerable amount of structural damage; and muscles that have once become weakened will always have a tendency toward disuse. Therefore, an athlete is never told that his or her shoulder function, following a short period of rehabilitation or after surgical intervention, will ever be 100%. Instead, if it is brought structurally within the 80% to 95% range, the athlete can possibly compensate for lack of complete structural integrity by muscular activity, flexibility, muscle toning, and training. It is the athlete's obligation to keep exercising on a permanent basis in order to retain a shoulder that is structurally capable of participation in athletic activity. The "shock absorbers" must be constantly "pumped up," and the joint kept flexible; otherwise, demand can lead to wearing and muscle imbalance that limit athletic performance, occupational endeavors, or daily activity. Lack of exercise can lead to new symptoms or recurrence of previous symptoms.

It is important for the physician to remember that the shoulder's main function is to position the hand through space. The combination of shoulder motion, body leaning, and use of all joints of the shoulder and surrounding structures that are linked together allows this to occur (Jackson & Ciullo, 1986; Nicholas et al., 1977). Surrounding structures, including the neck, temporomandibular joint, and back, interplay with shoulder rehabilitation. Dysfunction of one joint or one set of muscles of the body will lead to misuse or overuse of other joints or musculature throughout the body. Such misuse, or abuse, is a particular problem in the athlete for whom peak performance through repetitive training and activity is the goal. Again, accurate diagnosis is the key to proper management.

Once the proper diagnosis is made, therapy is initiated in three phases: healing, mobilization, and finally strengthening. These are the same stages that should be included in either conservative management or postoperative management. Modalities in therapy also progress in the same manner, discouraging inflammation and fibrosis initially and only then proceeding toward selective flexibility and concurrent selected strengthening exercises.

Exercises

Certain exercises have been found useful in rehabilitation and as preventative measures in dealing with athletic trauma (Ciullo, 1986b; Ciullo & Guise, 1981a, 1981b).

The following therapeutic and preventative exercises are suggested following shoulder injury or surgery.

Stage 1: Anti-Inflammatory and Healing Phase

Initially, anti-inflammatory medication (Figure 12.1) and ice (Figure 12.2) are found useful in

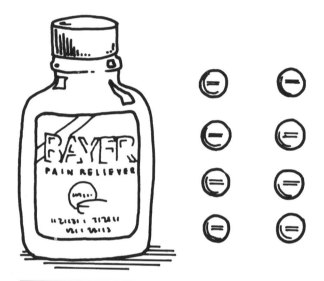

Figure 12.1 Stage 1: anti-inflammatory medication. Adapted from Ciullo 1986.

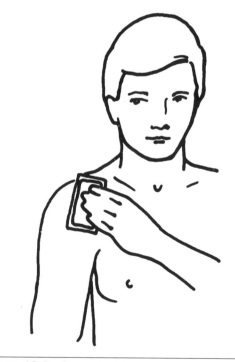

Figure 12.2 Stage 1: icing. Adapted from Ciullo 1986.

decreasing pain and swelling. A TENS unit or iontophoresis may be helpful at this stage.

A short period of rest or the use of a sling may be necessary after trauma or surgery, but pendulum exercises (Figure 12.3) must be started immediately to avoid stiffness. Passive assisted exercises, cane exercises, and the use of a shoulder pulley (Figure 12.4) can be initiated as muscle healing occurs.

Stage 2: Mobilization Phase

Posture and wall-climbing exercises (Figure 12.5), flexibility training (Figures 12.6 and 12.7), and weighted flexibility exercises (Figures 12.8 and 12.9) to stretch the posterior capsule and eliminate the decreased range of motion related to strength deficit are initiated at this stage.

Isometric and myostimulation (neuromuscular stimulation) may be utilized. A clavicular strap can be used for postural correction and to facilitate return of muscle balance.

Stage 3: Strengthening Phase

The isokinetic dynamometer can be used to identify specific strength deficits. Endurance rather than muscle hypertrophy is the key—aerobic training is emphasized. Advance to a home program of stretching and strengthening (Figures 12.10 and 12.11) in an effort to establish a lifetime maintenance program. This includes warm-up and

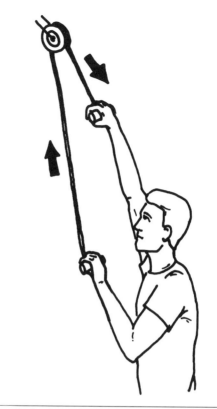

Figure 12.4 Stage 1: pulley exercises.

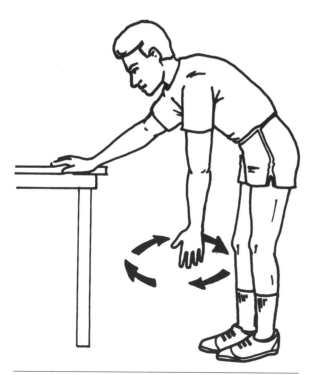

Figure 12.3 Stage 1: pendulum exercises.

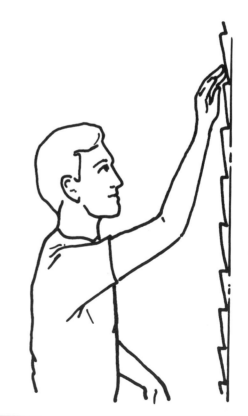

Figure 12.5 Stage 2: wall climbing.

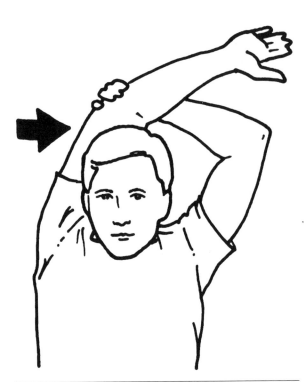

Figure 12.6 Stage 2: hyperabduction to break adhesions.

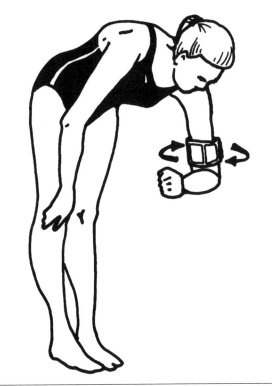

Figure 12.8 Stage 2: weighted Codman flexibility exercises.

Adapted from Ciullo 1986.

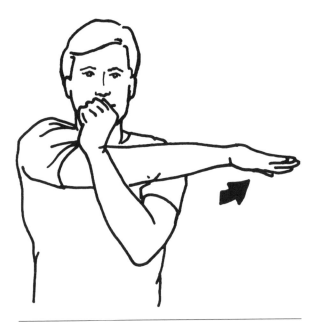

Figure 12.7 Stage 2: forced hyperabduction to break posterior capsular adhesions.

stretching prior to activity and cool-down and stretching following activity. Flexible tubing or cord (Figures 12.12 and 12.13), a light weight set, a stationary bicycle, or a ski machine is useful. Aerobic conditioning is mandatory.

Healing and Anti-Inflammatory Phase

With repetitive microtrauma, such as the progressive capsular tearing that occurs with subluxation, and after major trauma, such as a shoulder dislocation, the goals are the same. First inflammation and discomfort must be decreased so that selective therapeutic measures can become more effective. This is the reason for the short-term use of a sling after a major trauma such as dislocation and for decreased activity with microtrauma such as the progressive glenohumeral capsular stretching that occurs with throwing or swimming. In the latter case, when tendinitis is clinically present, decreasing activity by at least one half of what the patient found uncomfortable is usually sufficient. A swimmer's program may decrease from 18,000 m to 9,000 m per day. If he or she finds that this is still uncomfortable, decrease it by half again. Stopping activity altogether is not only unnecessary but quite dangerous if the athlete is to return to competitive sport activity. The athlete must maintain overall conditioning and aerobic capacity as much as possible; exercising all other parts of the body while decreasing activity of the injured extremity must be encouraged.

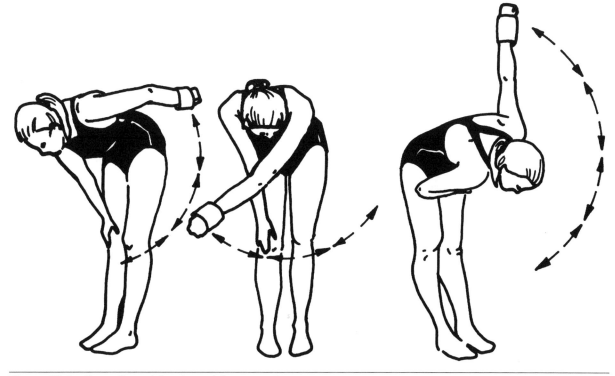

Figure 12.9 Stage 2: weighted pendulum exercises.
Adapted from Ciullo 1986.

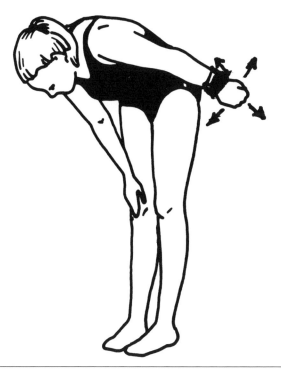

Figure 12.10 Stage 3: weighted short arc, short rotator strengthening exercises.
Adapted from Ciullo 1986.

Decreasing inflammation and pain by reducing activity or with the use of ice, nonsteroidal anti-inflammatory medication, or even a TENS unit (Roeser, Meeks, Venise, & Strickland, 1976) is important initially. Although athletic activity is diminished in this process, mobilization must be maintained through such activities as dependent pendulum exercises (Figure 12.3) and wall-climbing exercises (Figure 12.5). This phase may take 2 weeks with repetitive microtrauma and from 2 to 6 weeks after surgical intervention. What was done surgically will alter what can be done in early rehabilitation. If the standard deltopectoral interval approach to tighten the joint capsule was used in a standard Bankart procedure, mobilization may be initiated as early as at 2 weeks. When the deltoid is taken down to expose a rotator cuff tear, this must heal, which takes 4 to 6 weeks, prior to initiation of the next stage of activity. Nevertheless, dependent pendulum exercises are initiated 1 to 2 days postoperatively in either case to prevent stiffness that leads to muscle atrophy and imbalance and jeopardizes the surgical result.

Mobilization Phase

Once hemorrhage, inflammation, and pain have been minimized, more active motion is conceivable. The dependent pendulum exercises are replaced with passive assisted exercises, which the athlete can usually initiate him- or herself after

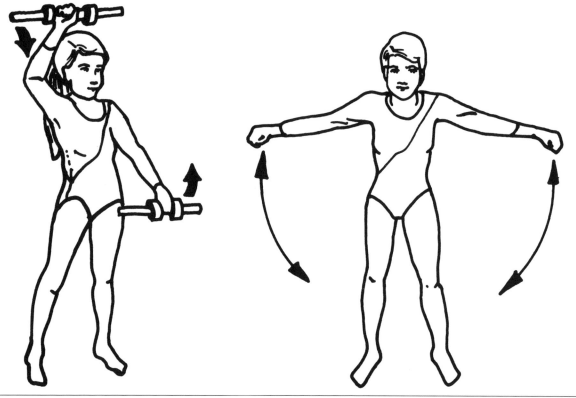

Figure 12.11 Stage 3: weighted deltoid strengthening exercises.
Adapted from Ciullo 1986.

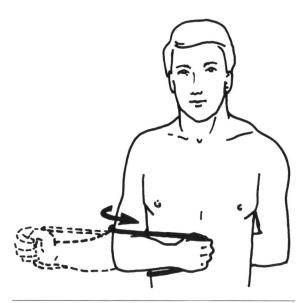

Figure 12.12 Stage 3: internal rotation strengthening.
Adapted from Ciullo 1986.

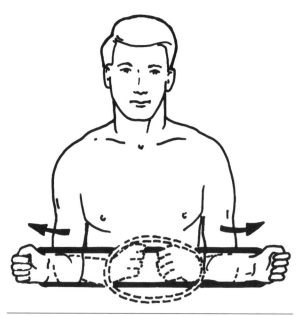

Figure 12.13 Stage 3: external rotation strengthening.
Adapted from Ciullo 1986.

training by using the opposite extremity to lift the affected arm. If the athlete has difficulty, a therapist may need to be involved, initiating passive range of motion in active hands-on therapy. At no time in any rehabilitative phase is the athlete to be left alone with weights or placed on a Cybex machine and expected to supervise his or her own rehabilitation. The therapist must apply hands on the patient; this is mandatory in the early phases of physical therapy.

More active muscular activity can be utilized at this time, but if the patient has symptoms of subluxation, pendulum exercises toward external rotation will be symptomatic, whereas those toward internal rotation are less likely to be symptomatic. External rotation mimics the abducted external rotation apprehension test. It is important at this phase to stretch out the posterior capsule and any other areas where motion is blocked (Figures 12.6 and 12.7).

Full motion is emphasized for muscular rehabilitation, because a muscle must be exercised through its full range to utilize the maximum amount of its fibers and to gain maximum power. The key to shoulder rehabilitation is the deltoid muscle. The use of a myostimulation unit for 15 min, three to four times a day, may be significantly useful to prepare the deltoid for lifting above 90° once motion begins to return (Figure 12.14). A secondary result of impulse stimulation working as a TENS unit appears to be effecting a neurologic blockade of pain fibers.

Active and passive stretching is emphasized, along with isometric short-burst activities, tightening each selected muscle group for 5 to 10 s with a 2- to 5-s rest in between until fatigue. This is not the time for isokinetic training with Cybex, Biodex, Kincom, or free-weight training. These should be avoided until motion has returned. Smooth scapulohumeral rhythm must be emphasized by the therapist or trainer to help achieve muscle balance and coordination.

While pain occurs, the shoulder tends to slump forward, throwing off normal dynamics. This may be a protective response but contributes to muscle imbalance. Changing postural habits is difficult but is mandatory to achieve muscle balance and avoid recurrence of symptoms (Figure 12.15, a-c). By reestablishing motion through the glenohumeral joint, acromioclavicular joint, and supraspinatus sliding mechanism, rather than shrugging the shoulder or rotating through the scapulothoracic joint, periscapular muscle spasm and neck pain can be markedly reduced. Merely changing posture back toward normal markedly diminishes pain.

The use of a clavicular strap to pull the shoulders back is often useful when thoracic outlet symptoms or periscapular muscle spasm occurs, either following trauma or after surgery (Figure 12.16). Motion, muscle balancing, and proper posture are necessary to regain proper glenohumeral and scapulothoracic rhythm.

Strengthening Phase

Once motion and posture have been corrected, selective strengthening of the short intrinsic muscles of the rotator cuff must be emphasized. Of prime importance is strengthening the humeral head depressors, that is, the subscapularis anteriorly and the infraspinatus and teres minor posteriorly. Pulling the humeral head downward will diminish stress on the supraspinatus and help prevent refibrosis of the posterosuperior subdeltoid area, bursa, and capsule. Minimizing impingement symptoms will maximize early recovery. Supraspinatus strengthening is *not* to be emphasized first, because this can accelerate impingement symptoms, continue the fibrosis in the posterior acromial area, and further stretch out the anterosuperior suspensory mechanism; the patient will complain that therapy is making him or her feel worse.

The principle of linkage must be remembered—the hand, elbow, shoulder, neck, and back must be rehabilitated concurrently. Fifty percent of shoulder strength in throwing or elevation comes from back musculature. Isotonic, isometric, and isokinetic activities are progressively phased in, but the basic stretching and body mechanics are maintained in the therapeutic setting. Aerobic activity, such as biking, use of a ski machine, use of upper body ergometers, and so on, becomes more important in helping the athlete to prevent fatigue and to get back into condition. At this point,

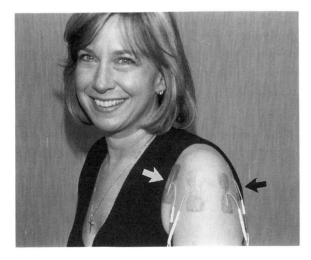

Figure 12.14 Application of a myostimulation unit along the path of the axillary nerve to restimulate unused deltoid muscle in preparation for therapeutic retraining.

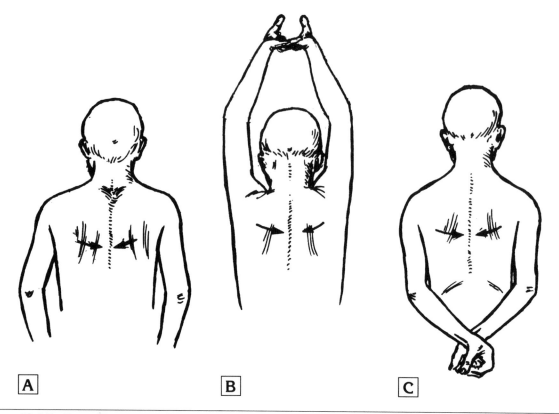

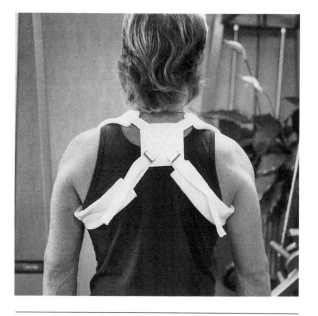

Figure 12.15 Postural retraining. Reestablishing posture is important to regain scapulohumeral rhythm and de-emphasize scapulothoracic overuse. This is accomplished by trying to bring the shoulder blades together by

[A] pushing them against a table in a supine position or against a wall in a standing position;

[B] stretching overhead; or

[C] locking the hands behind the back.

Figure 12.16 Clavicular strap to help restore posture and to aid in balancing muscles about the shoulder.

manual testers, such as the Nicholas-ISMAT, and isokinetic dynamometry, such as Cybex and Biodex, have their specific roles.

The manual muscle testers give a baseline to measure future progress. The isokinetic dynamometers help to identify specific deficiencies at slow-speed testing and test for endurance and coordination in high-speed testing. This equipment is to be used for testing purposes, not for rehabilitation. Dips in the isokinetic curve patterns identify specific areas that need to be rehabilitated with further isometric, eccentric, and controlled muscular activity or areas that structurally may be unable to recover further; they may need to be compensated for. Flexible cords and surgical tubing devices are specifically useful at this stage.

The goal is to obtain smooth motion and approach normal strength prior to the return to training. The athlete is not ready to return to sport training until the affected shoulder's strength deficit is less than 20% of what is considered normal for his or her height and weight and for the unaffected side. It may take endurance fibers longer to recover; it is not uncommon to take considerably more time (18 months or so) to overcome the final 20% deficit, especially in the recreational athlete. Nevertheless, if body mechanics are proper, the patient can return to training safely.

First the short intrinsic muscles are exercised, balancing the humeral head depressors prior to strengthening the supraspinatus. Once the supraspinatus is also strong, then the longer extrinsic deltoid and periscapular muscles must be trained, although they have been in effect trained by emphasizing normal scapulohumeral rhythm throughout the therapeutic period. The deltoid is the key to rehabilitation, and for this purpose neuromuscular stimulators may be of significant benefit. Application at the midpoint of the muscle where the neurologic innervation occurs (i.e., the course of the axillary nerve) for periods of 15 min, three to four times a day is advocated initially (Figure 12.14). This will help retrain the deltoid if overhead activity has been avoided, will speed therapeutic response once 90° of abduction has been actively regained, and in the long run will help prevent fatigue that could contribute to reinjury.

Interphasing Modalities

Therapeutic modalities must be used quite selectively in the rehabilitative process. In the initial phases when regaining motion and decreasing excess scar tissue are important, heat and ultrasound should be avoided. Heat can increase circulation, which may lead to hematoma, further muscle atrophy, and more overall scar in the healing process. Ultrasound is also believed to encourage excess healing scar deposition in early fibroblastic activity and for this reason should be avoided initially. Anti-inflammatory medication necessary in the early stage can possibly lead to increased clotting time and probably should be avoided for the first 3 days after injury or surgery so that bleeding can be minimized.

Modalities like iontophoresis are more beneficial in the early phases, along with ice to diminish inflammation. Phonophoresis is a process of introducing steroid anti-inflammatory molecules through the pores of the skin by ultrasound. The theory is that this allows much deeper penetration than can be accomplished by surface application alone. Iontophoresis goes one step further by breaking the anti-inflammatory medication into ions, which follow the electrical wave pattern even deeper. The ions then reorganize to accomplish a deeper anti-inflammatory response. As motion is increased, posture improved, and flexibility maintained, then selective tightening of maturing tissue through modalities like ultrasound may be more effective.

Following injury or surgery, ice is useful initially to diminish bleeding. Within a few days, as muscles attempt to exercise themselves in the healing

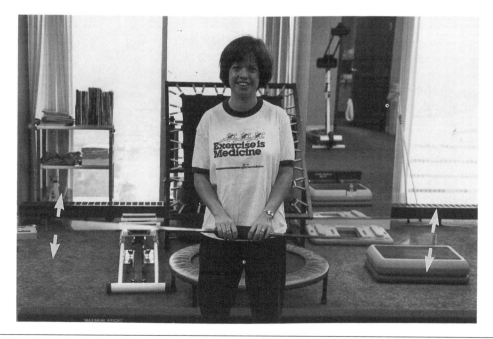

Figure 12.17 Open chain kinetic exercise using a Boggle Bar (Bruce Hymanson, Playa Del Rey, CA) to reestablish vibratory sense, proprioception, and coordinated neuromuscular motor patterns.

process, isometric contractures or spasm occurs, and heat, which diminishes spasm, has its role. As motion increases, scar tissue may break, leading to further bleeding, which necessitates reapplication of ice. This may be the basis of the effectiveness of contrast therapy, starting with ice, then using heat, and then ending with ice.

Again, ice is useful for decreasing inflammation, and heat is useful for decreasing muscle spasm. Therefore, the trainer or therapist is the best judge of which modality to utilize. Ultrasound is not always necessary, nor is heat; such therapeutic measures may even be contraindicated in certain phases of recovery. Modalities are useful if they are modulated by both the clinical presentation and therapeutic response and they will change through various phases of rehabilitation. The use of myostimulation, as outlined above, is occasionally useful.

Preparing for Performance

Regaining motion and strengthening muscles about the shoulder is not enough to ensure successful athletic performance. Throwing a ball, lifting a weight, or swinging a bat is not a function of shoulder activity alone, but a product of linked activity. Cybex muscle testing of cross-pattern motion while immobilizing the abdomen and chest demonstrates a 50% decrease in generated strength. In other words, 50% of the throwing force effected through the upper extremity is generated by the back. Reeducation or relinkage of unused parts requires special techniques.

Open and closed kinetic chain exercises and plyometrics can be useful to help increase performance in sport activities. They help prepare the injured individual for specific athletic activity. These exercise patterns increase neuromuscular recruitment and redevelop peak performance patterns.

Steindler (1973) described the *kinetic chain*, applying engineering principles to physical therapy. This was in effect another way of stating Nicholas et al.'s (1977) concept of *linkage*. Adjacent biomechanic segments are linked or connected at the joints, the entire construct forming a chain.

A *closed chain* occurs when both ends are immovable, essentially locked into a frame. A motion in one segment predictably will produce motion in all segments, because the two ends are locked in place. Isometrics thus are closed chain kinetic exercise. When the hand or foot does not meet

resistance, as in throwing a ball, this is an *open chain* activity. In most sport activity, open chain activity is emphasized, and therefore it should also be stressed in advanced rehabilitation (Figure 12.17).

Retraining proper biomechanics or neuromuscular coordination can be initiated with simple activities such as throwing a foam ball to a Velcro mitt, an open chain therapeutic exercise. The therapist has the opportunity to be creative here, developing novel equipment and exercise routines to keep the patient interested (Figures 12.18 and 12.19, a and b).

Athletic performance is achieved through proper neuromuscular coordination. The Golgi tendon apparatus and muscle spindles work through spinal reflex arcs to achieve balance and coordination. Muscles and tendons have innate

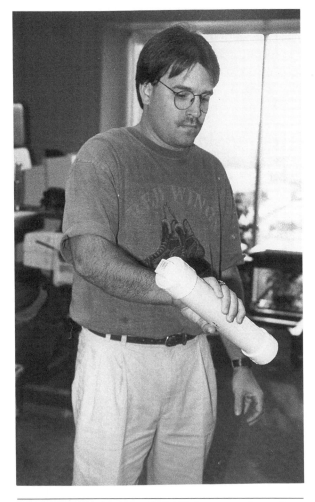

Figure 12.18 Rotating Tidal Tubes, proprioceptive dumbbells utilizing partially-fluid-filled PVC tubing, to reestablish proprioception is a method developed by athletic trainer, Jeff Rokop, at our facility, Sports Medicine Center of Metro Detroit, Troy, MI.

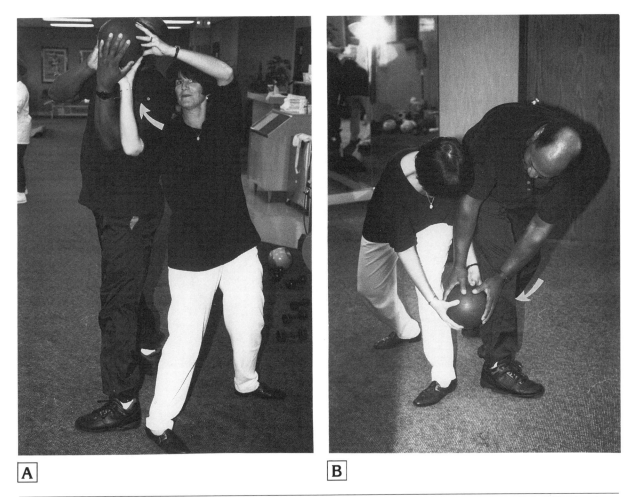

Figure 12.19 Functional facilitation to help regain neuromuscular balance following injury. Rehabilitation is occasionally tedious, and it is the therapist's job to help make it tolerable. Creativity will help in the rehabilitative process, as in this routine developed by our therapy director, Deborah Nadel, PT.

properties to store energy through viscoelastic means. A simple stretch can keep muscles warm for up to half an hour before athletic activity. Jumping twice in one spot while playing basketball allows one to jump higher on the second jump because of energy stored through the first jump (Ciullo & Zarins, 1983; Ciullo & Jackson, 1985). Such quick motion to prestretch or store energy through musculotendinous viscoelastic properties can be used to produce power. Prestretching the muscle can effectively shorten the stretch–performance cycle, the basis of reciprocal innervation and eccentric-concentric activity.

Teaching musculotendinous units to be maximally effective in specific athletic activity through the coordination of viscoelastic musculotendinous properties and neuromuscular reflex pattern reorganization is the basis of plyometric rehabilitation therapy. *Plyometrics* is the therapeutic modality that teaches the athlete how to preload the

muscle and make use of neuromuscular connections to result in an explosive, integrated athletic motion. Lowering then lifting a medicine ball, doing push-ups or dips, or pulling an arm back to preload the shoulder capsule prior to throwing are all plyometric exercises (Figure 12.20, a-c).

Summary

It must be emphasized to the athlete that once he or she has been through a successful course of rehabilitation, his or her therapy is not done. The athlete must maintain strength on a permanent basis. Structures that are injured are never 100% normal afterward; they must be compensated for by muscular activity. Muscles that have once been injured or atrophied will never be the same and need constant exercise to work at peak performance. Athletic activity for the athlete or industrial

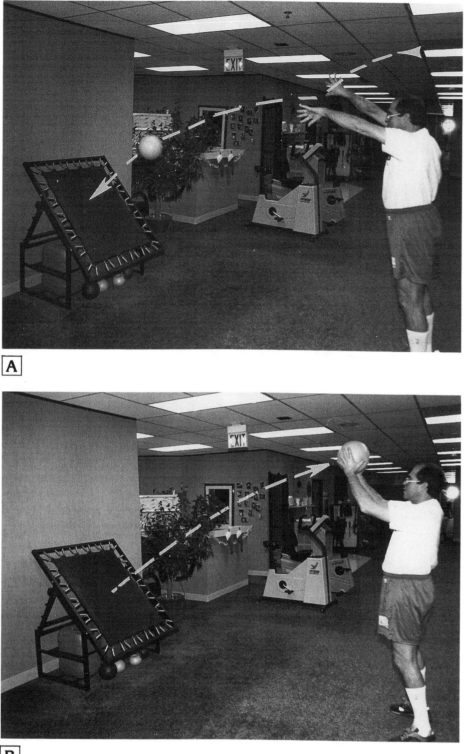

(continued)

Figure 12.20 Plyometric exercise for prestretching the capsule and muscles to utilize viscoelasticity and energy storage to assist in throwing power.

[A] Throw overhead to develop coordination.

[B] Retrieve to regain balancing and proprioception.

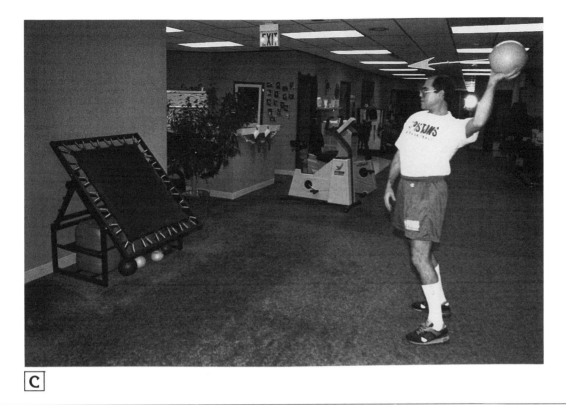

C

Figure 12.20   *(continued)*

[C] Throw from the side to reestablish more complex neuromuscular cross-patterns.

activity for the worker itself is not enough exercise to compensate after injury has occurred. Specific training activities as taught by athletic trainers or physical therapists, along with generalized conditioning, is the only way to prevent reinjury. A lifetime maintenance program using exercise equipment at home or in a health club setting should be taught by the therapist at discharge.

13

Return to Sport

It is most often the physician's responsibility to diagnose the problem. The trainer and therapist work together to rehabilitate the athlete's shoulder. In addition, the trainer may work with the coach to return the athlete to sport activity.

General Considerations

It is not the physician's role to return the competitive athlete to sport or the recreational athlete to full recreational activity. The doctor merely can suggest when the patient can return to training effectively, and it is the coach's responsibility to decide when the athlete is ready to actually participate and to retrain proper biomechanics of sport in an effort to avoid reinjury. An example is the return to pitching program in Table 13.1. The physician can release the athletic patient to training activity, but the coach and trainer are responsible for preparing the athlete to return to competition.

Most often, function can be restored nonsurgically. This assumes that the coach and athlete do not ascribe to the "no pain, no gain" attitude. Ideally, the coach knows the importance of the preparticipation physical, in that potential defects can be identified and corrected before competition and overuse cause injury. Fortunately, many acute and most overuse situations can be treated conservatively.

With extreme trauma or progressive overuse, conservative rehabilitation may not be feasible, and surgical intervention becomes more necessary. A surgeon cannot make extremely damaged tissue normal, but surgery can be most often used as a salvage technique to allow rehabilitation to compensate for remaining structural damage. Postoperatively, it is the therapist's role to help initiate motion and then progress toward strength, power, endurance, and the neuromuscular integration necessary for particular sport activities. Rehabilitation merely prepares the competitive athlete to return to the coach's tutelage prior to competitive activity.

It is true that many of the overuse situations common in sport activity are also seen in industrial injury. There are two advantages of taking care of

Table 13.1 Return to Competitive Throwing Program

Month 1

Week 1: Toss ball 30 to 40 feet without wind-up. Three to four 10-min sessions.

Week 2: Lob ball 30 feet playing catch without wind-up. Three to four 10-min sessions.

Week 3: Toss ball 40 to 50 feet with easy wind-up. Three alternate daily sessions of 20 min.

Week 4: Lob ball 60 feet with occasional straight throw. Three 20-min alternate-day sessions.

Month 2

Week 1: Long, easy throws from midoutfield, getting ball to home plate on five to six bounces. Alternate 2 days' practice with 1 day off for stretching and strengthening.

Week 2: Long throws from deep outfield. Five to six bounces to home plate; 30-min sessions for 2 days on and 1 day off for stretching and strengthening, then repeat.

Week 3: Stronger throws from midoutfield to home plate on three to four bounces; 30-min sessions, 2 days on, 1 day off, then repeat.

Week 4: Short, straight throws from short outfield to home on one bounce; 30-min sessions for 2 days on, 1 day off for stretching and strengthening, then repeat.

Month 3

Week 1: Throw daily and start *daily* strengthening and conditioning. Progress to next stage when painless.

Week 2: Pitch from mound or normal position with one-half to three-quarter effort, employing proper technique; 25-min sessions for 2 days on and 1 day off, then repeat.

Week 3: Throw with three-quarter to full effort; 30-min sessions for 2 days on and 1 day off.

Week 4: Six-inning game simulation includes warm-up and average number of pitches per inning with rest breaks simulating inning breaks, 3 to 4 days between pitching sessions simulating pitching rotation.

Return to full activity at discretion of pitching coach.

Assumes the goals of rehabilitative stages 1-3 have been met (see chapter 12). The athlete can progress faster than outlined sequence but only if pain-free prior to progression. Strengthening, stretching, and rehabilitation continues on off days.

Our program is a modification of the program developed by the Jobe and Kerlin Clinic, most recently described by Jobe, et al. (1990).

athletes. First, they tend to get better faster and seem more motivated than patients claiming worker's compensation. Second, the treating physician gains an appreciation of what can actually be achieved by surgery and subsequent rehabilitation. In most cases, 90% return of strength as determined by isokinetic testing is necessary prior to returning a professional athlete to the coach or trainer for further training. In the recreational athlete or industrial patient, who tends to wait longer for treatment and therefore has more atrophy, 80% is a more reasonable amount to allow safe return to former activity; further endurance strength can be expected to gradually increase with activity over time.

The recreational athlete's body must be his or her guide after being allowed to return to training by the doctor. Generalized conditioning is mandatory. Tissue that has been injured in the past is never normal, and in an effort to avoid reinjury, specific muscular activity and strengthening must be emphasized on a lifetime basis. If the shoulder hurts or fatigues, the athlete needs to back down and emphasize further endurance training. Even the recreational athlete should consider membership in a health club or procuring home exercise equipment and should not be discharged from a physical therapy program until he or she understands the home program well. Progression toward a home program is the goal of therapy in an effort to compensate for past injury and to avoid reinjury.

Summary

The shoulder's unique anatomic configuration leads to injury patterns that may overlap as the disease process progresses. History and physical examination are the keys to successful identification of injured anatomy that unlock the proper therapeutic doors. Although the end point of certain disease states may be the same, treatment of secondary symptoms alone without proper understanding of the underlying primary problem is not sufficient and in fact can make underlying problems worse; in this situation the patient will often state that he or she feels worse in therapy. Treatment is most predictable when correct diagnosis has been made.

Because of the shoulder's inherent instability, laxity is a major component of injury, due to either macrotrauma or microtrauma. Impingement or tendinitis is usually secondary to subluxation or postural change. The surrounding structures of the shoulder are linked together and can be overused when the linkage system is thrown out of phase. Although severe tissue damage can be the end stage of athletic shoulder injury, with luck it can be prevented by awareness, conditioning, proper treatment, and rehabilitation. Diagnosing the problem and rehabilitating the athlete's shoulder are a team effort.

Additional Reading

Codman, E.A. (1934). *The shoulder*. Boston: Thomas Todd.

Fu, F.H., & Stone, D.A. (Eds.) (1994). *Sports injuries: Mechanisms, prevention and treatment* (2nd ed.). Baltimore: Williams & Wilkins.

Nicholas, J.A., & Hershman, E.B. (1990). *The upper extremity in sports medicine*. St. Louis: Mosby.

Rockwood, C.A., & Matsen, F.A. (1990). *The shoulder*. Philadelphia: W.B. Saunders.

Rowe, C.R. (1988). *The shoulder*. New York: Churchill-Livingstone.

References

Adams, J.E. (1966). Little League shoulder: Osteochondrosis of the proximal humeral epiphysis in boy baseball pitchers. *California Medical Association Journal*, **105**, 22.

Andrews, J.R., Zarins, B., Carson, W.G., Nemeth, V., & Ciullo, J.V. (1983). *Shoulder arthroscopy*. An exhibit to the American Academy of Orthopaedic Surgeons, Anaheim, CA.

Basmajian, J.V., & Basant, F.J. (1959). Factors preventing downward dislocation of the adducted shoulder joint in electromyographic and morphological study. *Journal of Bone and Joint Surgery*, **41A**, 1182-1186.

Berg, E.E., & Ciullo, J.V. (1995). Heterotopic ossification after acromioplasty and distal clavicle resection. *Journal of Shoulder and Elbow Surgery*, **4**, 188-193.

Bigliani, L.U., Morrison, D., & April, E.W. (1986). The morphology of the acromion and its relationship to rotator cuff tears. *Orthopaedic Transactions*, **10**, 28.

Blazina, M.E., Kerlan, R.K., Jobe, F.W., Carter, W.S., & Carlson, G.J. (1973). Jumpers knee. *Orthopedic Clinics of North America*, **4**, 665-678.

Buckerfield, C.T., & Castle, M.E. (1984). Acute traumatic retrosternal dislocation of the clavicle. *Journal of Bone and Joint Surgery*, **66-A**(3), 379-384.

Burt, O.H. (1988). Personal communication, March. Past President, National Association of Watch and Clock Collectors.

Cahill, B.R., & Palmer, P.E. (1983). Quadrilateral space syndrome. *Journal of Hand Surgery*, **8**, 65-69.

Ciullo, J.V. (1986a, February). *Subscapular endoscopy in diagnosis and treatment of snapping scapula*. Exhibit to American Academy of Orthopaedic Surgeons, New Orleans, LA.

Ciullo, J.V. (1986b). Swimmer's shoulder. *Clinics in Sports Medicine*, **5**(1), 115-137.

Ciullo, J.V. (1989a, October 4-7). *Combined subacromial decompression, rotator cuff repair and capsular stabilization in one surgical procedure*. Exhibit to the 4th International Conference on Surgery of the Shoulder, New York, NY.

Ciullo, J.V. (1989b, February 12). *Relationship of rotator cuff "impingement" to glenohumeral "instability."* Paper read at American Orthopaedic Society for Sports Medicine, Interim Meeting of the American Association of Orthopaedic Surgeons, Specialty Day, Las Vegas, NV.

Ciullo, J., & Guise, E. (1981a). Coracoacromial impingement: Clinical presentation, radiographic findings, histologic evidence and therapy. *Orthopaedic Transactions,* **5**(3), 494.

Ciullo, J.V., & Guise, E.R. (1981b). Swimmer's shoulder: Adolescent manifestation and its treatment. *Orthopaedic Transactions,* **5**(1), 131-132.

Ciullo, J.V., & Jackson, D.W. (1985). Track and field. In R.C. Schneider, J.C. Kennedy, & M.L. Plant, *Sports injuries: Mechanisms, prevention and treatment* (pp. 212-246). Baltimore: Williams and Wilkins.

Ciullo, J.V., Koniuch, M.P., & Teitge, R.A. (1982). Axillary shoulder roentgenography in clinical orthopaedic practice. *Orthopaedic Transactions,* **6**(3), 451-452.

Ciullo, J.V., Koniuch, M.P., & Teitge, R.A. (1984). The axillary roentgenograph: A study of glenoid angle or hypoplasia in relationship to glenohumeral subluxation/dislocation and the use of axillary stress analysis in sports medicine. *Orthopaedic Transactions,* **8**(1), 74.

Ciullo, J.V., Koniuch, M.P., Teitge, R.A., & May, M. (1982). *Axillary shoulder roentgenography in clinical orthopaedic practice.* Exhibit to the Meeting of the American Academy of Orthopaedic Surgeons, New Orleans, LA.

Ciullo, J.V., & Stevens, G.G. (1989). The prevention and treatment of injuries to the shoulder in swimming. *Sports Medicine,* **7**, 182-204.

Ciullo, J., & Zarins, B. (1983). Biomechanics of the musculoskeletal unit: Relation to athletic performance and injury. *Clinics in Sports Medicine,* **2**(1), 71-86.

Codman, E.A. (1934). *The shoulder.* Boston: Thomas Todd.

Dunant, J.H. (1981). "Effort" thrombosis, a complication of thoracic outlet syndrome. *Vasa,* **10**, 322-324.

Estwanic, J.J. (1989). Levator scapulae syndrome. *The Physician and Sports Medicine,* **17**, 57-68.

Fisk, C. (1965). Adaption of the technique for radiology of the bicipital groove. *Radiological Technology,* **37**, 47-50.

Haber, E.C., & Storey, M.D. (1990). Effort thrombosis in a runner. *The Physician and Sports Medicine,* **18**, 76-84.

Hawkins, R.J., & Boker, D.J. (1990). Clinical evaluation of shoulder problems. In C.A. Rockwood & F.A. Matsen (Eds.), *The shoulder* (ch. 4). Philadelphia: W.B. Saunders.

Hawkins, R.J., & Kennedy, J.C. (1980). Impingement syndrome in athletes. *American Journal of Sports Medicine,* **8**(3), 151-158.

Hayes, J.M., & Zehr, D.W. (1981). Traumatic muscle avulsion causing winging of the scapula. *Journal of Bone and Joint Surgery,* **63A**, 495-497.

Hill, H.A., & Sachs, M.D. (1940). The grooved defect of the humeral head: A frequent unrecognized complication of dislocations of the shoulder joint. *Radiology,* **35**, 690-700.

Hirayama, T., & Takemitsu, Y. (1981). Compression of the suprascapular nerve by ganglion at suprascapular notch. *Clinical Orthopaedics and Related Research,* **155**, 95-96.

Hitchcock, H.H., & Bechtol, C.O. (1948). Painful shoulder, observation on the role of the tendon of the long biceps brachii and its causation. *Journal of Bone and Joint Surgery,* **30A**, 263-273.

Hovelius, L. (1982). *Anterior dislocation of the shoulder, a clinical study on incidence: Prognosis and operative treatment with a Bristow-Latarget procedure.* Linkoping University (Sweden) Medical Dissertations, No. 139.

Jackson, D.W., & Ciullo, J.V. (1986). Injury to the spine in the skeletally immature athlete. In J.A. Nicholas & E.B. Hershman (Eds.), *The lower extremity and spine in sports medicine* (pp. 1333-1372). St. Louis: Mosby.

Jakob, R.P., Kristiansen, T., Mayo, K., Ganz, R., & Müller, M.E. (1984). Classification and aspects of treatment of fractures of the proximal humerus. In J.E. Bateman & R.P. Welch (Eds.), *Surgery of the shoulder* (pp. 330-343). Philadelphia: B.C. Deckor.

Jobe, F.W., & Jobe, C.M. (1983). Painful athletic injuries of the shoulder. *Clinical Orthopaedics and Related Research,* **173**, 117-124.

Jobe, F.W., Tibone, J.E., Jobe, C.M., & Kvitne, R.S. (1990). The shoulder in sports. In C.A. Rockwood & F.A. Matsen (Eds.), *The shoulder* (pp. 962-982). Philadelphia: W.B. Saunders.

Kennedy, J.C. (1979). *The injured adolescent knee.* Baltimore: Williams and Wilkins.

Kennedy, J.C., & Willis, R.B. (1976). The effects of local steroid injection on tendons: A biomechanical and microscopic correlative study. *American Journal of Sports Medicine, 4,* 11-21.

Kessel, L., & Watson, M. (1973). The painful arc syndrome. *Journal of Bone and Joint Surgery, 59B,* 166-172.

Kohler, A., & Zimmer, E.A. (1988). *Borderlands of normal and early pathological skeletal roentgenology* (3rd American ed., S.P. Wilke, Trans.). New York: Grune and Stratton.

Kopell, H., & Thompson, W. (1959). Pain in the frozen shoulder. *Surgery, Gynecology, and Obstetrics, 109,* 92-96.

Leffert, R.D., & Gumley, G. (1987). The relationship between dead arm syndrome and thoracic outlet syndrome. *Clinical Orthopaedics and Related Research, 223,* 20-31.

Liberson, R. (1937). Os acromiale: A contested anomaly. *Journal of Bone and Joint Surgery, 19,* 683-689.

Lucas, D.B. (1973). Biomechanics of the shoulder joint. *Archives of Surgery, 107*(3), 425-432.

Matsen, F.A. (1988, September). *TUBS-AMBRI-pneumonics to differentiate traumatic instability from multidirectional instability.* American Academy of Orthopaedic Surgeons, Summer Institute, San Diego, CA.

McCarroll, J.R. (1985). Golf. In R.C. Schneider, J.C. Kennedy, & M.L. Plant, *Sports injuries: Mechanism, prevention and treatment* (pp. 290-294). Baltimore: Williams & Wilkins.

McMaster, W.C. (1986). Anterior glenoid labrum damage: A painful lesion in swimmers. *American Journal of Sports Medicine, 14,* 383-387.

Milch, H. (1950). Partial scapulectomy for snapping of the scapula. *Journal of Bone and Joint Surgery, 32A,* 561-566.

Neer, C.S. (1970). Displaced proximal humeral fractures: Part I classification and evaluation. *Journal of Bone and Joint Surgery, 52A,* 1077-1089.

Neer, C.S., II. (1983). Impingement lesions. *Clinical Orthopaedics and Related Research, 173,* 70-77.

Nicholas, J., Grossman, R.B., & Hershman, E. (1977). The importance of a simplified classification of motion in sports in relation to performance. *Orthopedic Clinics of North America, 8,* 499-532.

Nuber, G.W., Jobe, F.W., Perry, J., Moynes, D.R., & Antonelli, D. (1986). Fine wire electromyography analysis of muscles of the shoulder during swimming. *American Journal of Sports Medicine, 14,* 7-11.

Nuber, G.W., McCarthy, W.J., Yao, J.S., Schafer, M.F., & Suker, J.R. (1990). Arterial abnormalities of the shoulder in athletes. *American Journal of Sports Medicine, 18,* 514-519.

Osterman, A.L. (1988). The double crush syndrome. *Orthopedic Clinics of North America, 19,* 147-155.

Pappas, A.M., Goss, T.P., & Cleinman, P.K. (1983). Symptomatic shoulder instability due to lesions of the glenoid labrum. *American Journal of Sports Medicine, 11,* 279-288.

Pappas, A.M., Zawacki, R.M., & Sullivan, T.J. (1985). Biomechanics of baseball pitching: A preliminary report. *American Journal of Sports Medicine, 13,* 216-222.

Reeves, B. (1975). The natural history of the frozen shoulder syndrome. *Scandinavian Journal of Rheumatology, 4,* 193-196.

Richardson, A.B., Jobe, F.W., & Collins, H.R. (1980). The shoulder in competitive swimming. *American Journal of Sports Medicine, 8,* 159-163.

Rizk, T.E., Christopher, R.P., Pinals, R.S., Higgins, A.C., & Frix, R. (1983). Adhesive capsulitis (frozen shoulder): A new approach to its management. *Archives of Physical Medicine and Rehabilitation, 64,* 29-33.

Rockwood, C.A., & Green, D.P. (Eds.) (1984). *Fractures* (3 vols., 2nd ed.). Philadelphia: J.B. Lippincott.

Roeser, W.M., Meeks, L.W., Venise, R., & Strickland, G. (1976). The use of transcutaneous nerve stimulation for pain control and athletic medicine: A preliminary report. *American Journal of Sports Medicine, 4,* 210-213.

Roos, D.B. (1979). New concepts of thoracic outlet syndrome that explain etiology, symptoms, diagnosis and treatment. *Vascular Surgery*, **13**, 313-321.

Rowe, C.R. (1963). Anterior dislocation of the shoulder: Prognosis and treatment. *Surgical Clinics of North America*, **43**, 1609-1614.

Rowe, C.R., & Zarins, B. (1981). Recurrent transient subluxation of the shoulder. *Journal of Bone and Joint Surgery*, **63A**(6), 863-872.

Saha, A.K. (1983). Mechanism of shoulder movements and a plea for the recognition of "zero position" of glenohumeral joint. *Clinical Orthopaedics and Related Research*, **173**, 3-10.

Salter, R.B., & Harris, W.R. (1963). Injuries involving the epiphyseal plate. *Journal of Bone and Joint Surgery*, **45A**, 587-622.

Skyhar, M.J., Altcheck, D.W., & Warren, R.F. (1988). Shoulder arthroscopy in the seated position. *Orthopaedic Review*, **10**, 1033.

Smythe, H.A. (1981). Fibrosis and other diffuse musculoskeletal syndromes. In W.N. Kelly, E.D. Harris, S. Ruddy, & C.B. Sledge, *Text book of rheumatology* (pp. 485-493). Philadelphia: W.B. Saunders.

Snyder, S.J. (1989, November). Arthroscopy is only effective mode to diagnose superior labrum lesion. *Orthopaedics Today*, pp. 12-13.

Sonozaki, H., Azuma, A., Okai, K., Nakamura, K., Fukuoka, S., Tateishi, A., Kurosawa, H., Mannoji, T., Kabata, K., Mitsui, H., Seki, H., Abe, I., Furusawa, S., Matsuura, M., Kudo, A., & Hoshino, T. (1979). Clinical features of twenty-two cases with intersternal costoclavicular ossification. *Archives of Orthopaedic and Traumatic Surgery*, **95**, 13-22.

Steindler, A. (1973). *Kinesiology of the human body under normal and pathological conditions.* Springfield, IL: Charles C Thomas.

Symeonides, P.P. (1972). The significance of the subscapularis muscle and the pathogenesis of recurrent anterior dislocation of the shoulder. *Journal of Bone and Joint Surgery*, **54B**, 476-483.

Townley, C.O. (1950). The capsular mechanism in recurrent dislocation of the shoulder. *Journal of Bone and Joint Surgery*, **32A**, 370-380.

Tsairis, P., Dyck, P.J., & Mulder, D.W. (1972). Natural history of brachial plexus neuropathy: Report on 99 patients. *Archives of Neurology*, **27**, 109.

Warren, R.F. (1983). Subluxation of the shoulder in athletes. *Clinics in Sports Medicine*, **2**(2), 339-354.

Wood, V.E., Twitto, R., & Verska, J.M. (1988). Thoracic outlet syndrome. *Orthopedic Clinics of North America*, **19**, 131-146.

Zanca, P. (1971). Shoulder pain: Involvement of the acromioclavicular joint: Analysis of one thousand cases. *American Journal of Roentgenology, Radium Therapy, and Nuclear Medicine*, **112**(3), 493-506.

Index

About the Author

Jerome Vincent Ciullo, MD, is an assistant clinical professor in the Departments of Orthopaedic Surgery at Wayne State University in Detroit and Michigan State University in East Lansing. He has been Director of Sports Medicine and team physician for Wayne State University, where he has participated in research in exercise physiology, bioengineering, orthopedic implants, and surgical equipment. He has presented over 200 papers, published nine book chapters and approximately 20 journal and review articles, and has edited a book on swimming injuries. He has been team physician for the 1983 Michigan Panthers USFL Championship football team; and is presently an orthopaedic consultant for the Detroit Pistons (basketball); team physician for the Detroit Vipers (hockey) and Detroit Wheels (soccer); and serves on the medical staff of USA Swimming. He is a fellow of the American College of Surgeons and the American Academy of Orthopaedic Surgeons, and a member of the American Medical Association, the North American Arthroscopy Association, the International Arthroscopy As-

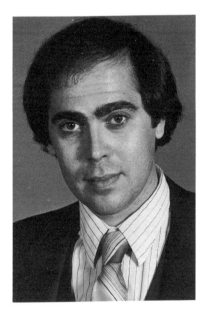

sociation, the American Orthopaedic Society for Sports Medicine, the American College of Sports Medicine, and the American Academy of Sports Physicians.